An Occupational
Perspective
of Health

An Occupational Perspective of Health

Ann A. Wilcock, PhD
Associate Professor of Occupational Therapy
University of South Australia

SLACK Incorporated, 6900 Grove Road, Thorofare, NJ 08086

Publisher: John H. Bond
Editorial Director: Amy E. Drummond
Senior Associate Editor: Jennifer J. Cahill
Creative Director: Linda Baker
Cover illustration by Shane O'Neil

Wilcock, Ann Allart.
    An occupational perspective of health/Ann Wilcock.
    p. cm.
    Includes bibliographical references and index.
    ISBN 1-55642-358-6
    1. Occupational therapy--Philosophy. 2. Industrial hygiene. I. Title.
        [DNLM: 1. Occupational Therapy. 2. Work--psychology. 3. Rehabilitation, Vocational. WB 555
W667o 1998]
    RM735.4.W55 1998
    616.8'515--dc21
    DNLM/DLC   98-5746
    for Library of Congress

Printed in the United States of America
Published by: SLACK Incorporated
                 6900 Grove Road
                 Thorofare, NJ 08086 USA
                 Telephone: 609-848-1000
                 Fax: 609-853-5991
                 Website: www.slackinc.com

Dedication

This book is dedicated to Molly Jones, Peggy Jay, Betty McIntyre, Rosemary Donald, and Cecilie Bearup, and to the continual development of a discipline based on the understanding of humans as occupational beings.

Contents

Dedication v

Acknowledgments ix

About the Author xi

Foreword *by Josephine C. Moore, PhD, OTR, FAOTA, DSc(hon.)²* xv

Foreword *by Elizabeth J. Yerxa, EdD, LHD(hon.), DSc(hon.), OTR, FAOTA* 1

Chapter 1: Introduction...2

Chapter 2: An Occupational Theory of Human Nature.............................20

Chapter 3: Biological Characteristics and Capacities: The Foundation for Occupational Behavior..40

Chapter 4: Occupational Evolution 70

Chapter 5: Health: An Occupational Perspective 96

Chapter 6: Ill Health: Occupational Risk Factors 130

Chapter 7: The Genesis of Occupational Therapy....................................164

Chapter 8: Occupational Therapy's Relationship with Occupation and Health 186

Chapter 9: Occupational Therapy and Public Health 220

Glossary...253

Index 261

Acknowledgments

My sincerest thanks go to:

- Dr. Neville Hicks, Reader, University of Adelaide, for patient persistence in developing my scholarship, for enriching my ways of thinking, and for ongoing interest and support in this work
- My husband, Derek, for his encouragement, time, and practical help
- Jan Heath, Librarian, University of South Australia, and Peter Newnham, Librarian, University of Adelaide
- Bob Hall, Senior Lecturer in Mathematics, University of South Australia, for his advice on statistical matters; Dr. Matt Gaughwin for his advice on "evolution"; and Dr. AD Hunt for his clarification of theological history
- Professional colleagues from throughout my career, who have contributed (in many ways) to my work and ideas
- Occupational therapy staff and students at the University of South Australia who have shared my ongoing struggles, enthusiasms, frustrations, and interest in the development of occupational science

About the Author

Ann A. Wilcock (née Ellison), PhD, DipCOT, BAppSciOT, GradDipPH, was born in the United Kingdom, and was brought up in the Lake District. She graduated as an occupational therapist from the Derby School in 1961. She learned early of the need to think about the purpose of the profession as, in order to obtain some financial assistance for her training, at 16 years of age she had to convince the Westmorland Education Authority of the merits of the profession, and the reason they should support her tertiary education in this field. No occupational therapists were employed in Westmorland at that time.

Before leaving for Australia in 1964, Ann worked at Black Notley Hospital in Essex, and at Farnham Park Rehabilitation Centre in Buckinghamshire, with Peggy Jay and the late Mary S Jones, both well-known occupational therapists, researchers, and authors in the field of rehabilitation and activities of daily living. Ann worked on the original research for the book *Help Yourselves: A Handbook for Hemiplegics and their Families* by Jay, Walker, and Ellison, which was published by Butterworths in 1966.

Ann was married shortly after her arrival in Australia, and she and her husband settled in Newcastle, New South Wales. At the Royal Newcastle Hospital she practiced in acute and long-term rehabilitation with tuberculous, stroke, hand-injured, quadriplegic, cerebral palsied, orthopedic, geriatric, and mentally ill patients. In the early 1970s, she moved to Southern Tasmania and worked at the Royal Hobart Hospital, mainly with neurological, geriatric, and hand-injured patients. In 1976, she moved to Adelaide to work at the School of Occupational Therapy. During her years there she has taught most subjects, both of an academic and practical nature, but developed particular expertise in the rehabilitation of stroke. Her book *Occupational Therapy Approaches to Stroke* was published in 1986 by Churchill Livingstone. Between 1986 and 1993, Ann was head of the school, and during that time post-graduate teaching was established. Since then she has been involved principally in post-graduate education toward coursework and research degrees. These are offered by the University of South Australia in flexible (distant) teaching mode. Students, including those undertaking research PhDs, can be found throughout Australia and New Zealand and, a few, in more distant parts of the world.

Work with graduate students has focused on recent interests in occupational science and health promotion. Her commitment to the establishment of occupational science began in 1988 when a visiting professor first said those words to her with regard to an initiative occurring "somewhere in the USA." Before the first written accounts of this science reached Australia in 1990, from what turned out to be the University of Southern California, Ann had given two papers on the topic at occupational therapy conferences, including one at the World Federation of Occupational Therapists Congress in Melbourne. This was later published in the *British Journal of Occupational Therapy*. At the Congress, and later in South Australia, it was a thrill for Ann to meet Elizabeth Yerxa, who was the prime mover in establishing the science at the University of Southern California, and they spent many exciting hours talking about the emerging discipline. In 1993, Ann established and became founding editor of the *Journal of Occupational Science: Australia*, an international and interdisciplinary publication which is now supported by the University of Southern California, as well as the University of South Australia and the Auckland Institute of Technology. Ann is currently the executive editor, and Clare Hocking from New Zealand the editor of what, from this year, is known simply as *Journal of Occupational Science.*

A principle aim behind the establishment of the journal was to bring to the attention of a wide range of disciplines the need to understand better humans as occupational beings. Ann believed that a lack of understanding and awareness were partly to blame for many of the vexed and urgent problems which face most people in the post-industrial world. From the point of view of occupational therapists, it is partly to blame for the limited understanding of what the profession has to offer. Ann's commitment to the establishment of the science was recognized by the University of Southern California by the award of the Wilma West Lecture in 1995. Her own personal direction within the science is exploration of the relationship between people's occupational natures and health. This was firmly established as Ann undertook graduate studies in public health, and was the subject of her PhD thesis.

At present, Ann is undertaking a two-volume history of the profession commissioned by the British College of Occupational Therapists. This year she is giving keynote addresses at the World Federation of Occupational Therapists Congress in Montreal where she will talk about *doing, being, and becoming,* and at the British Occupational Therapist's Conference in Belfast on *health through occupation.*

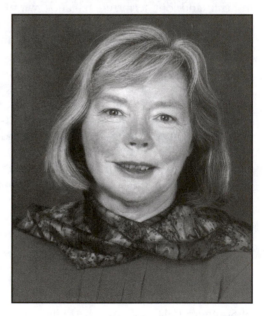

Foreword

The focus of this book, *An Occupational Perspective of Health*, could become the central, unifying bond for occupational therapists in the development of approaches to all aspects of their work. For one, this publication provides an extensive background on which to base practice and concurrently it makes a therapist feel confident about the importance and relevance of one's practice. It also conveys to others in the health field, as well as the wider community, the importance of a little understood concept—that of the place of occupation in health.

The author, Dr. Ann Wilcock, brings together many scientific, sociological, psychological, and anthropological ideas which support the central theme of occupational science, that is, that humans are occupational beings, and shows that there is a three-way link between survival, health, and occupation. It is clear from the argument put forth in this text that occupation is necessary to health and well-being. Conversely, if the drive to be occupied and fulfilled is not adequately met, humans become prey to ill health, and may engage in many deviant behaviors, such as using drugs and alcohol, becoming violent, or simply "giving up," all of which are part of an ill health syndrome. The nature versus nurture debate, and the human versus nature debate, which has led to alienation being perpetuated over time, are central to the health themes being drawn out of this historical exploration of "occupational health."

The sections on Darwin and neo-Darwinism, and the relationship between brain and behavior, are extremely interesting. The discussions, which are up-to-date and well referenced, link a range of topics and cover unexpected aspects such as studies about sexual dimorphism as it relates to the brain, hormones, and behavior, which I believe are very important. The section on occupational evolution is fascinating and also touches on my sphere of interest, in that it flows from prehistoric times into the future, linking the biological and neurological with sociological and anthropological thought.

The chapters which refer to the history and development of occupational therapy as a basis for the proposition that this discipline has something distinct and relevant to offer the field of public health does so by considering the sociopolitical contexts of its changing directions. For example, there is excellent discussion of Dunton's work and its effects in terms of occupational therapy concepts versus those of medical science, and the paradox of the history of the profession's advances and retreats according to societal change and medical technology. These discussions are nicely linked with the coverage of the ongoing debate about the place of occupational science within occupational therapy.

If health care practices were to adopt some of the broader concepts within this text, it might be possible to effect change for the good of all toward the fulfillment of personal and community needs, and acceptance of these ideas within the public health arena. Indeed, it may help humankind create a culture or environment that would not only be fair to each individual but to many different types of communities and to ecology.

Josephine C. Moore, PhD, OTR, FAOTA, DSc(hon.)[2]
Professor Emeritus
Department of Anatomy
University of South Dakota Medical School
Vermillion, South Dakota

Foreword

In 1962, one of our profession's seminal thinkers, Mary Reilly, proposed occupational therapy's great hypothesis: "That man, through the use of his hands as energized by mind and will, can influence the state of his own health."[1] This book provides scholarly support for Reilly's prediction by synthesizing relevant ideas from an array of disciplines into a fresh configuration.

Dr. Wilcock and I met in Australia for the first time several years ago. It was a joy to discover that we could converse immediately in the language of occupation, finding substantial similarities in our thinking, in spite of distance and differences in culture. I felt as though I had discovered an "alter ego" down under.

This impressive work contributes to the profession of occupational therapy by increasing its understanding of occupation while revealing the potential of occupational therapy practice to affect individuals and communities positively via occupation. A bona fide profession is expected to develop and evaluate its own practice which is based on a unique set of ideas.[2] In the current world climate of reductionism and oversimplification, occupational therapy needs substantive knowledge that will enable it to define its own knowledge-based scope of practice and thereby serve humankind in ethical and responsible ways under changing environmental conditions. This book contributes to such substantiation, supporting a self-defined profession.

The book also speaks to other relevant disciplines such as public administration, public health, and social ecology. It reveals that occupation, rather than being trivial or mundane, is a universal phenomenon worthy of serious study since it is essential to adaptation and survival. Dr. Wilcock courageously tackles the complexity of occupation and relates it to another challenging concept—health. By explicating these two rich constructs, she delineates new roles and capacities for the occupational therapy profession demonstrating its potential impact on society as a whole, including achieving social justice for disadvantaged people and contributing to a sustainable ecology.

This work will be an invaluable resource for students, academics, and clinicians who seek a deeper understanding of occupation and its essential contribution to human life. It is instructive in both its content and scholarly process. It presents a set of ideas whose time has come to a world that desperately needs occupation even if it has not recognized that. It will soon.

Elizabeth J. Yerxa, EdD, LHD(hon.), DSc(hon.), OTR, FAOTA
Distinguished Professor Emerita
Department of Occupational Therapy
University of Southern California
Los Angeles, California

References
1. Reilly M. Occupational therapy can be one of the great ideas of 20th century medicine. *American Journal of Occupational Therapy.* 1962;16:300-308.
2. Etzioni A. *The Semiprofessions and Their Organization: Teachers, Nurses, and Social Workers.* New York, NY: Free Press; 1969.

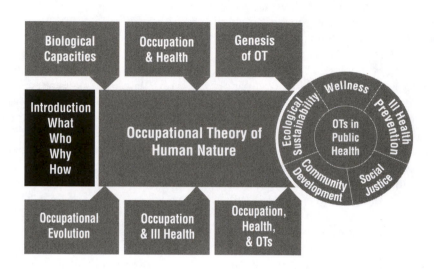

Chapter 1
Introduction

This chapter presents the reader with ideas about:
- The purpose of this book
- The background to the author's perspective
- The "history of ideas" approach used in the research and writing of this book as a way to consider already known information in a different light
- Occupation, health, health care, and the ideologies which surround them
- The need to consider biological and sociocultural issues when exploring health and occupation
- An outline of the story told in this book about occupation and health, occupational therapy, and public health

This book explores the relationship between occupation and health, how this relationship is addressed by occupational therapists, and its importance to public health. Throughout the text, "occupation" is used to mean "all purposeful human activity."

Four specific issues are addressed:
1. The importance of occupation in human life
2. Occupation as a positive influence on health
3. The potential of occupational therapy to be a health promoting profession
4. The compatibility of occupational therapy with current public health and World Health Organization (WHO) objectives

The benefits that a greater emphasis on the relationship between occupation and health may yield are discussed, with the recommendations that there should be greater recognition of the potential role of occupational therapists in programs initiated by primary health care and public health organizations.

The exploration, which has led to the development of an occupational view of human nature and health, was prompted by documents from the WHO and the Better Health Commission of Australia, which called for an acceptable level of health for all by the year 2000.[1,2] These documents stressed the need for the reorientation of all health professions toward the pursuit of health. For each profession, particular perspectives of health and illness are somewhat different, and for each professional, there are also slight differences according to underlying beliefs, values, and experiences. Nevertheless, there is scant acknowledgment that basic ideas about what health is may not be constant between professions or even within the general population. There is little appreciation that in order to meet professional, community, and individual goals, health care workers, including occupational therapists, need to be able to define clearly what they, their clients, and the communities they serve mean by health and illness.

This does not imply that a standard definition is required by all health professionals. In fact, because ideas about "health and well-being" do differ between individuals, communities, professions, societies, and cultures, it is important to search for factors common to the experience of "health" and for those that may have been overlooked. It is also necessary for occupational therapists, along with other professionals, to describe clearly their profession's particular views and their own underlying views and values. With this in mind, it becomes necessary to provide a brief history of my own professional views.

Trained as an occupational therapist in England between 1958 and 1961, my training was based on physical and mental health care concepts according to the medical model. An example of the influence of the medical model on occupational therapy at that time is provided by the following quote:

> *Occupational therapy is the term given to the use of activities of many kinds, medically prescribed, for the distinct purpose of contributing to recovery from disease or injury, or for the maintenance of function when complete recovery is not possible. It is directed to ultimate re-establishment of the patient in home and employment, or in work or recreation under sheltered conditions.*[3]

A commitment to and interest in rehabilitation, established during World War II, was still dominant within this model. Students learned about anatomy, physiology, psychology, and medical, surgical, and psychiatric disorders, along with practical training, such as woodworking, weaving, recreation, dance, household maintenance, gardening, and process work to a level of competence enabling graduates to teach or use these in the treatment of patients. The relationship between these occupations and health was hardly considered in philosophical terms, and theoretical considerations were directed to the prescriptive use of occupation to remedy physical, mental, and, occasionally, social disorders. At the time, information sharing was didactic and authoritarian, rather than participatory, so the teaching and learning environment did not encourage questioning or self-directed study. This resulted in an occupational therapist who was competent to practice within a wide range of medical services, with a strong belief in the efficacy of occupation to influence health status, but little ability to articulate its rationale. This made it difficult to defend the value of occupation to health when medicine adopted an increasingly reductionist, scientific, and technological stance from the late 1960s onward.

This did not result in a decrease of my belief in the influence of occupation on health because experience had provided evidence that this was the case. Experience had also broadened my concept of health to incorporate the notion of maximizing individual potential and well-being. Three case histories illustrate the point.

Case 1

In 1961, Harriet was a 45-year-old woman who had been disabled with rheumatoid arthritis since her late teens. She was unable to sit at all, spending her time lying in bed or standing for brief periods, having reached this upright position with the mechanical aid of a tilting mechanism. She had minimal shoulder, elbow, and finger movement, to the extent that she could not touch her face, feed herself without aids, or attend to even simple self-care. Because of this restricted mobility and tremendous pain, throughout her adult life she had suffered gross occupational deprivation. During the course of our professional association, she mentioned, by chance, that she envied those who could paint and by inference that this, for her, was beyond the realms of possibility. As this was before the days of rehabilitation and education aid catalogs, much to her surprise a "Heath Robinson" device, which enabled her to paint tiny areas of a pre-drawn canvas, was concocted and set up across her bed. With a master painting to follow for color, she completed piece by painful piece a small landscape, which to her was the equivalent of a "Constable." There is no way to describe her joy as she went on to her next masterpiece or the disappointment she expressed in a letter she wrote after a move to another treatment facility where she was unable to continue her new-found occupation.

Case 2

A man in his 30s lived, more or less permanently, in a hospital following spinal injuries that left him quadriplegic. Peter had had an unusual and deprived childhood: he was brought up in an institution with intellectually handicapped children following abandonment as an infant. As a result, he had experienced minimal education and poor job opportunities. Following his accident, Peter was taught by an occupational therapist to do tapestry embroidery, in which he became very interested and skilled. He entered and won competitions in local shows and became a local celebrity as a result. He regularly glowed with well-being following his occupational achievements being recognized and applauded.

Case 3

Sharon was 17 when her nightgown caught fire. She was badly burned over her face, neck, chest, arms, and hands. Ultimately, she lost several fingers and suffered facial disfigurement. At first meeting, early in the medical and functional restoration process, it was obvious to her that she would be unable to follow her previous long-term plan, which was to join the armed forces. To provide the greatest choice for her future, it was suggested that she could, if she wished, use the years of treatment as a time to rebuild her future. She chose to undertake external matriculation studies between bouts of surgery. It was hard work and took a long time, but resulted in entry to a university and successful graduation into a profession. This course of action facilitated a new way of life and enabled Sharon, despite physical loss, to use capacities that had previously been untapped.

These people who, despite residual disability, were enabled to reach higher levels of well-being through maximizing untapped potential are examples of "growth models of health" advocated by psychologists such as Maslow. Ideas based on this belief are central to the notions about occupation and health discussed in this book.

Other important health-related functions of occupation became apparent during my 4 years' experience in a small, acute psychiatric unit during the late 1960s and early 1970s. This unit was run as a therapeutic community, which used the community's social processes as treatment for those admitted. The strategies included group therapy, in which feedback was given on individual behavior by others in the group, encouragement of frank expressions of thoughts and feelings about the here and now, and peer group pressure.[4] Group therapy was not restricted to discussion, but included action and community occupation. The idea upon which the 7-days-a-week occupational therapy sessions was based was that when people are "well" and are together in a group, they formulate plans quite quickly for how they will spend their time together, and having decided on a course of action will engage in what they have chosen to do.[5] Therefore, the program planners held a positive and stated expectation that members of the group would spend 2 to 3 hours each morning together in what was known as "the practical relationship room" and that they would engage in group activity of their choice. The staff's role was to encourage such activity, but not to initiate it.

What happened in these sessions was, of course, a major topic for consideration in other parts of the program. For days, weeks, and, occasionally, months, very little in the way of group occupation was done, but a great deal was accomplished in terms of identifying difficulties experienced by members of the group in initiating occupation. Staff discovered many ways to encourage activity, often tapping unexpected capacities in themselves in their efforts to overcome occupational deprivation resulting from the patients' lack of mental health. It was a difficult role for staff who tended, erroneously, to equate the patients' reduced engagement in purposeful occupation as a reflection of their own techniques being ineffective. The staff members themselves had to contend regularly with their own frustration as well as the extremely demanding work of helping the patients explore what was happening. As this challenging process was worked through, the patients eventually arrived at a state in which their drive for occupation was restored. It usually occurred for most of the group at about the same time and resulted in some dynamic, exciting, and different activity. The group held art shows, made movies, built brick barbecues, and even group knitted with group-turned 10-foot-long knitting needles. Completion of a major community occupation was almost a signal for discharge: health, well-being, and self-initiated occupation appear to be inseparable, just as lack of health results in poverty of occupational engagement.[6]

More recent interest concentrated on neurological rehabilitation,[7] with some time spent undertaking post-graduate study in neuropsychology at Flinders University. A principle text recommended by my professors was *Fundamentals of Human Neuropsychology* by Kolb and Whishaw,[8] which contains material relevant to many of the issues addressed in this book. Interest in neuroscience has led to an appreciation of the role of the central nervous system in evolution and all aspects of human life, including the promotion of health, and in understanding humans as occupational beings, because as Edelman proposes:

In the course of evolution, bodies came to have minds. But it is not enough to say that the mind is embodied: one must say how. To do that we have to take a look at the brain and the nervous system and at the structural and functional problems they present.[9]

A second major interest has been in public health and health promotion, influenced by post-graduate studies in public health at the University of Adelaide, introducing me to the concepts of social medicine and social health.

My interest in studying the occupational nature of humans was precipitated by the emergence of a new generic discipline—namely, occupational science. This sparked a professional revelation of the need to understand more fully the apparent human need for occupation as a basis for the practice of occupational therapy. Occupation, to date, has received little attention within the conventions of medical scientific inquiry. Those who have considered it have usually regarded aspects of occupation as observable human behavior that can be used as a surrogate measure for other criteria they wish to research. In the past 20 years, occupational therapists, prompted by the work of Mary Reilly at the University of Southern California in the 1960s,[10] have begun to develop an interest in the study of human occupation in a holistic sense,[11,12] but Dr. Elizabeth Yerxa from the University of Southern California was most responsible for the "naming and framing" of occupational science as the study of humans as occupational beings.[13,15] Interest in this new science has prompted me to bring together a history of ideas surrounding the relationship between occupation, health, public health, and occupational therapy.

The ideas presented in this text, therefore, represent an exploration based on observations and reflections of professional experience in clinical practice and education in occupational therapy and the health care system over three decades. The rationale for this approach is an appreciation that every person holds a view of human nature formed as a result of life experiences and extensive and ongoing contact with people, cultures, and communities. This provides an often unacknowledged source from which to draw a theoretical model.

However, developing a perspective centered on humans as occupational beings is particularly difficult because occupation is such an integral part of life and of already accepted, but different, perspectives on life. To rethink issues from this different, yet familiar, focus demands that "the ways of thinking which seem so natural and inevitable that they are not [usually] scrutinized with the eye of logical self-consciousness" be identified and analyzed, and, following scrutiny, re-synthesized.[14] Even a background in occupational therapy has not foreshortened, for me, the development of a sense of competence in processing problems from an occupational viewpoint. Despite the difficulty, tentative ideas from this perspective have broadened my ways of looking at vexed problems in health care and education and for social problems at a global-political level. Examples include ecological degradation, paid employment, resource allocation, street kids, or the destructive behavior of youth gangs, which appear to be unresponsive to present initiatives formulated within the context of primarily "market economy" or social perspectives.

Another difficulty encountered is the prevailing reductionism of traditional scientific methods. Human engagement in occupation is complex and varied and almost impossible to explore according to methods that are essentially reductionist and contextually controlled. To reduce engagement to component parts would diminish its study as it is the integrated complexities that require the most rigorous investigation.[15] Indeed, the complexities of human characteristics and the variety of occupational environments are often seen by traditional experimental researchers as contaminants to research design.[16] Gergen, a social psychologist, is one of many who criticize using traditional science methodology for studying human beings, because techniques do decontextualize, are atemporal and deterministic, and lead to inadequate and distorted findings.[17] Open-minded consideration of different research methodologies, such as those used in developmental and social psychology, anthropology, sociology, history, and evolutionary biology, which study people contextually, view their activities diachronically, and recognize individual will, are more suitable as a means of building a knowledge base for a science of occupation.[15] Additionally, methods advocated by critical social scientists as appropriate for interdisciplinary research about the "conditions which make possible the reproduction and transformation of society, the meaning of culture, and the relationship between the individual, society, and nature" are valuable to consider as tools in understanding the occupational nature of humans.[18] A synthesis of ideas from a wide range of disciplines is required for the broad issues being explored in this text; therefore, the exploration takes the form of a history of ideas.[19] The next section discusses this approach.

A History of Ideas Approach

Burke explains in *The Fontana Dictionary of Modern Thought* how Arthur Lovejoy coined the term "history of ideas" in the 1920s to cover study approaches that center on concepts and how changes in their meaning and associations change according to history.[20] Lovejoy proposed that the task of the history of ideas is to:

Attempt to understand how new beliefs and intellectual fashions are introduced and diffused, to help to elucidate the psychological character of the processes by which changes in vogue and influence of ideas have come about; to make clear, if possible, how conceptions dominant or extensively prevalent in one generation lose their hold upon men's minds and give place to others.[14]

He described the viewing of ideas "from the standpoint of a particular purpose," made possible by considering and dividing "in great part...the same material as the other branches of the history of thought," so that "new groupings and relations" emerge. He argued for the history to be concerned with "ideas which attain a wide diffusion, which become part of the stock of many minds," which "disregard national and linguistic boundary lines," and cross barriers between different disciplines and thinking, so demonstrating that ideas that emerge at any one time usually manifest themselves in more than one direction.

The particular purpose here is the exploration of the meaning and associations between concepts of occupation and health within the framework of an occupational theory of human nature and in relation to occupational therapy and public health. It groups and relates already "known" thoughts and facts in a different way, contending that the concept and meaning of occupation and of health has changed with occupational technology and subsequent sociocultural evolution, ideas, and expectations. This text reviews material from other disciplines, from several cultures, and from ideas and artifacts of the people, as well as known experts, in a new light from the standpoint of the proposed occupational theory. Like other histories of ideas it "aims at interpretation and unification and seeks to correlate things" that, in our present structures and reductionist ways of thinking, may appear unconnected. At first glance, it may appear to be "a strange combination of incongruences: general but detailed, straightforward but intricate, pragmatic but abstract," and because it tells a story, the rigor of the research effort is easily overlooked.[21]

The rigor is demonstrated by my early presumption that humans have always engaged in occupation, before I realized that I had to discover if this was generally held to be so. This led to a voyage of discovery through evolutionary texts, anthropology, sociology, philosophy, ethology, sociobiology, genetics, labor studies, psychology, ecology, and neural Darwinism; in no place did I find a direct answer. Engagement in occupation is so fundamental it is taken for granted. As I plowed backward and forward through these, as well as texts from other disciplines, issues emerged and fresh connections were made. Ideas disregarded at one stage became important at a later stage. As immersion led to saturation, themes and, eventually, a major hypothesis about occupation and health developed. The history of ideas process also facilitated a critical viewpoint because it enabled me to look at the world through a different lens. It generated a belief in the necessity for political and social change to improve occupational experience, health, and well-being, along with sustaining the ecology, and, unexpectedly, the need for occupational therapists to become social activists.

The writing was also an essential aspect of the research process. As Laurel Richardson suggests, writing can be "a way of 'knowing'"—a method of discovery and analysis. Historical research, in contrast to most other forms of qualitative inquiry, depends upon the quality of a reasoned argument, which is considered of more importance than particular methodological steps or stages that are in accord with scientific conventions.[22] Learning this art has been the most difficult part of this exploration.

Apart from misunderstanding the nature, depth, and rigor of the exploration and analysis, histories of ideas carry another risk:

Because the historian of an idea is compelled by the nature of his enterprise to gather material from several fields of knowledge, he is inevitably, in at least some parts of his synthesis, liable to the errors which lie in wait for the non-specialist.[19]

For this reason, secondary and tertiary sources of information as well as primary works were used. Primary sources of literature are generally considered preferable, but secondary sources, which are accounts "reacting to the ideas of a primary author," can further illuminate the original ideas and point the novice toward new or different sources of evidence. Tertiary sources, such as current books and articles, are also useful for suggesting lines of inquiry and other historians' viewpoints. The story, which emerges from this process, though, must open up "new avenues of investigation, criticism, and reflection, not simply recreate another author's interpretation of the past."[21]

Relevant material for this research is wide ranging, from works pertaining to those disciplines noted earlier, as well as human anatomy and physiology, public health and health promotion, archaeology, occupational evolution, philosophy, economics, and research that considers occupation or relates to the human need for occupation. The latter required an extensive "meta-review" of occupational therapy journals and texts, viewing historically and collectively, rather than in the ahistorical, sequentialist way in which journal articles are necessarily published. For exploration outside the health field, specialist dictionaries and encyclopedias, such as *The Cambridge Encyclopedia of Human Evolution*,[23] Tom Bottomore's *A Dictionary of Marxist Thought*,[24] and Kuper's and Kuper's *The Social Science Encyclopedia*,[25] were useful as first ports of call for new lines of inquiry as they emerged. Electronic searches were used for particular topics such as sleep, alienation, well-being, community development, bipedalism, deprivation, and so on, although only a fraction of the available material could be used to illustrate the arguments being pursued. Choice was made according to my interpretation of their relevance to the questions being explored and to the importance given to a particular point of view by other historians, scientists, time, or culture, all within the confines imposed by a huge amount of material.

Because the topic is so broad ranging, mention is made of many issues or themes that, to do them justice, could be expanded. However, I have had to be content with raising them as relevant and choosing to provide some lengthier, but still brief, discussion on a few outstanding examples, as in Chapter 4, where a number of particular human characteristics or capacities are examined, or the several times the ideas of Konrad Lorenz, Karl Marx, or Gerald Edelman are raised.

Some of the central or emerging concepts have been supported with ideas that arose out of many small empirical studies conducted, mainly using questionnaires, employed with a variety of people from the community, as well as occupational therapists and students. The sampling employed in these differed. One study used random sampling, others used cluster sampling, and still others used total populations in particular situations, such as students or participants at a seminar or conference. Questionnaires were also used in a pilot study that accessed a convenience sample of people known to the group of students taking part in the research. All of these studies were exploratory in nature, seeking to expand understanding of the relationships between health and occupation, and beliefs, values, perceptions, and ideas that people, including occupational therapists, hold about this relationship.

Having discussed the way in which this topic was explored, a few important concepts need to be introduced about health, occupation, and biological and sociocultural approaches to studying health and occupation, which provide a backdrop to the book; all are revisited later in the text.

Background Concepts
Influence of Medical Science

First, in seeking to clarify people's beliefs, values, perceptions, and ideas about the relationships between health and occupation, it is important to recall that, presently, in post-industrialized societies, health care is dominated by medical science. This is based mainly on contemporary understanding of physiology, biochemistry, pathology, and biostatistics, and societal acceptance of modern technological, surgical, and pharmaceutical advances. Medical science values are so integral to post-industrial culture's thinking, it is difficult for those brought up in such a society to perceive health from other than a medical science perspective. To some extent, this limits the study of health to ideas, beliefs, and approaches that are valued, advocated, and deemed important by medical science.

Even the growing behavioral-health, social-health, and health science professions, different and distinct from medicine, are still influenced by medical science values and perspectives in that they challenge or use medical science categories and theories, accept many medical science priorities, and are concerned with strategies to diagnose or analyze, reduce, or prevent illness resulting from physical, behavioral, or social factors. Because of this emphasis, the major preoccupation in health research is to uncover the causes of ill health and disease. Notwithstanding the holistic philosophy of the Ottawa Charter for Health Promotion,[26] which has been adopted by the "new public health" movement,[27] health research remains preoccupied with reducing the incidence of ill health at the expense of detailed exploration of the causes of good health and well-being. Recent interest in social determinants of health, health promotion, and wellness has centered to a large extent on the prevention of illness, many people using the terms "prevention" and "health promotion" synonymously. Preventive approaches, which dominate health promotion just as medicine dominates health care, generally take for granted a medical science explanation of the cause of disease and the mechanisms for prevention.

The new public health is also influenced by a post-industrial debate between the values of economic rationalism and social equality. Caught between medical science and the debate about social values, public health has largely failed to consider how basic human needs relate to health, unless the needs can be reduced to obvious physiological functioning or monetary terms. Rather like "instinct theory," the idea of human needs is unfashionable and to a large extent ignored, being associated with "naturalistic fallacy"[28] and out of step with the dominant notions of behaviorism and cultural relativism. This stance ignores many of the needs and potential of humans, which are part of their "hard-wired" neuronal structure, and, as Doyal and Gough maintain in their award-winning book *A Theory of Human Need*, even if needs are not identical with drives or a "motivational force instigated by a state of disequilibrium...neither are they disconnected from 'human nature.'" These authors state that "to argue for such disconnection would be to identify humanity with no more than human reason and to bifurcate human existence from that of the rest of the animal world."[29]

It is argued here that health is related to the meeting of biological needs and potential, to learning "how nature intended human beings to live,"[30] and that the needs of any living organism are related to health from the point of view of "how a specimen" of that kind of organism "can be recognized as flourishing."[28]

Human Need for Occupation

The second major concept maintains that humans have "occupational needs" that go beyond the instinctive patterned behaviors of many other animals and that these needs are related to health. In fact, they are the species' primary health mechanism, motivating the provision of other basic requirements as well as enabling individuals to use their biological capacities and potential, meet sociocultural expectations, and thereby flourish. The adaptive capacity of the human brain allows the innate drive for purposeful activity to respond to cultural forces and values that add a social dimension to the relationship between occupation and health. I explore health from an occupational perspective by considering how biological and sociocultural needs influence each other.

Although in recent times occupation, in its own right, has not been a focal point of study, socialist reformers in Europe who recognized the value of human labor and pragmatist philosophers in the United States in the late 19th and early 20th centuries did recognize the centrality of occupation to life. Since then, sociology, economics, technology, and medical science have so dominated thinking that occupation has been considered from these perspectives rather than in its own right. It is interesting to note that socialist and pragmatist recognition of the importance of occupation in life grew from the results of huge social change from a technology of human labor based on agriculture to one based on industry and that occupational therapy originated as a result of this occupational interest. The current resurgence of interest in occupation by occupational therapists may well be a response to a particular need to reconsider human occupational requirements afresh at another time of change.

Combining Biological-Sociocultural Issues

Third, in order to understand health and occupation, both biological and cultural issues require exploration. This history of ideas focuses on combining two different approaches—an evolutionary, biological approach and a modern, culture-concept approach. This is not an unusual combination for occupational therapists, although it is uncommon for biological and sociocultural determinants of human behavior to be studied together today.

This exploration of the innate evolutionary aspects of health and occupational behavior and those determined by experience, learning, and cultural evolution involves ideas similar to those of modern ethologists seeking to discover, among other ideas, the survival function of the behavior under study. Ethology has emerged over a period of approximately 75 years, the term having been initially applied in a variety of contexts, overlapping at one extreme with ecology and at the other with psychology.[31] The current view of ethology that behavior demonstrates the interactions between the inborn, natural aspects of behavior and those determined by experience and learning contrasts with the "ultra-environmentalism" of modern anthropology and sociology.[32] Durant argues that the "idea of innate character in animals [and man] was central to the work" of Konrad Lorenz.[31] Lorenz (1903-1989), an Austrian zoologist, explained ethology as the process of examining:

> *Animal and human behavior as the function of a system owing its existence, as well as its special form, to a development process that has taken place in the history of the species, in the development of the individual and, in man, in cultural history.[33]*

In line with Lorenz's perspective, I consider prehistoric occupational traits alongside "natural" health behaviors of early hominids, before they were affected by millions of years of acquired health and occupational values, the assumption being that human traits resulting from biological evolution will have affected occupational evolution, just as changes in social values and occupational technology will have affected natural health behaviors. However, making inferences about occupational behavior and health by considering early human lifestyles is difficult because of the lack of written records. Historians, anthropologists, and the like have had to make do with hypotheses about human evolution informed by archaeological fragments and by inference from 20th century cultures, which appear similar to those of early humans. I use accounts of such work in order to pursue the evolution of occupation and its relationship to health.

Outline of Chapters

The book has four main sections, which address the particular questions explored: Chapter 2 proposes a theory of human nature, and Chapters 3 and 4 consider the importance of occupation in human life according to that theory; Chapters 5 and 6 suggest the positive influence of occupation on health and the negative effects of occupational alienation, deprivation, and imbalance; Chapters 7 and 8 inquire into the potential of occupational therapy to be a health promoting profession; and Chapter 9 explores a role for occupational therapy with current WHO and public health objectives.

Each chapter will now be outlined. Chapter 2 defines occupation as a central aspect of the human experience because it covers the whole range of purposeful human activity whether work, play, or rest, obligatory or chosen, biological or sociocultural in origin. Occupation is so much a part of the ordinary fabric of life that it is taken for granted, despite the fact that it provides the mechanism to fulfill basic human needs essential for survival and to enable people to adapt to biological, social, and environmental changes. A theory of human nature based on the human need to engage in occupation is proposed. It takes an evolutionary and humanist view, which also has the advantage of bringing reductionist presumptions into question.[34] It also advocates for ecological sustainability, because, although the humanist/ecological mix may seem somewhat incompatible, a line taken argues that because of our occupational natures, humans now dominate the ecological chain yet tend to see themselves as separate from it. They degrade the environment, in part, in response to the materialism resulting from occupational "progress" and, in part, because they do not appreciate the consequences of meeting their occupational needs.

Many existing views of human nature have influenced or are integral to the theory that humans are occupational beings. For example, from Plato comes the notion that humans are fitted by nature for different activities because of their particular aptitudes and interests. From Freud and the psychoanalysts comes agreement that all mental entities have some physiological basis, but that we are not aware or conscious of them all. From existentialist theories comes the concept of the uniqueness of individuals and that meaning, purpose, and choice in human life is as important as scientific or metaphysical truths. From outside the Occidental tradition comes the need for balance, which is central to many Eastern views and is seen as important to occupational well-being. These as well as modern biology, sociology, and behavioral and neuropsychology offer a variety of views, which, collectively, sustain an occupational view of the nature of humans.

Chapter 3, based mainly on biological and neurosciences, explores, from an occupational perspective, the particular mix of human characteristics and capacities that have enabled us to survive healthily and successfully as a species. In the latter half of the 20th century, evolutionary theories regarding biological determinants of behavior have been dominated by postulates that human actions are determined by sociocultural environments, rather than inherited characteristics. Human capacities are indeed developed according to individual utilization, experience, and sociocultural environments, as sociologists postulate. However, it is also true that there are particular neuronal systems genetically endowed with the capacity for particular behaviors, such as bipedalism, dexterity, speech and language, body image, or visual perception.[8] Chapter 3 provides a basis for the later argument that the human drive for purposeful use of capacities, through occupation, is a biological endowment, but that the purpose is the result of sociocultural values and forces.

To understand the relationship between occupation and the sociocultural environment, Chapter 4 traces "occupational evolution," comparing the lifestyles of early and modern humans in order to discover basic occupational drives and how engagement in occupation has changed throughout time. Human occupation has become extremely complex because of the never-ending development of occupational technology and the social structures and values that accompany it. People's occupational nature is evidenced by the diversity of activities that are culturally valued, as well as the diversity of values given to the many ways of dividing and classifying occupation.

The exploration covered by Chapters 2 through 4 leads me to propose that the evolutionary functions of occupation are integral to survival and health, but that the basic occupational needs of people are now obscured by the values imposed by the cultures and societies in which they live and by prevalent philosophies. This leads naturally to Chapter 5, which explores positive health from an occupational perspective. I argue that there is an integrated biological and sociocultural construct of health that relates to survival of the species, enables individuals and communities to flourish, and has built-in flexibility in that it can change according to context. The chapter is founded on the WHO's 1946 definition of health and well-being and how the Ottawa Charter for Health Promotion describes health.

In the search for links between occupation and health, the biologically endowed relationship between needs of humans and health is considered by focusing on health issues for hunter-gatherer peoples and views held about "natural" health. Just as concepts of occupation have changed throughout history, so have changes to major occupational structures and foci distorted early health behaviors so that they no longer serve their original purpose effectively. The importance to health of balanced use of capacities through engagement in occupation, according to individual need, emerges as a primary consideration from this exploration.

I make an unexamined assumption that aiming health care toward good health and well-being is a laudable and desirable objective. As part of this aim, the need to prevent illness is recognized. This being so, Chapter 6 discusses the relationship between occupational structures and illness at population levels and goes on to consider evidence from existing studies about ill health resulting from occupational deprivation, alienation, and imbalance. I argue that there is inadequate consideration of underlying sociocultural determinants, which lead to occupational deprivation, alienation, or the need for balanced utilization of capacities, in health care, education, or social and political policies, strategies, and programs. This should be a concern for public health.

Current fascination with health, driven both by personal vitalism and by economic doctrines, is associated with much rhetoric published by health professionals and political authorities about the importance of developing health promotion programs. There may be some health professionals who do not perceive good health as their concern. Whether or not this is the case, there are few opportunities available for established health services to either evaluate services or to undertake major program changes toward facilitating good health and well-being. Indeed, for one of occupational therapy's traditional client groups, the chronically disabled, programs with that aim seem to be disappearing.

To address these issues and others, an original exploration of occupational therapy's role and potential in promoting health is offered. Occupational therapy has not been thoroughly reviewed from a perspective of the relationship between occupation and health. The profession developed from ideas generated by the work of 19th century social reformers and philosophers as mentioned earlier, and has been one health profession intimately concerned with occupation. Despite a common assumption that it is similar to other medically accepted health sciences, most applicable to the remediation of ill health, occupational therapy's philosophical base relates to the facilitation of good health and well-being through engagement in purposeful occupation. Occupational therapists have long held a belief that health can be enhanced by occupation that is beneficial to human well-being. However, present social and political thinking fails to acknowledge a human need for occupation for its own sake, apart from paid employment for monetary reasons. Occupational therapy's appreciation of a basic value of occupation is therefore out of step with dominant values. The next two chapters ask how occupational therapy's focus on occupation and on health has changed historically as a result of both external and internal pressures.

Chapter 7 describes and analyzes the origins of occupational therapy in North America at the beginning of the 20th century. Notions about occupation and the development of human potential surfaced then as themes common to philosophies and policies proposed by industrialists, educators, philosophers, and social and health workers. This mélange of themes culminated, in the health arena, in the formation of occupational therapy. Occupational therapy is, in fact, different from many other health professions in that it began with a philosophy that is not based on physical science; its growth was a response to social problems stemming from widespread industrialization, to a growing appreciation of the value of human labor, and to ideas central to "moral treatment" of mental illness in the 19th century. This difference has made it hard for others to understand. Occupational therapists tried to reduce the difference by conforming to physical science presumptions of other health professions. The conformity achieved some useful outcomes, but at the cost of devaluing and almost losing many of occupational therapy's distinctive features. Because of the uncertainties caused by a shifting foundation and by medical science directives that encouraged reductionist rather than holistic approaches, occupational therapists have experienced many difficulties in explaining their contribution to health care and have suffered some loss of overall direction of professional aspirations.

Chapter 8 analyzes the historical relationship between occupational therapy and occupation. Although the 20th century has been an era of rapid change in occupational technology, occupational issues have, on the whole, been addressed through legislation and procedures aimed at social equity or the economy. In response to these forces, plus advances in medical science and, frequently, in the organization of health care services, occupational therapists have altered substantially, if temporarily, the value and importance given to occupation. This led eventually to serious consideration being given by the profession to re-identifying its ideological foundation and theory base. An exploration of this theoretical soul-searching in recent years demonstrates that occupational therapists are developing a greater appreciation of their profession's original philosophy, with most now identifying occupation as their particular focus in health care.

Chapter 8 also considers the relationship between occupational therapy and health promotion. Occupational therapy's philosophical base, even when aimed at remediating ill health, relates to the promotion of health. Practice is founded on the notion that health can be improved by people being enabled to reach their "occupational" potential. However, occupational therapy's contribution to health promotion is not recognized for many reasons, including its long association with the medical model, which, to an extent, deflected some of occupational therapy's initial purpose. Other important factors in the lack of recognition are:

- The poorly understood relationship between occupation and health
- Differing views of health and the promotion of health between health care workers
- Differing models of practice within professions
- The fact that views of occupational therapists do not necessarily agree with changing cultural values of the most influential health care workers and policy makers

The chapter explores these issues as well as occupational therapy's particular contributions to health promotion. Key concepts important in health promotion rhetoric are integral to the aims of occupational therapy, such as being primarily responsive to client participation and goals, facilitating quality of life, and enabling people to maximize potential, independence, self-growth, and actualization. Current difficulties and problems that prevent the achievement of these aims are identified. One source of empirical data for the exploration is a national survey of Australian occupational therapists undertaken to evaluate their interest and current professional direction toward and in health promotion.

Although I concentrate on exploring health from an occupational perspective, in the process, I also attempt to clarify different approaches to health. Such clarification is required to provide a foundation for considering the actual and potential relationship between public health and occupational therapy. Based on the assumption that occupation is important to the health of individuals and communities, Chapter 9 proposes an actual and potential role for occupational therapy in public health. It structures this proposal around five different health approaches that, together form an integrated view of health promotion. The approaches span wellness within conventional medicine, preventive medicine, social justice, community development, and ecological sustainability. This view, should it be implemented, would enable systematic and logical integration of the WHO health objectives into health care. Priority health strategies could be encouraged and reinforced, and noncompetitive recognition and encouragement of different values, approaches, and contributions may be more possible than at present. The current, non-integrated, structure of health care is arbitrarily divided, for example, in terms of acute versus long-term, individual versus community, or medical versus social health. The "new public health" direction toward "health for all" is relevant to all aspects of health care from illness to wellness and cannot be seen to start where conventional medicine, for example, is assumed to leave off.

Within these approaches, occupational therapists, attending to the relationship between occupation and health, can make special and particular contributions toward public health. The chapter outlines a new synthesis of occupational therapy using action-research approaches compatible with its philosophical and theoretical base as well as subsequent development. It is proposed that an occupational perspective on health would allow occupational needs to be integrated with medical science approaches. Preventive medicine and health and wellness education would expand to address issues such as the importance of balancing and making use of human capacities, and community development and social justice initiatives would cast occupational deprivation issues and inequalities in a new light. In all approaches, a stronger focus on the development of services aimed at disadvantaged people is required. Finally, I propose that an occupational perspective of health will assist ecologists in a better understanding of how to harness or adapt human occupational traits to sustain rather than destroy the earth.

Because of the historical nature of the exploration, this book tells a story. It is designed to be read from beginning to end as each chapter builds upon the ideas discussed in earlier ones. If used in this way, readers can trace the origins and argument for the occupational approaches to public health that have grown from this exploration. Figure 1-1 is a diagrammatic representation of the storyline. At the start of each chapter it is used to indicate the chapter's contribution to this occupational perspective of health.

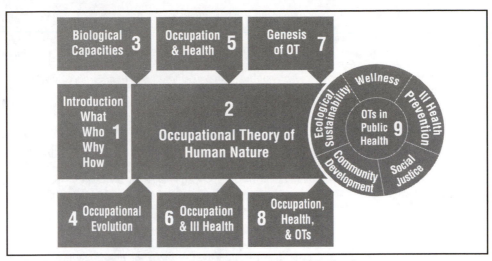

Figure 1-1. Diagrammatic representation of the storyline of the book.

References

1. World Health Organization. *Primary Health Care.* Report of the International Conference on Primary Health Care, Alma Ata, USSR, 1978.
2. Better Health Commission of Australia. *Looking Forward to Better Health.* Canberra: Australian Government Publishing Service; 1986.
3. MacDonald EM, ed. *Occupational Therapy in Rehabilitation.* 2nd ed. London, England: Bailliere, Tindall and Cassell; 1964:2.
4. Levy BS. Therapeutic community. In: Kuper A, Kuper J, eds. *The Social Science Encyclopedia.* Rev ed. London, England: Routledge; 1989.
5. Johnson H. Psychiatrist, Shortland Clinic, Royal Newcastle Hospital, professional communication, 1968.
6. Wilcock AA. *Shortland Clinic Memoirs.* Unpublished document written at the time of the author's transfer to another post, 1972.
7. Wilcock AA. *Occupational Therapy Approaches to Stroke.* Melbourne, Australia: Churchill Livingstone; 1986.
8. Kolb B, Whishaw IQ. *Fundamentals of Human Neuropsychology.* 3rd ed. San Francisco, Calif: WH Freeman and Co; 1990.
9. Edelman G. *Bright Air, Brilliant Fire: On the Matter of the Mind.* London, England: Penguin Books; 1992:15.
10. Reilly M. The education process. *American Journal of Occupational Therapy.* 1969;23:299-307.
11. Christiansen C, Baum C, eds. *Occupational Therapy: Overcoming Human Performance Deficits.* Thorofare, NJ: SLACK Inc; 1991.
12. Kielhofner G, ed. *A Model of Human Occupation, Theory and Application.* Baltimore, Md: Williams and Wilkins; 1985.
13. Yerxa EJ. Occupational science: a new source of power for participants in occupational therapy. *Journal of Occupational Science: Australia.* 1993;1(1):3–10.
14. Lovejoy AO. The study of the history of ideas. 1936. In: King P, ed. *The History of Ideas.* London, England: Croom Helm; 1983:179-194.
15. Yerxa EJ, Clark F, Frank G, et al. An introduction to occupational science: a foundation for occupational therapy in the 21st century. *Occupational Therapy in Health Care.* 1989;6(4):1–17.
16. Yerxa EJ. A mind is a precious thing. *Australian Occupational Therapy Journal.* 1990;37(4):170–171.
17. Gergen K. *Towards Transformation in Social Knowledge.* New York, NY: Springer-Verlag; 1982.
18. Held D. Frankfurt School. In: Bottomore T, ed. *A Dictionary of Marxist Thought.* 2nd ed. Oxford, UK: Blackwell Publishers; 1991:209.
19. Lovejoy AO. *Essays in the History of Ideas.* Baltimore, Md: The Johns Hopkins Press; 1948:195.
20. Burke P. History of ideas. In: Bullock A, Stalleybrass O, Trombley S, eds. *The Fontana Dictionary*

of Modern Thought. 2nd ed. London, England: Fontana Press; 1988:388.

21. Hamilton DB. The idea of the history and the history of ideas. *Image: Journal of Nursing Scholarship.* 1993;25(1):45–48.

22. Richardson L. Writing: a method of inquiry. In: Denzin N, Lincoln Y, eds. *Handbook of Qualitative Research.* London, England: Sage; 1994:516-529.

23. Jones S, Martin R, Pilbeam D, eds. *The Cambridge Encyclopedia of Human Evolution.* New York, NY: Cambridge University Press; 1992.

24. Bottomore T, ed. *A Dictionary of Marxist Thought.* 2nd ed. Oxford, UK: Blackwell Publishers; 1991.

25. Kuper A, Kuper J, eds. *The Social Science Encyclopedia.* Rev ed. London, England: Routledge; 1989.

26. World Health Organization, Health and Welfare Canada, Canadian Public Health Association. *Ottawa Charter for Health Promotion.* Ottawa, Canada; 1986.

27. Ashton J, Seymour H. *The New Public Health: The Liverpool Experience.* Milton Keynes: Open University Press; 1988.

28. Watts ED. Human needs. In: Kuper A, Kuper J, eds. *The Social Science Encyclopedia.* Rev ed. London, England: Routledge; 1989:367-368.

29. Doyal L, Gough I. *A Theory of Human Need.* London, England: Macmillan; 1991:35-36.

30. Coon CS. *The Hunting Peoples.* London, England: Jonathan Cape Ltd; 1972:393.

31. Durant JR. Innate character in animals and man: a perspective on the origins of ethology. In: Webster C, ed. *Biology, Medicine and Society 1840-1940.* New York, NY: Cambridge University Press; 1981:164-165.

32. Webster C, ed. *Biology, Medicine and Society 1840-1940.* New York, NY: Cambridge University Press; 1981:3.

33. Lorenz K. *Civilized Man's Eight Deadly Sins.* Latzke M, trans. London, England: Methuen and Co Ltd; 1974:1.

34. Stevenson L. *Seven Theories of Human Nature.* 2nd ed. Oxford, UK: Oxford University Press; 1987:143.

Suggested Reading

Hamilton DB. The idea of the history and the history of ideas. *Image: Journal of Nursing Scholarship.* 1993;25(1):45–48.

Lovejoy AO. The study of the history of ideas. 1936. In: King P, ed. *The History of Ideas.* London, England: Croom Helm; 1983.

Richardson L. Writing: a method of inquiry. In: Denzin N, Lincoln Y, eds. *Handbook of Qualitative Research.* London, England: Sage; 1994.

World Health Organization. *Primary Health Care.* Report of the International Conference on Primary Health Care, Alma Ata, USSR, 1978.

World Health Organization, Health and Welfare Canada, Canadian Public Health Association. *Ottawa Charter for Health Promotion.* Ottawa, Canada; 1986.

Yerxa EJ. Occupational science: a new source of power for participants in occupational therapy. *Journal of Occupational Science: Australia.* 1993;1(1):3–10.

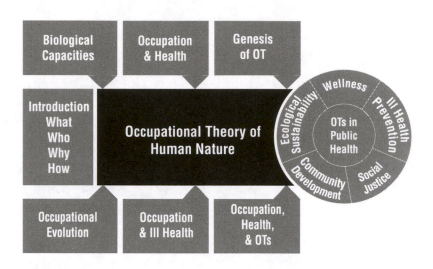

Chapter 2
An Occupational Theory of Human Nature

This chapter presents the reader with ideas about:
- Theories of human nature
- An occupational theory of human nature which takes an evolutionary, humanist, and ecological view based on the human need to engage in occupation
- Occupation as a central aspect of the human experience
- A three-way link between occupation, health, and survival

In this chapter, occupation is introduced as a central aspect of the human experience and is defined by occupational therapists and others. The discussion leads to the proposition that, from an evolutionary perspective, there is a three-way link between survival, health, and occupation, in that occupation provides the mechanism for people to fulfill basic human needs essential for survival, to adapt to environmental changes, and to develop and exercise genetic capacities in order to maintain health.

As a particular focus for the history of ideas explored in this text, a theory of human nature is proposed, based on the idea that defines the emerging discipline of occupational science—that humans are occupational beings.[1] In this chapter, the main direction of the theory is set out, but the details are explored in Chapters 3 through 6. A theory, in the sense it is used here, is a system of ideas held to explain a group of facts or phenomena. It includes a "related set of principles" that "tie two or more concepts together, usually in a correlational or causal way," such as those in the paragraph above relating to survival, health, and occupation.[2] According to Lewin's three stages of theory development—the speculative, the descriptive, and the constructive—this theory is at the second stage of development, which is a time for testing. In this case, throughout the text, the concepts, relationships, and principles will be measured against a broad range of ideas and against known research from other theories.[3]

That the theory is concerned with human nature is ambitious, but it is addressed in this way to emphasize the extent of the complexity and of the influence engagement in occupation has had upon cultural evolution, upon our present circumstances, and upon the health of individuals and communities. "The notion of human nature involves the belief that all human individuals share some common features" and characteristics that are innate.[4] Accepted by many Marxist theorists, this is a concept central to humanist and critical theorists also in that it provides the grounds for aiming toward growth models of health and for critical analysis of social or health environments that inhibit human potential. It should be noted that Marx made valuable contributions to a social and occupational view of human nature, which is dismissed in the official ideology of socialist countries and by Marxist structuralism.[5]

Apart from Marx's view, well-articulated examples of differing theories of human nature range as widely as those proposed by Plato, Freud, or Sartre, as well as those embraced in creeds as diverse as Christianity or Taoism. In addition, each person thinks and acts according to a personal view of human nature, but seldom attempts to articulate or to test this view, preferring instead to profess allegiance to a socio-culturally accepted view. These diverse theories about human nature provide the context for beliefs about the meaning and purpose of life, about visions of the future, and about what humans should or should not do.[6]

The theory of human nature proposed here is based on the idea that we have an innate need to engage in occupation. This need has, on the whole, been over-looked in scientific inquiry and in most theories of human nature because it is so mundane. That engagement in occupation is innate, inborn, or natural is indicated by the fact that people spend their lives almost constantly engaged in purposeful "doing" even when free of obligation or necessity. They "do" daily tasks including things they feel they must do and others that they want to. Human evolution has been filled with ongoing and progressive doings that, apart from enabling the species to survive, has stimulated, entertained, and excited some people and bored or stressed others according to what was done. Doing is so much a part of every-day life that within Western cultures people frequently identify themselves and each other by what they do. For example, common forms of introduction name occupa-tional pursuits, such as, "May I introduce Fred Jones? He is a computer operator." Many family names from England and Europe reflect long past occupations of their members, such as Smith and Barber. Children frequently are asked, "What are you planning to do when you grow up?" or "What have you been doing?" It is as if the occupational background, present, or future of people is a major reflection of every individual, that what they do, in some ways, is what or who they are. The things people do are described as occupations.

Defining Occupation

Because occupation is a central theme of this text, it is necessary to clarify, as far as is possible, what is meant by the word in this particular context. It will be used here as occupational therapists use it, in the generic sense, perhaps reflecting com-mon usage of the word when their profession was developing in the first decades of this century. In *The Concise Oxford Dictionary of Current English* of 1911, occu-pation was defined as "occupying or being occupied, what occupies one, means of filling up one's time, temporary or regular employment, business, calling, pursuit."[7] In *Webster's Revised Unabridged Dictionary of the English Language* of 1919, the definition includes "that which occupies or engages the time and attention."[8]

Occupation also has several meanings in contemporary dictionaries. *The Oxford English Dictionary* of 1989 defines the aspect of occupation central to this text as "being occupied or employed with, or engaged in something."[9] Despite this gener-ic meaning, occupation is currently commonly used to refer to paid employment, specifically. The adjective "occupational" is particularly used in this way, as in "occupational health and safety" and "occupational diseases." The use of occupa-tion to refer, as it does in this text, to all purposeful human activity is sometimes misunderstood. It may, therefore, be useful to consider other words with similar meaning in order to justify the continued generic usage. These include praxis, which is used in various ways in scholarly or academic circumstances, but seldom as part of common usage, and words in common use such as work, labor, leisure, and activity.

Praxis

"Praxis," from the Greek for "of action," according to Lobkowicz "refers to almost any kind of activity that a free man is likely to perform; in particular, all kinds of business and political activity."[10] In *Roget's Thesaurus,* praxis is given as a synonym for action,[11] but it is such a specialized word that it does not appear in all dictionaries. In *The Oxford English Dictionary,* it is defined as "doing, acting, action, practice," yet in another dictionary, it is defined as "accepted practice or custom."[9]

In neurorehabilitation, apraxia (no action) is a common sequela of stroke or head injury. In that instance, it refers to a lack of ability to carry out purposeful activity or skilled movement when there is no physical, cognitive, or emotional reason for difficulty. This disorder was first defined by Hughlings Jackson in the 1860s, named by Steinthal in 1871, but detailed analysis is attributed to Leipmann from 1900 onwards.[12] At the opposite end of the skill continuum, "praxiology"—the science of efficient action—is a discipline "dealing with methods of doing anything in any way...from the point of view of its effectiveness."[13]

Marx's use of praxis is perhaps the most similar to occupation as it is used in this text. To him, praxis was "the free, universal, creative, and self-creative activity through which man creates (makes, produces) and changes (shapes) his historical, human world and himself."[14] Marx usually opposes "labor" to "praxis," but in *Economic and Philosophical Manuscripts* is sometimes inconsistent, using labor synonymously with praxis.[15] Praxis, as action, is used in the present day as a descriptor for many types of action-research, such as critical praxis research or critical feminist praxis.[16,17] Its many different meanings, and its obscurity despite increased usage since the 1960s following translation and availability of Marx's early writings, preclude praxis as the most appropriate word for all purposeful activity.

Work

Dictionary definitions of "work" describe it as "action involving effort or exertion, especially as a means of gaining livelihood."[18] Work derives from an Old English word, "Weorc," and is described by Williams as the most general word for "doing something and for something done," however, its current predominant use is, like "occupation," for "regular paid employment."[19] Its usage in this way is even more specialized than "occupation." Williams notes that "the specialization of work to paid employment is the result of the development of capitalist productive relations," which in part shifted the meaning "from the productive effort itself to the predominant social relationship." "Work (in its widest sense, including labor)," observes Parker, is "independent of any particular form of society." It "is a basic condition of the existence and continuation of human life."[20] It is also the antithesis of play, leisure, rest, and recreation, implying an element of compulsion or necessary toil, so earning a description as "everything we do to keep body and soul together."[21]

Labor

"Labor," like work, is used for activities that are, for some reason, necessary or enforced. Williams suggests it has a "strong medieval sense of pain and toil" and that it is a harder word than work, with manual workers being described as labor-ers from the 13th century.[19] Labor is described by Marx as:

> *A process in which both man and Nature participate, and in which man of his own accord starts, regulates, and controls the material reactions between himself and Nature. He opposes himself to Nature as one of her own forces, setting in motion arms and legs, head and hands, the natural forces of his body in order to appropriate Nature's productions in a form adapted to his own wants.*[22]

Ruskin, an English 19th century socialist, described it as the "contest of the life of man with an opposite; the term 'life' including his intellect, soul, and physical power, contending with question, difficulty, trial, or material force."[23] Harry Braverman, a contemporary socialist, in his 1974 book addressing the degradation of work in the 20th century, writes that labor "represents the sole resource of humanity in confronting nature...whether directly exercised or stored in such products as tools, machinery, or domesticated animals" and cites Aristotle's description of labor being "intelligent action."[24]

Despite these very broad concepts, labor, like work, is not used for activities that are restful or playful, and although neither means only paid employment, like occupation, they are used frequently in this way. Both describe an aspect of what can be meant by "occupation," that is, work and labor are an integral part of "occupation."

Leisure

Time other than that spent in paid employment is described as "leisure" from the Latin "licere," meaning permit, and from the 14th century meaning of opportunity or free time. An alternative is a "holiday, the old word for religious festival,"[19] although this has implications of a contained time, such as a "day" or "week" and, "in countries affected by the Hebrew tradition," the Sabbath "is not so much a day of leisure as a day of ceremonial inactivity, a day of restraint."[20] Leisure, holiday, and religious pursuits are also occupations.

Activity

"Activity" is defined as "the state of being active; the exertion of energy, action"[9] and, like occupation, describes specific deeds or actions. It is often used inter-changeably with occupation, even by occupational therapists, but activity is seldom used to imply paid employment, despite its derivation from Latin "agere," to do.[25] Of these choices, despite its frequent limited use, occupation remains the only word that can be used for all types of activity and is therefore the most appropriate word to use.

Occupation is so much a part of everyday life that it is reasonable to make empir-ical statements about it. It can be said, therefore, that humans engage in occupa-tion, with individuality of purpose; they think about the effects, conceptualize, and plan before undertaking activity; and they are able to reflect and mentally alter future behavior as a result of outcomes. Occupations demonstrate an individual's culturally sanctioned intellectual, moral, and physical attributes. It is only by what they do that people can demonstrate what they are or what they hope to be. Accolades for individual achievement are often surrounded with ritualized activities, such as graduations, ticker-tape parades, and initiation ceremonies. Awards and rituals are highly valued as demonstrations of the appreciation of occupational achievement.

In order to satisfy their need to exercise their capacities, humans seek out various and sometimes novel ways to pass the time. Without occupation, time appears to pass extremely slowly, as any long distance air traveler can attest, even with the frequent meals, drinks, and movies. Occupation is a natural user of time, which provides a sense of purpose, and without which humans are apt to be bored, depressed, and sometimes destructive. Even the stylite, the eremite, or the monk passes the time in a way purposeful to him or her, despite the purpose perhaps appearing obscure to others. People so commonly express a need to "do something to pass the time," that we have a word for this in the English language—"pastime." Exploring how and why people use time the way they do provides a rich source of data on many different sociocultural and health-related issues, and thus this perspective of occupation has been subject to scrutiny. Time-use surveys originated early this century, with most studying large population groups for comparative purposes, to inform social planners at national and international levels. Today, many time-use studies provide an important source of empirical information for occupational scientists and therapists.[26-30]

Adolph Meyer, an American psychiatrist, eminent in the first half of this century and credited with providing a philosophy to occupational therapy, also proposed that how people use time is very important. He asserted that in order to maintain and balance the organism that is a person, there is a need to act in time with bodily and natural rhythms and that timely activity and rest are vital components of healthy living. He observed to an historic meeting of occupational therapists in 1922 that:

> *Human ideals have unfortunately and usually been steeped in dreams of timeless eternity, and they have never included an equally religious valuation of actual time and its meaning in wholesome rhythms. The awakening to a full meaning of time as the biggest wonder and asset of our lives and the valuation of opportunity and performance as the greatest measure of time; those are the beacon lights of the philosophy of the occupational worker.[31]*

(Meyer is the subject of a brief biographical note included in Chapter 7.)

Despite this early pointer, it was not until about the 1970s that occupational therapists seriously began to recognize the value of time-use research and the study of human temporality.[32-39]

Occupation also provides the mechanism for social interaction and societal development and growth, forming the foundation of community, local, and national identity, because individuals not only engage in separate pursuits, they are able to plan and execute group activity to the extent of national government or to achieve international goals for individual, mutual, and community purposes. Anthropologists describe this unique human trait as "culture" and suggest:

> *It is the unique blend of biology and culture that makes the species* Homo sapiens *a truly unique kind of animal...Humans are different, not so much for what we do...but rather the fact that we can do more or less what we want. That is what having a highly developed culture really means.[40]*

Statements by occupational therapists suggest a view within the profession that occupation is central to the human experience. In the professional literature, occupation has been described as "a natural human phenomenon" that is taken for granted because it forms "the fabric of everyday lives,"[41] more specifically, as purposeful "use of time, energy, interest, and attention"[42] in work, leisure, family, cultural, self-care, and rest activities. It includes "activities that are playful, restful, serious, and productive," which are "carried out by individuals in their own unique ways" based on societal influences; their own needs, beliefs, and preferences; "the kinds of experiences they have had; their environments; and the patterns of behavior they acquire over time."[43] Occupation that is culturally sanctioned is seen by some as "a primary organizer of time and resources," enabling humans to survive, control, and adapt to their world; be economically self-sufficient[1]; and to experience social relationships and approval, as well as personal growth.[44] This view of occupation is applicable to communities at local to global levels and should not be seen as referring only to individuals. All aspects of this description will be integral to the meaning given to occupation throughout this text and will provide a base for the occupational theory proposed.

An Occupational Theory of Human Nature

The occupational theory of human nature will now be introduced. This provides the idea around which the story proceeds to unravel the relationship between health and occupation. This theory, being based upon few arbitrary elements derived from multiple and ongoing observations, meets the criteria of empirical accuracy and predictive capacity required by contemporary canons of science, such as Stephen Hawking. It can also definitely predict that, in the future, people will continue to engage in occupation, although the form of the occupation will change according to sociocultural evolution.

The occupational theory set out also meets Stevenson's requirements for a theory of human nature. In *Seven Theories of Human Nature*, he sets his requirements as:

1. A background theory of the nature of the universe
2. A basic theory of the nature of man
3. A diagnosis of what is wrong with man
4. A prescription for putting it right[6]

Stephen W. Hawking suggests that:

A theory is a good theory if it satisfies two requirements; it must accurately describe a large class of observations on the basis of a model that contains only a few arbitrary elements, and it must make definite predictions about the results of future observations.

Hawking SW. *A Brief History of Time.* Toronto, Canada: Bantam Books; 1988:10.

The theory is set within generally accepted scientific theories of the evolution of the universe and the species that inhabit it. Its basic concept of the nature of humans is that, as a result of their biological evolution and enculturation, humans are occupational beings. That is, the need to engage in occupation forms an integral part of innate biological systems aimed at survival and health, that the varying potential of individuals for different occupations is a result of their genetically inherited capacities, and that the expression and execution of occupation is learned and modified by the ecology and sociocultural environments. "As natural selection acts on phenotypes, not genotypes, and as phenotypes always include an environmental component, it is of course fallacious to oppose genes and environment."[63] This con-

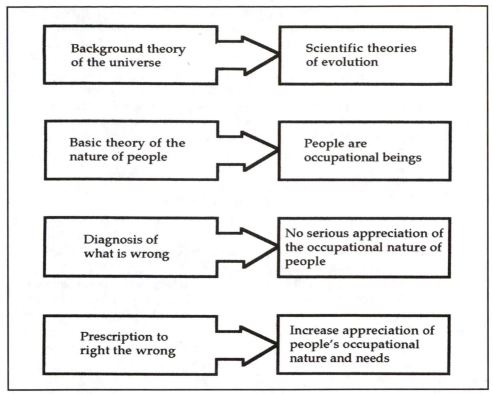

Figure 2-1. Occupational theory of human nature outlined according to Stevenson's requirements for theories of human nature.

cept is in accord with Csikszentmihalyi's view that human action is shaped by genetic, cultural, and self teleonomies,[45,46] and is supported by Snell's proposal that the making of "humans" is about 50% genetics and 50% culture.[47] The theory provides a simple diagnosis and prescription—namely, that humans have not seriously considered the implications or requirements of their occupational nature; that this has caused deleterious effects to individual, community, and ecological health; and that addressing this lack of awareness has the potential to result in major and beneficial changes to social, political, economic, ecological, and health policies and outcomes (Figure 2-1). Having outlined the theory, it will now be discussed in some detail.

Background

The background of the occupational theory of human nature discussed in this book can be seen in the following brief account of biological and cultural evolu-

Early speculation, interest, and theory about evolution of humans and the universe are demonstrated by geologist James Hutton's *Theory of the Earth* published in 1795; clergyman TR Malthus's book *An Essay on the Principle of Population* published in 1798; French naturalist Jean Baptiste Lamarck's theory of organic evolution *Systeme des Animaux* published in 1801; and Charles Lyell's *Principles of Geology* published between 1830 and 1833.

tionary theory. Current scientific thought generally accepts that living matter evolved naturally from nonliving matter in the form of single-celled creatures. Over a period of perhaps a billion years, some electrons, protons, and neutrons combined to form atoms, which formed molecules. Some of these became "more or less well-organized aggregates," one class of which is organic matter. In turn, some original micro-organisms went through a "comparable hierarchical evolution" to primitive plant forms to invertebrates to vertebrates, and, in the past 60 million years, to mammals.[48]

Against a background of geologist and naturalist speculation, interest and theories that were out of step with dominant Christian beliefs, Darwin's *Origin of the Species by Means of Natural Selection (1859)*[49] and *The Descent of Man and Selection in Relation to Sex (1871)*[50] are recognized as the works that brought theories of evolution to public debate and inquiry in the Occident. Darwin's evidence did not come from human beings, and only his conclusion suggested that his theory would shed light on the origin of man. Nonetheless his theories were received with moral shock, fear, and derision in the lay community, although accepted rapidly in biological science, at least until the return of the creationists.[51]

Dawkins suggests that although it is difficult to explain "how even a simple universe began," Darwin's theory of evolution by natural selection demonstrates a way in which "simplicity could change into complexity" and how collections of stable molecules could eventually, through "high longevity/fecundity/copying-fidelity," evolve into complex living beings.[52] Darwin's theory is based on the empirical observations that there is a tendency for parental traits to be passed to their offspring; that despite this, there are considerable and noticeable variations between individuals; and that species are capable of a rate of generation that cannot be supported by available natural resources. That is, more are born than can survive, requiring a struggle for existence. This leads to survival by natural selection of those with "certain inherited variants which increase the chances of their carriers surviving and reproducing."[53] Spencer termed this "survival of the fittest," in an often-quoted phrase that is frequently misconstrued to mean survival of those physically fit and strong, rather than those with "expected reproductive success," because it is taken literally and out of context.[54] Natural selection results in the accumulation of favored variants that will effect gradual adaptive change in every generation and, over extended periods, produce new forms of life. Diversity and individual uniqueness is the consistent message of evolutionary studies from Darwin's time to the present.[53]

Individual uniqueness, particularly in relation to biological characteristics and capacities influencing engagement in occupation, is a focal concern of occupational therapists, but not of political, social, or health planners for whom population and group similarities rather than individual diversity are the focus. Humans, because their biological capacities enable flexible, adaptable, and wide-ranging occupations, are fitted for almost any environment and are dispersed across the globe. Cultural and occupational evolution such as tool use, agriculture, and modern medicine have broken through natural population restraints that maintained population size of species more or less constant over long periods of time and as a result have reached a point where humans dominate ecological systems, many believe, to the extent of natural resources not being sufficient to maintain predicted population growth.[53,55]

Working at almost the same time as Darwin, the Austrian monk Gregor Mendel studied and experimented with plant species, which led to his formulation of biological laws of heredity. Virtually ignored at the time, his work was rediscovered in 1900 by three scientists working separately—De Vries, Correns, and Tschermak—all within a 3-month period. Mendel's work provided the answer to the "causes of the variations on which natural selection acts."[55] Darwin's theory, modified in light of Mendelian genetics,[56] is now known as neo-Darwinism[57] or synthetic evolution.[58] In recent times, "the discovery of the structure and function of DNA has made clear the nature of the hereditary variations upon which natural selection operates."[59] It is now acknowledged that humans are mammals with much in common with other animals and that like other species humans have "a certain genetic constitution that causally explains not only the anatomical features...but also our distinctive...behavior."[6] As Bronowski explains so succinctly:

> *The evolution of the brain, of the hand, of the eyes, of the feet, the teeth, the whole human frame, made a special gift of man...faster in evolution, and richer and more flexible in behavior...he has what no other animal possesses, a jigsaw of faculties which alone, over three thousand million years of life, make him creative.*[60]

Bronowski's description of human difference is a useful bridge between Darwinist theories of evolution and the occupational nature of humans, which will be introduced here and explored more fully in the next two chapters.

Central Concepts

The next stage of the argument relies on three related sets of principles. First, all people (unless prevented by congenital or acquired dysfunction, such as brain damage) engage in complex and self-initiated occupational behavior because of their species' common combination of biological features, such as consciousness, cognitive capacity, and language. Although it is higher cortical adaptations such as these that have generated and made possible the complex occupational behavior that sets humans apart from other animals, anatomical and physiological characteristics of the body, such as bipedalism, upright posture, and hand dexterity, are vital instruments in the execution of occupation. Because of the integrated function of each, the mind and body are not seen as separate entities, but "simply one and the same."[61] Lorenz contends that this is the only possible view "tenable for the evolutionary epistemologist" and that "the razor-edge demarcation" seen as existing between them by some disciplines is only for the purpose of understanding them.[61] Certainly, because Descartes, in the 17th century, separated the body from the mind epistemologically, generations of scientists, up to the present day, have fed the assumption that mind and body can and should be considered separately. (Consider, for example, how the treatment of people with mental disorders is separated from those with physical disorder.) This separation has hindered the growth and understanding of humans as occupational beings who, because of mind-body unity, are able to engage in occupation.

Second, engagement in occupation is indispensable to survival, as well as being an integral part of complex health maintenance mechanisms. The latter point will be explored further in Chapters 5 and 6. This hypothesis is in line with another of Lorenz's suggestions—that the principal purpose of both anatomical characteristics and behavior patterns is survival[61]—and with Ornstein's and Sobel's proposition that

Figure 2-2. Human life expectancy during evolution.

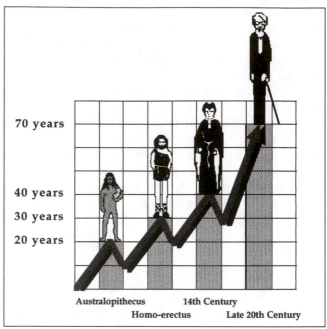

"the major role of the brain is to mind the body and maintain health."[62] My theory of occupation combines these views, maintaining that a primary function of human anatomical characteristics, particularly the brain, is to facilitate healthy survival and that occupation is a primary mechanism for this function. To this end, the whole of the brain is involved in survival and health, and the whole of the brain is involved in engagement in occupation. This notion is complementary to a predominant view that genomic reproduction is the principal goal of evolution, contending that, as reproduction can only occur during a particular stage of the life cycle, to reach reproductive age, individuals have to survive and resist disease and death and that positive health enhances survival and reproductive success. After reproduction, off-spring require nurturing and education so that they, too, can eventually reproduce. Engagement in occupation is not only required for survival to the point of repro-duction, but also for a long time after to provide support for the immature of the species. Views held about "kin selection" or "gene selection," which develop the concept of Darwinian "fitness" to include reproductive success of individuals who share genes,[55] accounts, at least in part, for social and altruistic behaviors and occu-pations. Given the short life expectancy of humans until fairly recently, support, beyond that provided by biological parents, was often necessary because human young have lengthy childhoods. See Figure 2-2 for a diagrammatic representation of human life expectancy during evolution.

Third, the theory recognizes as important that, in large part, genetic traits or capacities are inherited and that there is considerable variation between individuals because of genetic recombination, which "theoretically...can create nearly an infi-nite number of different organisms simply by reshuffling the immense amount of genetic differences between the DNA of any two parents."[58] The differences between humans are discussed further in the next chapter, and the importance of considering the exercise of the particular range of capacities of each individual is also raised in later chapters as an important issue in terms of positive health and well-being and in preventing illness.

Integral to the three principles are ideas about the biological and sociocultural bases of behavior, the haphazard nature of evolution, the similarities and differences between species, brain size and capacities, and the impact of occupational humans upon cultural change. While acceptance of a biological basis for occupational behavior may be criticized by those who claim that human behavior depends on culture rather than genetics, modern sociobiologists and ethologists contend that:

> *Within [a] gene-environmental action model, culture can be seen as the man-made part of the environment, preselected by the specifically human genome...Culture can have no empirical referent outside of the human organisms that invent and transmit it, and, therefore, its evolution is inevitably intertwined with the biological evolution of our species.*[63]

Such contention provides "a factual background for a middle view"[47] that is in accord with the theory of human nature proposed here because it "demonstrates the importance of evolutionary origins in the behavior of the species,"[64] but also maintains that, because of their biology, humans' occupational behavior, as sociologists claim, is, in large part, socioculturally determined.

Evolutionary biologists believe that the origin of the human species was not inevitable but a consequence of "a long series of events, each depending on the other, and each unpredictable and unique."[65] As Lorenz explains, species have evolved in "unforeseeable ways" not "predetermined and directed toward some purpose."[61] This notion is fundamental to a humanist approach that recognizes freedom of choice and self-responsibility. Because humans are goal-directed and committed by their nature to purposeful occupation, it is difficult to appreciate that evolution may not have an ultimate purpose. The notion of predestination has led many theories of human nature, such as Marxism, to maintain that advances in cultural evolution must progress to the enhancement of human nature. In fact, the occupational nature of humans may not be progressive in terms of ultimate "good" for the species. It may lead to less desirable outcomes for health and well-being, with occupational technology, for example, having the potential to destroy the earth's environment and the species.

In this theory, the need to "do" is not species specific, because all living things carry out survival activities. For example, birds build nests, decorate bowers to attract mates, and dive from great heights for fish or small prey. Domesticated dogs can learn that certain activities will be rewarded with food or praise or will run or play with a ball for no apparent reason except for fun, which coincidentally maintains their level of physical fitness and acuity. What animals do and how much freedom they have in the choice of occupations depends upon the size, structure, and capacities of their nervous systems, as well as upon environmental opportunities and constraints. In the evolution of the human brain, through the processes of natural selection, many pathways and connections remain from earlier developmental stages, and few structures have been discarded, although there may be alterations in size and function. Current evidence suggests that new brain functions are the result of "systematic reorganization, elaboration, or reduction of existing structures or shifts in proportions of existing connections."[66] In fact, except for the neocortex, all cerebral regions have a rudimentary equivalent in reptilian brains.[67] Bronowski

Figure 2-3. Size differences of association areas of the brain between humans and other mammals. Adapted from Rose S. *The Conscious Brain*. Rev ed. London, England: Penguin Books; 1976:170 and Deacon TW. Primate brains and senses. In: Jones S, Martin R, Pilbeam D. *The Cambridge Encyclopedia of Human Evolution*. New York, NY: Cambridge University Press; 1992:110.

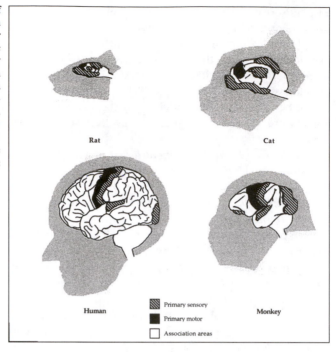

observes that while "every human action goes back in some part" to animal origins, an important distinction remains: "What are the physical gifts that man must share with the animals, and what are the gifts that make him different?"[60]

All animals appear to have some special attributes that are paramount to their survival and that influence their regular occupations. This varies between and within species. For some, it is speed; for others, it is the ability to camouflage; and for yet others, it is highly developed visual or auditory capacities. Many animals possess qualities and characteristics once thought unique to humans, which is not surprising as all mammalian brains have neuronal circuitry and systems that enable them to receive, attend to, interpret, communicate with, and act upon information from the environment. In fact, "there is no strong evidence of unique brain-behavior relationships in any species within the class *Mammalia*."[68]

> *Our brain is not so much different from other brains, it is bigger. We are not a whole new experiment in the evolutionary process, but a superprimate. A quantitative change in the evolving human brain, however, has produced a qualitative change of extraordinary significance.*[55]

The gifts that make humans different are particular adaptations that evolved with increased brain size and, more specifically, association areas of the cortex.

The degree of difference is manifested in the size of the human brain, which is "the largest primate brain that has ever existed."[66] It is 6.3 times larger than expected for mammals of the same body size.[69] Deacon suggests that the structure, configuration, and architecture is typical of other primates, despite unique anatomy and functions for special human adaptations, such as "symbolic communication, speech, tool usage, and culture," and that "comparative size of brain may not be as important as its internal organization." He puts a case that "language abilities may be the 'special intelligence' of humans," that the "brain has been shaped by evolutionary processes that elaborated the capacities needed for language, and not just by a general demand for greater intelligence," and that "when all such species-specific biases are taken into account, 'general intelligence' will be found to be less variable among species than once thought."[66] Others attribute the difference to an increase in association areas of the cortex. The difference is clearly indicated in Figure 2-3.

The association areas are responsible for complex communication and emotional tone, language, thinking, humor, forward planning, problem-solving, analysis, judgment, and adaptation, and Lorenz has noted that:

Among humans...perceptions of depth and direction, a central nervous representation of space, Gestalt perception and the capacity for abstraction, insight and learning, voluntary movement, curiosity...exploratory behavior [and] imitation...are more strongly developed than any of them is among an animal species, even if they represent for those animals a fulfillment of the most vital, life-furthering functions.[61]

These highly developed capacities, along with consciousness and particular physical characteristics, such as bipedalism, are the special survival mechanisms of humans, in that they endow unprecedented flexibility, enabling them to adapt to and meet the challenge of many different environments and dangers. The "intelligence and skills of our forebears do not only manifest themselves in the evolutionary transformations of the brain; they can also be seen in the results of their activity."[70]

The differences in degree of capacity, which frees people from the instinctive and functional constraints of most animals, are central to the particular occupational nature of humans, giving them their apparently strong drive to engage in daily, new, or adventurous occupations and to undertake unwelcome or unenjoyable activities according to sociocultural expectations. Indeed, popular writers such as Desmond Morris and Lyall Watson contend that most people enjoy a challenge and are neophilic in that they "actively pursue the new and different."[71,72] Bruner suggests it is only human adults who "introduce" their offspring to challenging and sometimes frightening new experiences,[73] while among both birds and other mammals the presence of mothers is required to reduce fear of novel stimuli to enable their offspring to explore.[74] If Bruner's suggestion is true, perhaps such learning experiences are a necessary precursor for people to take risks to create environments in which they feel comfortable and to brave exploration of the unknown.

Some suggest that humans appear to go beyond survival needs in their pursuit of occupation.[75] The range of capacities available to humans certainly allows them to pursue many options that may not appear to have an obvious relationship to survival, but much deliberation about this point has determined that this extended ability is an integral part of healthy survival mechanisms, in that engagement in wide-ranging occupations enables people to hone their skills, their capacities, and their flexibility so that they are competent to deal with novel situations as they occur, as well as providing exercise to maintain the "well working of the organism as a whole."[76] This freedom and flexibility has, along with genetic and biological variability, resulted in humans from different regions of the world appearing "different." A large part of the difference can be attributed to the occupations in which their forebears have engaged over time and the value given to them by the culture in which they live, because as anthropologist Richard Leakey observes:

The most pronounced differences are the way in which people do things: their dress, their architecture, their myths, their songs, their ideals and so on...The earth is populated by one people living many different styles of life because of a unique cultural capacity. And the mind that expresses this unique capacity is the one that also universally seeks beyond itself for explanations of man himself and the nature of the world around him.[77]

Indeed, from birth, children, through their predominant occupation of play, seek beyond themselves for explanations of the world and their place within it. As they do this, they develop their innate capacities through learned behaviors, through practicing skills and using their minds and bodies to enable them to survive, to interact with others, and to choose future roles. In going beyond obvious survival needs in their pursuit of occupation, people evolve and adapt as occupational beings according to their environment and cultural values. The brain's capacity to adapt to social environs different from those in which humans evolved has led to "culture itself" creating "norms of human behavior that, in a certain sense, can step in as substitutes for innate behavior programs."[61]

The ability of humans to adapt socioculturally enables infants at a very early age to assimilate and retain information from the environment, before a conscious appreciation of meaning or significance is possible. This early absorption of observed behaviors enables ontogenetic development to be in step with sociocultural expectations. In fact, the complexity of the human brain as the species' survival mechanism means that human babies are not able to reach a stage where they can take care of themselves before birth, and they require social support for many years to assume "full humanness." As part of this process, attitudes, as well as occupational behaviors, are absorbed and adopted, and it is those formed before intellectual capacities are sufficiently advanced to allow for adequate understanding or refuting that have the strongest, albeit unconscious, hold on individuals. This mechanism was central to early humans' healthy survival because it allowed essential learning to occur from birth and stimulated the development of capacities. Their view of the strength of such learned attitudes and behaviors led founding behavioral psychologists Watson[78] and Skinner[79] to argue that only physiological reflexes are inherited, Watson going so far as to claim:

Give me a dozen healthy infants, well-formed, and my own specific world to bring them up in and I'll guarantee to take any one at random and train him to become any kind of specialist I might select—doctor, lawyer, artist, merchant-chief, and yes even beggar-man and thief regardless of his talents, penchants, abilities, vocations, and race of his ancestors.[78]

Sociologists might not accept Watson's exaggerated language but a similar understanding by them has led to one of sociology's fundamental postulates: human actions are limited or determined by past and present environments, and humans are the products and the victims of their society.[80] Sociologists, in contrast to sociobiologists, also reason that "human beings are made, not born" because "even if someone argues that human endowments such as soul and rationality are innate, these gifts are not sufficient to ensure that an infant will become a truly functional human being, capable of ethical and cultural responsibility," and that "the infant has to be learned...in short, we enact, rehearse, work, and play our way into the human condition."[81] However, this implies that people have the genetic and biological capacity to learn, which is also part of being human. My occupational theory of human nature holds that, because of their particular mix of biological characteristics and capacities, humans are receptive to the process of enculturation and socialization to the extent that they can indeed be considered products of their particular culture.

It is also held in my theory that societies are the products of humans acting on their environment. As people engage in occupation, the physical and social environment is altered. Often, the more sophisticated the occupation, the greater the change to the environment, which in turn causes further change to and development of people. Karl Marx suggests that "by thus acting on the external world and changing it, [man] at the same time changes his own nature,"[22] and Braverman, in the same vein, proposes that people are the special product of purposeful action. He argues that occupation that "transcends mere instinctual activity is the force which created humankind and the force by which humankind created the world as we know it."[24] Neff agrees that the most revolutionary force in human history is technological change associated with the way people "wrest their living from nature."[82] He argues that social institutions are merely mirrors of technological levels. This idea, apparently well accepted in archaeological circles, as well as Marxist sociology, supports the theory that humans are occupational beings, that occupation has the potential to change the world or the species, and that it provides the mechanism to enable people to survive and to adapt to biological, sociological, and environmental demands. This view points to the need to consider humans' occupational nature from an ecological as well as a sociological perspective.

The many models of cultural evolution based on occupational technology are sometimes said not to address sufficiently the influences of other variables, such as local environments, ecology and climate, war and conquest, spiritual beliefs and social struggles, or the complexities of the interactions between them.[82] From my standpoint, there is some truth in the criticisms, because such views have been limited to economic "work" or "labor" perspectives, neglecting a holistic view of occupation, which, of necessity, integrates many factors. Other criticisms have been leveled at the notion of cultural evolution itself, particularly as postulated by Victorian anthropologists such as Tylor[83] and Morgan,[84] in that it seems to imply progress in the sense that advanced technological societies are somehow "better" or "higher up the evolutionary ladder" than older cultures with less technical economies.[82] However, the notion of cultural superiority is called into question by the argument that cultures can vary independently of race and that no one culture is superior to another.[85] Similarly, the occupational nature of humans is not seen to be more evolved in technologically advanced societies in contrast to hunter-gatherer or agrarian societies but, rather, expressed differently according to each culture's history and technological development.

Diagnosis and Prescription

Having outlined the main concepts of this occupational theory of human nature, two points of Stevenson's notion must be considered: any such theory has to include a diagnosis of "what is wrong with humans" and a prescription of how to "right the wrongs" from its particular perspective.

As to diagnosis, although the occupational behavior of early humans was in tune with self-sustaining "natural" health and ecological balance, the current direction of occupational behavior is out of step with humans' animal heritage, natural behaviors, and the ecology. This echoes a sentiment expressed by Alexis Carrel, in 1935, that modern civilization "does not suit us," being "born from the whims of scientif-

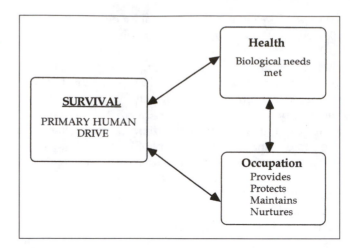

Figure 2-4. Three-way link between occupation, health, and survival.

ic discoveries, from the appetites of men, their illusions, their theories, and their desires" but "without any knowledge of our real nature." He argued for a science of human individuals that views them as "an indivisible whole of extreme complexity."[86] It could be suggested that, in the present day, knowledge of human nature remains rudimentary and that Carrel's science is still necessary despite an avalanche of research in various disciplines in recent decades. The knowledge is certainly fragmentary, and, without a real appreciation of the human need to engage in occupation, it is incomplete.

As for a prescription of how to "right the wrongs," addressing the lack of awareness of our occupational natures has the potential to influence social, political, economic, and health policies so that they are more in tune with our occupational natures, self-sustaining "natural" health and ecological balance. More concrete solutions do not seem advisable, as theories of human nature that are prescriptive, such as "Marxist Communism," do not allow sufficient flexibility to allow solutions to be responsive to contextual and evolutionary change.

Gaining an increased understanding of an occupational perspective of human nature is worthy of further extensive inquiry as it appears appropriate to many of the problems the world faces today and in the future, namely how to maintain health and ensure human survival in an economic and self-sustaining way, which meets the biological, sociocultural, and occupational needs of people as well as redressing ecological degradation. Because of the nature of the approach taken, the exploration that follows can only touch on these wide-ranging issues, although it is acknowledged that each requires study in its own right.

Three-Way Link: Occupation, Health, Survival

At the center of this occupational theory of human nature is the proposal that the superprimate brain of the human species has "healthy survival" as its primary role. It is a brain that continually activates humans' particular mix of characteristics and capacities through engagement in occupation. It is an occupational brain and a healing brain. Our occupational nature is the result of evolution/phylogeny, genetics, ontogeny, ecological and sociocultural environments, and opportunity, all of which are centered or integrated in the brain. Engagement in occupation forms a three-way link with health and survival, which is illustrated in Figure 2-4.

Survival is recognized as the primary drive of humans, as of all other animals. Survival of individuals is the outcome of the use of capacities through occupations that provide for essential needs of the organism, including supportive social, ecological, and material environments. The extent and quality of survival for individuals, communities, and societies depends on their health and physical, mental, and social well-being; health is the outcome of each organism having all essential sustenance and safety needs met and of having physical, mental, and social capacities maintained, exercised, and in balance. This is achieved through occupation. Engagement in occupation depends, in turn, on a level of health and its specific components, which are able to provide the energy, drive, and functional attributes necessary for engagement.

Additionally, the survival of healthy species depends on a human's capacity to live in harmony within an environment that can continue to provide basic requirements, ensure the continued acquisition of these requirements, and provide safety and education for the next generation.

The integrative functions of the central nervous system, which process external and internal information, activated by engagement in occupation, are focal to survival, the maintenance of homeostasis, and facilitating health and well-being. The next four chapters, which consider biological characteristics and capacities, occupational evolution, health and well-being, and the prevention of illness, explore the ideas behind this view of human nature.

References

1. Yerxa EJ, Clark F, Frank G, et al. An introduction to occupational science. A foundation for occupational therapy in the 21st century. *Occupational Therapy in Health Care*. 1989;6(4):1-17.
2. Duldt BW, Giffin K. *Theoretical Perspectives for Nursing*. Boston, Mass: Little, Brown and Co; 1985:47.
3. Lewin K. *Principles of Topological Psychology*. New York, NY: McGraw Hill; 1947.
4. Markovic M. Human nature. In: Bottomore T, ed. *A Dictionary of Marxist Thought*. 2nd ed. Oxford, UK: Blackwell Publishers; 1991:209.
5. Althusser L. *For Marx*. Paris, France: F. Maspero; 1965. Translated by Brewster B. London, England: Allen Lane; 1969.
6. Stevenson L. *Seven Theories of Human Nature*. 2nd ed. Oxford, UK: Oxford University Press; 1987:9,137.
7. *The Concise Oxford Dictionary of Current English*. Oxford, UK: Clarendon Press; 1911.
8. *Webster's Revised Unabridged Dictionary of the English Language*. London, England: G Bell and Sons Ltd; 1919.
9. *The Oxford English Dictionary*. 2nd ed. Vol XII. Oxford, UK: Clarendon Press; 1989:130,633.
10. Lobkowicz N. *Theory and Practice: History of Concept from Aristotle to Marx*. London, England: University of Notre Dame Press; 1967:9.
11. Roget PM. *Roget's Thesaurus of Synonyms and Antonyms*. London, England: The Number Nine Publishing Company; 1972.
12. Leipmann H. *Drei Aufsatze aus dem Apraxiegebiet*. Berlin, Germany: Springer; 1908.
13. Kotarbinski T. The goal of an act and the task of the agent. In: Gasparski W, Pszczolowski T, eds. *Praxiological Studies: Polish Contributions to the Science of Efficient Action*. Dordrecht, Holland: D. Reidel Publishing Co; 1983:22.
14. Petrovic G. Praxis. In: Bottomore T, ed. *A Dictionary of Marxist Thought*. 2nd ed. Oxford, UK: Blackwell Publishers; 1991:435.
15. Marx K. Economic and philosophical manuscripts, 1844. In: Livingstone R, Benton G, trans. *Karl Marx: Early Writings*. New York, NY: Penguin Classics; 1992.
16. Comstock D. A method of critical research. In: Bredo E, Feinberg W, eds. *Knowledge and Values in Social and Educational Research*. Philadelphia, Pa: Temple University Press; 1982:370-390.
17. Lather P. Research as praxis. *Harvard Educational Review*. 1986;56(3):257-277.
18. Work. *The Standard English Desk Dictionary*. 2nd ed. Sydney, Australia: Bay Books for Oxford University Press; 1976:975.
19. Williams R. *Keywords*. London, England: Fontana Press; 1983.
20. Parker S. *Leisure and Work*. London, England: George Allen and Unwin; 1983:13,17.

21. Smith R. *Unemployment and Health: A Disaster and a Challenge.* Oxford, UK: Oxford University Press; 1987.

22. Marx K. *Capital.* Vol 1. Hamburg, Germany: Otto Meissner; 1867:179-180.

23. Ruskin J. Preface. In: Yarker PM, ed. *Ruskin: Unto This Last.* London, England: Collins Publishers; 1970.

24. Braverman H. *Labor and Monopoly Capital: The Degradation of Work in the Twentieth Century.* New York, NY: Monthly Review Press; 1974.

25. *Word Finder, The Australian Thesaurus.* Sydney, Australia: Reader's Digest; 1983.

26. Castles I. *How Australians Use Their Time.* Catalog No. 4153.0. Australian Bureau of Statistics, 1992 (embargoed to 1994).

27. Harvey AS. Quality of life and the use of time theory and measurement. *Journal of Occupational Science: Australia.* 1993;1(2):27-30.

28. Andrew C, Milroy BM, eds. *Life Spaces: Gender, Household, Employment.* Vancouver, Canada: University of Vancouver Press; 1988.

29. Robinson JP. *How Americans Use Time: A Social-Psychological Analysis of Everyday Behaviour.* New York, NY: Praeger Publishers; 1977.

30. Szalai A. *The Use of Time: Daily Activities of Urban and Suburban Populations in Twelve Countries.* The Hague: Mouton; 1972.

31. Meyer A. The philosophy of occupational therapy. *Archives of Occupational Therapy.* 1922;1:1-10.

32. Mackinnon J, Avison W, McCain G. Rheumatoid arthritis, occupational profiles and psychological adjustment. *Journal of Occupational Science: Australia.* 1994;1(4):3-10.

33. Stanley M. An investigation into the relationship between engagement in valued occupations and life satisfaction for elderly South Australians. *Journal of Occupational Science: Australia.* 1995;2(3):100-114.

34. Yerxa EJ, Locker SB. Quality of time used by adults with spinal cord injuries. *American Journal of Occupational Therapy.* 1990;4:318-326.

35. Pentland W, McColl MA, Harvey A, do Rozario L, Neimi I, Barker J. *The Relationship Between Time Use and Health, Well-Being, and Quality of Life.* Proceedings of a multidisciplinary research meeting. Kingston, Canada: Queens University; 1993.

36. Kielhofner G. The temporal dimension in the lives of retarded adults. *American Journal of Occupational Therapy.* 1979;33:161-168.

37. Neville A. Temporal adaptation: application with short-term psychiatric patients. *American Journal of Occupational Therapy.* 1980;34:328-331.

38. Rosenthal LA, Howe MC. Activity patterns and leisure concepts: a comparison of temporal adaptation among day versus night shift workers. *Occupational Therapy in Mental Health.* 1984;4:59-78.

39. Weeder TC. Comparison of temporal patterns and meaningfulness of daily activities of schizophrenics and normal adults. *Occupational Therapy in Mental Health.* 1986;6:27-45.

40. Leakey R, Lewin R. *People of the Lake: Man: His Origins, Nature, and Future.* New York, NY: Penguin Books; 1978:38-39.

41. Cynkin S, Robinson AM. *Occupational Therapy and Activities Health: Towards Health Through Activities.* Boston, Mass: Little, Brown and Co; 1990.

42. Occupational therapy: its definitions and functions. *American Journal of Occupational Therapy.* 1972;26:204.

43. Kielhofner G, ed. *A Model of Human Occupation, Theory and Application.* Baltimore, Md: Williams and Wilkins; 1985.

44. Wilcock AA. *Occupational Therapy Approaches to Stroke.* Melbourne, Australia: Churchill Livingstone; 1986.

45. Csikszentmihalyi M, Csikszentmihalyi IS. *Optimal Experience: Psychological Studies of Flow in Consciousness.* New York, NY: Cambridge University Press; 1988.

46. Csikszentmihalyi M, Massimini F. On the psychological selection of bicultural information. *New Ideas in Psychology.* 1985;3(2):115-138.

47. Snell GD. *Search for a Rational Ethic.* New York, NY: Springer Verlag; 1988:140.

48. Stavrianos LS. *The World to 1500: A Global History.* 4th ed. Upper Saddle River, NJ: Prentice Hall; 1988:4.

49. Darwin C. *Origin of the Species by Means of Natural Selection (1859).* Cambridge, Mass: Harvard University Press; 1964.

50. Darwin C. *The Descent of Man and Selection in Relation to Sex (1871).* New York, NY: Appleton; 1930.

51. Ridley M. Creationism. In: Bullock A, Stallybrass O, Trombley S, eds. *The Fontana Dictionary of Modern Thought.* 2nd ed. London, England: Fontana Press; 1988.

52. Dawkins R. The replicators. In: Dixon B, ed. *From Creation to Chaos: Classic Writings in Science.* Oxford, UK: Basil Blackwood Ltd; 1989:39-44.

53. Jones S. The nature of evolution. In: Jones S, Martin R, Pilbeam D, eds. *The Cambridge Encyclopedia of Human Evolution.* New York, NY: Cambridge University Press; 1992:9.

54. Spencer H. *Principles of Biology.* Vol 1. New York, NY: Appleton; 1864:444.

55. Campbell BG. *Humankind Emerging.* 5th ed. New York, NY: Harper Collins Publishers; 1988:60-69,90-91,366.
56. Stern C, Sherwood ER, eds. *The Origin of Genetics.* San Francisco, Calif: WH Freeman; 1966.
57. Medawar P. Darwinism. In: *The Fontana Dictionary of Modern Thought.* 2nd ed. London, England: Fontana Press; 1988.
58. McHenry HM. Evolution. In: Kuper A, Kuper J, eds. *The Social Science Encyclopedia.* Rev ed. London, England: Routledge; 1989:280.
59. Dyson F. The argument from design. Disturbing the universe 1979. In: Dixon B, ed. *From Creation to Chaos: Classic Writings in Science.* Oxford, UK: Basil Blackwood Ltd; 1989:49.
60. Bronowski J. *The Ascent of Man.* London, England: British Broadcasting Corp; 1973:31.
61. Lorenz K. *The Waning of Humaneness.* Boston, Mass: Little, Brown and Co; 1987:5,21,57-58,93,124.
62. Ornstein R, Sobel D. *The Healing Brain: A Radical New Approach to Health Care.* London, England: MacMillan; 1988:11-12.
63. van den Berghe PL. Sociobiology. In: Kuper A, Kuper J, eds. *The Social Science Encyclopedia.* Rev ed. London, England: Routledge; 1989:795-798.
64. Edelman G. *Bright Air, Brilliant Fire: On the Matter of the Mind.* London, England: Penguin Books; 1992:40.
65. Pilbeam D. What makes us human. In: Jones S, Martin R, Pilbeam D, eds. *The Cambridge Encyclopedia of Human Evolution.* New York, NY: Cambridge University Press; 1992:1.
66. Deacon TW. The human brain. In: Jones S, Martin R, Pilbeam D, eds. *The Cambridge Encyclopedia of Human Evolution.* New York, NY: Cambridge University Press; 1992:115,119,123.
67. Rose S. *The Conscious Brain.* Rev ed. London, England: Penguin Books; 1976.
68. Kolb B, Whishaw IQ. *Fundamentals of Human Neuropsychology.* 3rd ed. San Franscico, Calif: WH Freeman; 1990:106.
69. Jerison HJ. *Evolution of the Brain and Intelligence.* New York, NY: Academic Press; 1973.
70. Jelinek J. *Primitive Hunters.* London, England: Hamlyn; 1989.
71. Morris D. *The Human Zoo.* London, England: Jonathan Cape; 1969.
72. Watson L. *Neophilia: The Tradition of the New.* Great Britain: Hodder and Stoughton Ltd; 1989.
73. Bruner JS. Nature and uses of immaturity. *American Psychologist.* 1972;August:687-708.
74. King DL. A review and interpretation of some aspects of the infant-mother relationship in mammals and birds. *Psychological Bulletin.* 1966;65:143-155.
75. Morris D. *The Human Animal.* BBC TV Production, England, 1994.
76. Kass LR. Regarding the end of medicine and the pursuit of health. In: Caplan AL, Englehardt HT, McCartney JJ, eds. *Concepts of Health and Disease: Interdisciplinary Perspectives.* Reading, Mass: Addison-Wesley Publishing Co; 1981.
77. Leakey R. *The Making of Mankind.* London, England: Michael Joseph Ltd; 1981:248.
78. Watson JB. *Behaviourism.* New York, NY: WW Norton; 1970:104.
79. Skinner BF. *Science and Human Behaviour.* New York, NY: Macmillan; 1953.
80. Shils E. Sociology. In: Kuper A, Kuper J, eds. *The Social Science Encyclopedia.* Rev ed. London, England: Routledge; 1989:799-810.
81. Driver T. *The Magic of Ritual.* San Francisco, Calif: Harper Collins Publishers; 1991:16.
82. Neff WS. *Work and Human Behavior.* 3rd ed. New York, NY: Aldine Publishing Co; 1985:20.
83. Tylor EB. *Anthropology: An Introduction to the Study of Man and Civilization.* Ann Arbor, Mich: University of Michigan Press; 1960.
84. Morgan LH. *Ancient Society.* Cambridge, Mass: Belknap; 1964.
85. Hatch E. Culture. In: Kuper A, Kuper J, eds. *The Social Science Encyclopedia.* Rev ed. London, England: Routledge; 1989:179.
86. Carrel A. *Man the Unknown.* London, England: Burns and Oates; 1935:14.

Suggested Reading

Bronowski J. *The Ascent of Man.* London, England: British Broadcasting Corp; 1973.
Bruner JS. Nature and uses of immaturity. *American Psychologist.* 1972;August:687-708.
Campbell BG. *Humankind Emerging.* 5th ed. New York, NY: Harper Collins Publishers; 1988.
Carrel A. *Man the Unknown.* London, England: Burns and Oates; 1935.
Darwin C. *Origin of the Species by Means of Natural Selection (1859).* Cambridge, Mass: Harvard University Press; 1964.
Lorenz K. *The Waning of Humaneness.* Boston, Mass: Little, Brown and Co; 1987.
Snell GD. *Search for a Rational Ethic.* New York, NY: Springer Verlag; 1988.
Stevenson L. *Seven Theories of Human Nature.* 2nd ed. Oxford, UK: Oxford University Press; 1987.
Watson L. *Neophilia: The Tradition of the New.* Great Britain: Hodder and Stoughton Ltd; 1989.

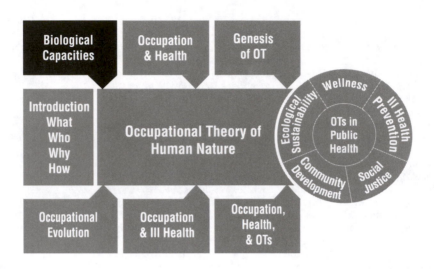

Chapter 3
Biological Characteristics and Capacities: The Foundation for Occupational Behavior

This chapter presents the reader with ideas about:
- An occupational perspective of evolution, and the structure and function of the brain
- Biological characteristics and capacities which provide a foundation for humans' occupational natures
- Genetic variation in capacities from research about twins, race, gender, and ontogenesis
- The particular mix of human characteristics and capacities which have enabled humans, through occupation, to survive healthily and successfully as a species, namely bipedalism, hand function, vision, language, consciousness, creativity, sleep, and homeostasis

To substantiate one aspect of the theory, in this chapter, ideas concerning biological characteristics and capacities that appear to make considerable contributions to occupational behavior are explored. Some capacities and characteristics that have been identified as important by evolutionary scientists, archaeologists, and anthropologists will be discussed because they are adaptations that set humans apart from other mammals. As these are explored, ideas about the potential role of these capacities in survival, health, and well-being, and how they can be used in occupation for self-maintenance, development, and growth will also be considered.

The central nervous system is the major focus, because it is the brain that coordinates and controls humans' engagement in occupation. However, it is important to recall that, according to this theory, the central nervous system cannot be studied in isolation because, as Gerald Edelman explains, "the shape of an animal's body is as important to the functioning and evolution of its brain as the shape and functioning of the brain are to the behavior of that body," and in evolutionary terms "the shape of cells, tissues, organs, and finally the whole animal is the largest single basis for behavior."[1] (Gerald Edelman's work, centered on his theory called "neural Darwinism," has been described as "the first biological theory of individuality and autonomy" by Oliver Sachs in the *New York Review of Books*, and as such is very relevant to the themes in this book.) Sources for much of the material in this chapter come from the neurosciences, along with that from archaeologists and anthropologists who explore the biological development of humans through brain size and structure, physiological capacities, such as bipedal locomotion and hand function, and evidence of intellectual function, such as language, all of which are prerequisite to complex occupational behavior, such as tool manufacture.

Defining Capacity

To consider the links between use of capacities, engagement in occupation, health, and survival, it is necessary to first define what is meant by "capacity." Texts and articles reviewed in the course of exploration of "capacity" use words such as "genetic potential, characteristic, trait, talents, and ability" interchangeably. Both academic and popular dictionaries and thesauruses use words such as "faculty," "capability," and "trait" to describe capacity. These in turn extend our understanding, with capability defined as "power of undeveloped faculty" and faculty as "aptitude for any special kind of action; power inherent in the body or an organ; [and] mental power."[2] Trait has synonyms, such as "characteristic quality, distinguishing mark, attribute, feature, peculiarity, speciality, and idiosyncrasy,"[3,4] but in most instances implies an observable rather than a potential aptitude. Capacity, then, in this context, is used to mean the innate and perhaps undeveloped potential, aptitude, ability, talent, trait, or power with which each individual is endowed.

Species' characteristics and range of capacities express the essential difference of one species of animal from another. Complex occupational behavior differentiates humans from others and allows humans to adapt to and survive healthily in many different environments, and it is:

Expansion of a standard primate brain [that has provided humans with] behavioral possibilities undreamed of in other even closely related species. This brain...gives us the human potential for making tools, talking, planning, dreaming of the future, and creating an entirely new environment for ourselves.[5]

This point leads us to consideration of the evolution, structure, and function of the brain.

Evolution, Structure, and Function of the Brain

The "rather haphazard and seemingly disorganized set of structures"[6] in the brain evolved in "archaeological" layers as animals adapted to different habitats, climates, and subsistence demands. Each layer maintained stability and health of the organism as conditions changed, and each layer added a new dimension to occupational behavior. Herbert Spencer (1820-1903), an evolutionist social philosopher, was the first to argue that "the brain evolved in a series of steps, each of which brought animals the capacity to engage in a constellation of new behaviors," and John Hughlings-Jackson (1835-1911), an English neurologist who based his work on Spencer's theory, recognized that the cortex has a special role in purposeful behavior, which is supported by subcortical areas concerned with more elementary forms of the same behavior.[7]

Although in the 1990s it is generally accepted that the brain is organized according to systems, some neuroscientists still refer to the human brain's functional hierarchy based on phylogenic evolution. The brainstem is the oldest part of the brain, which developed before the advent of mammals. It controls the simplest life support systems such as breathing, heart rate, and general alerting to predators or prey. The limbic system evolved to ensure stability of the organism on land, which called for structures to maintain internal temperatures, fluid levels, and emotional reactions, such as those concerned with self-protection. The cerebellum was probably the first area to specialize in sensorimotor coordination and is integral to efficiency of skilled movement. The cerebral cortex is the most recent layer. It is here that the processes occur that make humans most different from other animals, such as their capacity to analyze, organize, understand, produce, judge, plan, activate, sense, formulate, and execute complex occupation.[7] Some of these processes, such as "the perceptual systems of seeing, hearing, and language comprehension," are more structured than others, such as "thinking and imagining, learning, and judging," so although "we can perceive the world only in certain modes, we can think about the finished products of perception, embellish them, and manipulate them in many different ways." Such cortical functions give humans the "capacity to adapt culturally...enabling [them] to insulate themselves from the environment and to exploit the environment."[5]

The growing knowledge about the relation of brain structure to behavior demonstrates "...enormously intricate brain systems at...molecular levels, cellular levels, organismic levels (the whole creature), and transorganismic levels (i.e., communication of some sort or other)," all of which interconnect. In the cerebral cortex alone, it has been estimated that there are between 20 and 100 billion neurons and about 1 million billion connections, all of which are capable of many combinations so that "the sheer number and density of neuronal networks in the brain" reaches "hyperastronomical" figures and "the brain might be said to be in touch more with itself than with anything else." Indeed, "the kinds of unique individuality in our brain networks make that of fingerprints or facial features appear gross and simple by comparison."[8] Many neurons, each of which is "unusual in three respects: its varied shape, its electrical and chemical function, and its connectivity," have specific potential.[1] In fact, "very specific patterns of behavior are determined by very specific brain areas," with "each behavioral system probably [having] its own underlying neurophysiological mechanisms."[9] Different brain areas have different cell formations that have been described in functional and cytoarchitectonic maps.[10,11] "Mapping is an important principle in complex brains," and the fibers that connect maps with each other "are the most numerous of all those in the brain."[1]

Mapped areas of the brain that have been identified with specific functions do relate to occupational behavior, although the "complexity of the brain's structure makes it incredibly difficult to relate its components to individual capacities."[7] This is also because capacities themselves are incredibly complex systems. In fact, the complexity of brain organization, as it relates to occupation and to capacities, is one factor in the difficulty experienced throughout history in understanding what happens where. For example, Kolb and Whishaw report in a history of neuropsychology that while Alcmaeon of Croton (c. 500 BC), Hippocrates (430-379 BC), and Plato (420-347 BC) subscribed to a view that located mental processes in the brain, Empedocles (c. 490-430 BC) and Aristotle (384-322 BC) believed the heart to be the source of mental functions.[7] Galen (129-199 AD) refuted Aristotle's view after experiments in which he applied light pressure to heart and brain and found pressure to the brain stopped voluntary behavior. Eighteenth-century anatomists Franz Joseph Gall and Johann Casper Spurzheim are credited with originating the localization of function argument. They developed a theory of phrenology, in which specific capacities of the brain were attributed according to the bumps and depressions apparent on the surface of individual skulls. However, in large part, because they assigned capacities derived from a value-laden philosophical view, such as "veneration" and "secretiveness" rather than from observable behaviors, their contribution was rejected. In recent years, localization theories have been substantiated with the proviso that any area with a specific function does not work in isolation. In fact, the complexities of the interactive nature of specific areas of the brain have been demonstrated by the "zenon 133" studies of brain activity in which a two-dimensional measure of regional blood flow (following inhalation of radioactive gases) was taken during performance of tasks as compared

Figure 3-1. The interactive nature of brain function demonstrated by various means during communication processing tasks: a) by electrical stimulation, b) by zenon 133, and c) by PET scans. From Deacon TW. The human brain. In: Jones S, Martin R, Pilbeam D, eds. *The Cambridge Encyclopedia of Human Evolution*. New York, NY: Cambridge University Press; 1992:121. Reprinted with the permission of Cambridge University Press.

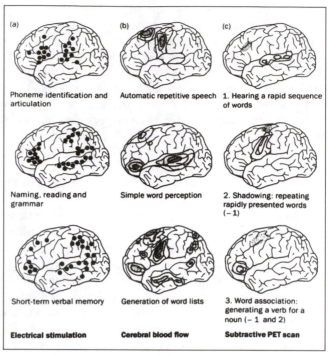

(a) Phoneme identification and articulation

(b) Automatic repetitive speech

(c) 1. Hearing a rapid sequence of words

Naming, reading and grammar

Simple word perception

2. Shadowing: repeating rapidly presented words (− 1)

Short-term verbal memory

Generation of word lists

3. Word association: generating a verb for a noun (− 1 and 2)

Electrical stimulation   **Cerebral blood flow**   **Subtractive PET scan**

to a resting state. It was found that the frontal lobes were relatively active bilaterally even at rest and that just simple movement of the fingers involved activity of many different areas.[12,13] Such complexity has been confirmed by three-dimensional positron emission topography, which has been used to image the neuronal activity of both hemispheres and deeper brain structures during use (Figure 3-1).[14-17]

Complex and integrative neuronal activity at many levels and the notion of localization of function are not incompatible; and if the former is kept very much in mind, it is possible to accept that:

> *Inside the cortex lie separate centers with specific functions, which we like to call talents. Mathematical ability is a separate talent from the ability to move gracefully; verbal agility is distinct from the previous two. There is a range of different functions, for smelling, for thinking, for moving, for calculating that the brain possesses.*[6]

However, talents "are not given equally to all of us; people are not as consistent as we might have imagined" and recognizing this, Ornstein and Sobel contend that to understand the brain's operation, as well as its concern with health, it is necessary to study the collage of "specialized neural systems each of which possesses a rich concentration of certain abilities" that are talents of a specific nature or of generic organization or tendency.[6] One such study led Gagne to propose a "differentiated model of giftedness and talent," which identifies giftedness as "aptitude" and talent as "fulfillment or activity performance," with aptitude being translated into talent via environmental and intrapersonal catalysts. Gagne groups aptitudes and talents into aptitude domains, such as intellectual, creative, socio-affective, and sensorimotor, and fields of talents, such as academic, technical, artistic, interpersonal, and athletic.[18] He also groups primary capacities, such as seeing, standing, perceiving color, or touching, which are complex physiological processes in their own right; there are other more complex capacities, such as problem-solving, exploration, consciousness, creativity, and so on. These more complex capacities do not appear to be based on specific maps but are examples of the integrative workings of many independent and interdependent systems.

Genetic Variation in Capacities

To corroborate the idea that individual variation in capacities is genetically endowed, the next few pages will consider ideas and evidence from studies relating to genetics, including those on twins, race, gender, and ontogenesis.

In common with other animals, the range of human capacities is, on the whole, common to the species, but individual variation is the rule. For example, in an early classic experiment on fowls, JBS Haldane (1892-1964), who is credited with the first case of genetic linkages in mammals, found that when he mated fowls weighing an average 1,300 grams with bantams averaging 750 grams there was a tendency for the weight of their hybrid offspring to split the difference between their parents' weight. When hybrid mated hybrid, the variations that ensued produced birds with a range of weights from much greater to much smaller than the grandparents. Inheritance is "cooperative" in that genes as part of a "gene complex" combine or interact, and it is usually more than one gene that produces a single trait. Haldane estimated, in his experiment, that if 10 genes had an effect on weight, they could produce 59,049 variations.[19] Now, as geneticists and biologists have come closer to understanding the structure and function of genes by using biochemical technology, ranging from electrophoresis of proteins to very sophisticated analysis of DNA structures, "they have uncovered inherited variation, or polymorphism, at almost every level of organization" to the extent that "it is certain that every human being who has lived or ever will live is genetically unique."[20] The biological processes that have increased genetic variability throughout evolution are "mutation, sexual recombination, genetic drift, gene flow, and increase in population size,"[5] so that except for identical twins every individual carries different genetic material.

Twin Studies

Despite some methodological flaws that discredited early findings in some twin studies that sought to explore the relative roles of nature and nurture in behavior, there is now abundant evidence from these that capacities are part of our genetic inheritance. In studies of genetically identical twins compared with fraternal, or non-identical, twins, Plomin, DeFries, and McClearn found that the general cognitive ability of identical twins was more alike than those of fraternal twins in 17 of 18 studies, which included more than 6,000 identical and non-identical twin pairs.[21] Other traits such as schizophrenia, drinking habits, homosexuality, criminal tendencies, prosocial behavior, and personality characteristics have consistently been found more similar in identical twins.[9] In a study of 850 pairs of twins, Loehlin and Nichols concluded that "genes and environment carry roughly equal weight in accounting for individual variation in personality,"[22] although Vandenberg suggests that the relativity of heredity and environment varies according to specific capacities.[23]

With regard to variation in neurophysiological processes, not even identical twins have "the exact pattern of nerve cells...at the same time and place,"[1] nor have they exactly corresponding numbers of branches of any one neuron because of "the stochastic nature" of the "topobiological and epigenetic developmental driving forces provided by cellular processes such as cell division, movement, and death."[1] (Topobiology ["topos" meaning place] is a term used by Edelman in his theories about brain evolution because many transactions between cells leading to "shape" and "function" are place dependent, only occurring when a cell is surrounded by other cells in a particular place. According to *Dorland's Illustrated Medical Dictionary*, 25th ed., epigenesis is the development of an organism from an undifferentiated cell, consisting in the successive formation and development of organs and parts that do not pre-exist in the fertilized egg.)

In evolutionary terms, factors that increase or decrease individual variability include contentious issues relating to race and gender. These will be briefly considered, because increased awareness and encouragement of the unique potential of individuals are important. If there are differences according to race or gender, apart from individual genetic inheritance or cultural learning, this should not be overlooked in "socially just" research or intervention aimed at individual or community health and well-being through engagement in occupation.

Race

The biological processes in question for race are those that decrease variability within particular groups, such as when "natural selection and reduction in population size" results in the "founder effect" in which different gene frequencies are perpetuated in isolated communities.[5] Examples of this type lead to speculation that some differences in capacities may well be found in people of different races, who, particularly because of geographical isolation over a long period of time, inherit variations fitted to their environment through the processes of natural selection.[24,25]

While the "overwhelming majority of genes of *Homo sapiens* are shared by all mankind, a relatively small percentage is believed to control those features which differentiate the races from each other."[26] Anatomical differences that are adaptations to past or present environments, such as hair, eyelid, breast, or lip form; pigmentation; frequencies of balding; and body build are easily demonstrated. There are also physiological differences, such as in blood groups, basal metabolic rate, bone growth, age and order of tooth eruption, and subtle variations that give rise to diseases like "sickle cell anemia, phenylketonuria, favism, or familial Mediterranean fever."[5] It is possible, of course, that such differences may, in the future, be found to result from environmental factors, such as nutrition. Anatomical and physiological differences may account for some particular skills more prevalent in one racial group than another, such as in athletics. As well, differences in the occupational behaviors characterizing some cultures may result, in part, from particular genetic inheritance. Despite suggestions that there may be racial differences in IQ, mechanical and abstract reasoning, form discrimination, color sense, and tonal memory,[27,28] some investigators stress that race is based on genetic physical traits rather than mental traits.

Indeed, the race concept itself has been challenged.[29] Littlefield, Lieberman, and Reynolds found that of 58 texts that appeared between 1932 and 1979, only 25 accepted the race concept, while 17 did not. The remaining 16 were non-committal, said there was no consensus, or did not mention the subject. There was, in fact, an evident swing away from the concept of race in more recent texts.[30] While this may reflect data from new studies, it may also reflect changes of ideas and values about racial differences and concerns about discrimination. Many scientists working in this area express concern about differences being viewed as evidence of superiority or inferiority. To counter possible racism, some investigators have developed an environmental hypothesis that suggests that differences, particularly concerning IQ scores, are attributable to cultural factors,[31,32] and Tobias observes that "at this stage of our ignorance, it is unjustified to include intelligence, however tested, among the validly demonstrated, genetically determined differences among the races of mankind."[26]

As IQ tests measure ideas and intelligence values of the societies who devise them, they are only valid in that environment. What is deemed intelligent and valued by other cultures may not be the same capacities. One capacity is not more valuable than another outside a particular context, they are just different and the notion of difference in capacities due to racial "fitness" does not imply racial superiority or inferiority, but rather a cause for celebration and pride of particular capacities and human adaptability to environmental circumstances. However, as world travel, migration, multiculturalism, and interracial marriages increase, what differences there are between racial groups will decrease, as gene flow decreases variation between populations but increases variation within them.[5] Appreciating possible differences in capacities between individuals from different racial backgrounds may be as important to health and well-being as recognizing species' similarities and cultural diversity, if it assists in recognizing and enabling expression of the unique range of capacities of each individual that will enhance individual and community experiences of health and well-being.

Gender

Similarly, there may be differences in capacities between genders because of the evolutionary pressures of natural selection and hormonal differences, which are under the control of genetic influences. Not only do levels of testosterone, estrogen, and progesterone account for differences in male and female behavior, but, in addition, Kolb and Whishaw report, after an examination of behavioral, anatomical, and neurological studies, there are significant gender differences in cerebral organization, including cerebral maturation rates, cerebral laterality, language, and spatial capacities.[7] For example, it is thought that the gene for spatial ability is recessive on the X (female) chromosome, that males require only one X chromosome but that females require both X chromosomes to carry the gene before spatial ability is demonstrated. With this model, it is possible to predict that while 50% of men would possess the trait, only 25% of women would, although some women would demonstrate greater ability than average men.[33] As well, it seems that differences in cerebral maturation rate can result in different capacities. It has been proposed that men generally mature physically and mentally more slowly than women and that maturation rate is a critical determinant of cerebral asymmetry. Although there must be, or have been, some adaptive advantage in laterality, such as more storage space with the subsequent potential for a greater range of skilled capacities, there are no compelling theories as to purpose, and, indeed, theories of laterality, as they were proposed 20 or so years ago, are being challenged by some neuroscientists in the 1990s.[7] Waber has demonstrated that regardless of gender, adolescents who mature early perform better in verbal tasks, and those who mature later perform better on spatial tasks.[34]

Ontogenesis

Waber's material supports the idea that just as capacities can differ between individuals, races, and genders, so are there differences because of age, as discrete neurophysiological mechanisms start functioning at specific times during ontogenesis.

This can be observed when infants become responsive, often quite suddenly, to specific external stimuli.[35] In fact, because "connections among the cells are...not precisely prespecified in the genes," epigenetic processes start in embryo when "key events occur only if certain previous events have taken place."[1] After birth, apart from obvious physical capacities, such as crawling, walking,[36] and talking, whose appearances are well documented:

> *At a certain point in ontogenesis, each individual begins to realize his or her own powers to direct attention, to think, to feel, to will, and to remember. At that point a new agency develops within awareness. This is the self.[37]*

With knowledge of the self comes an increased need to conform with others of the species and to demonstrate particular skills and capacities that are socioculturally valued. Capacities, therefore, also vary between individuals as they:

> *Change in various ways as an individual grows up, since every competence need [has] not appeared fully formed at birth. Some competencies improve with learning and practice during childhood and youth, and all do not improve at the same rate, or necessarily are perfected during a lifetime.[36]*

Particular Human Capacities and Characteristics

Capacities are the building blocks of unique occupational natures and personalities, despite the remarkable sameness in the range of capacities available to human beings. Subtle variations between humans lead to amazing differences in occupational interest, competence, and satisfaction, which grow or diminish according to environmental demands, enculturation, and individual opportunity. "No two mixes of the inner and outer factors are just alike."[9] The external variables increase individual differences in capacity, in part, because of structural change, which results from the neuronal demands of activity, so it is not surprising that the "brains of individuals vary in features just as the faces of individuals vary."[7]

Purposeful use of time is also part of our biological heritage, as Selye observes: "our brain slips into chaos and confusion unless we constantly use it for work that seems worthwhile to us," however much "the average person thinks he works for economic security or social status,"[38] and the human need to make use of capacities is evident from very early in evolution. (This need will be discussed further in Chapter 5.) Because the type of purpose and nature of occupation depends upon humans' particular capacities, the chapter will now turn to consider some of those capacities that are critical to complex, self-initiated occupational behavior and that are also focal points in debates about evolution and about humanness. The human capacities of upright walking, hand dexterity, stereoscopic vision, language, and social nature are prime examples. Campbell suggests that these particular capacities have "overwhelming significance" and when "added together separate all humans from all other animals."[5] The first four of these will be discussed now, and the social nature of humans will be discussed in the next chapter.

Bipedalism

Upright posture seems to be one of the most ancient of the species' particular features "associated with the ecological adaptations of early hominids."[39] Evidence, such as fragments of a 4-million-year-old thigh bone found in Ethiopia, and the discovery in Laetoli of a trail of footprints left by three hominids in volcanic ash more than 3.5 million years ago, leads to anthropological opinion that hominids stood

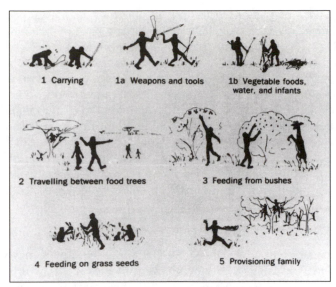

Figure 3-2. Some theories of the origin of bipedal locomotion. From Fleagle JG. Primate locomotion and posture. In: Jones S, Martin R, Pilbeam D, eds. *The Cambridge Encyclopedia of Human Evolution*. New York, NY: Cambridge University Press; 1992:79. Reprinted with the permission of Cambridge University Press.

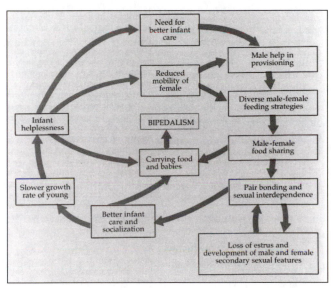

Figure 3-3. Pliocene adaptations of early hominids according to Lovejoy, drawn as a feedback system. *Humankind Emerging*. 5th ed. Campbell BG. Copyright 1988. Reprinted by permission of Addison-Wesley Educational Publishers Inc.

like humans before they could think like humans. Lewin suggests that the explanation of bipedalism, which currently enjoys the most scientific support, is that upright walking was a biological adaptive response to accessing traditional foods in a changing environment, that a more energy-efficient mode of walking was required because food sources became dispersed with climatic and subsequent environmental changes.[40] Another explanation is based on the fact that human young, who take a long time to mature, are dependent on their parents to carry them, unlike other primate offspring who are able to cling to their parents' long body hair. Erect standing and bipedal locomotion enabled mothers to move about while using arms and hands to support their children.[41] However, these are only two of several plausible explanations, all of which may have influenced bipedal evolution (Figures 3-2 and 3-3).

Although other animals have the ability to walk upright, humans have developed bipedalism into an adaptation as specialized as flight in a hovering hawk, while also developing versatility.[42-44] Humans can run, jump, dance, climb, swim, and cope with almost any terrain, and the health advantages of bipedal occupations, such as running, walking, and swimming, particularly with regard to the cardiovascular system, are well researched and applauded, even if not all epidemiologists agree about which form of activity is most valuable. Skilled use of bipedal locomotion varies among all humans, as evidenced by the number of sports and athletic pastimes that are based on different aspects of it. Not everyone can triple jump, dance like Fonteyn, or run a 4-minute mile, and while many climb, only a few pursue this occupation to the ultimate achievement of climbing to the summit of Mount Everest. However, despite the fact that bipedal locomotion is slower than quadrupedal, humans have thrived from the occupational advantages of having the forelimbs free.

Hand Function

Hand dexterity is also so characteristic that Benjamin Franklin is reputed to have observed that "man is a toolmaking animal." Although other primates are known to use tools (Jane Goodall and others have demonstrated how chimpanzees in the wild, with great care and skill, use grasses to extract termites from their nest),[45,46] the *Homo* genus is said to have begun with the ancestors who are credited as being the first manufacturers of stone tools. They lived about 2.5 to 1.6 million years ago and are known as *Homo habilis* (handy man, so named by Leakey, Napier, and Tobias in 1964), and although it is believed their tools were meager, "statistical studies of these tools have shown that their makers...had a concept of symmetry...and...a planned technique."[41] *Homo habilis* is also credited with building the first known stone shelters in Olduvai and of carrying food to such camp sites for processing and sharing.[41] These occupations were facilitated by a hand structure similar to our own, with a thumb positioned for opposition, essential for tool handling and manufacture, facilitated by a wrist joint that pronated and supinated.[47]

The anatomical advantage of hands capable of many types of prehension enabled them to be used as tools in their own right. This endowed early humans with the capacity for manipulative skill, which was facilitated by a refinement of specialized brain centers within the primary sensory and motor areas of the cortex, coordinated with other brain centers, such as the basal ganglia and the cerebellum.[48,49] As Sir Charles Bell observed, in his 1833 *Bridgewater Treatise* (one of a number of treatises sponsored by The Right Honorable Francis Henry, Earl of Bridgewater) on the hand, which related the hand's structure and function to environment:

> *This difference in the length of the fingers serves a thousand purposes, adapting the hand and fingers, as in holding a rod, a switch, a sword, a hammer, a pen or pencil, engraving tool, in all which a secure hold and freedom of motion are admirably combined.*[50]

Such a hand structure, along with the capacity to walk upright, thus freeing the hands for activity, is one of the special human attributes important to the unique occupational history of the species. Jelinek suggests this attribute was pre-adaptive to tool use, and it is probable that this pre-adaptive period was characterized to some extent by playful occupation.[41] Psychologist Jerome Bruner, for example, argues that "play...can produce the flexibility that makes tool using possible," citing the laboratory studies of Birch and of Schiller, which indicate that play with materials is necessary

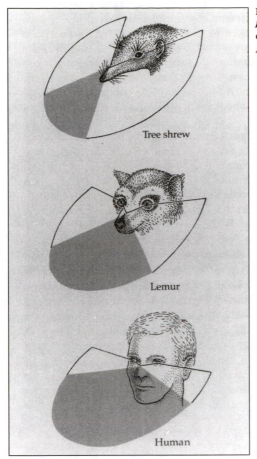

Figure 3-4. Stereoscopic vision in primates. *Humankind Emerging*. **5th ed. Campbell BG. Copyright 1988. Reprinted by permission of Addison-Wesley Educational Publishers Inc.**

Tree shrew

Lemur

Human

prior to using it for "instrumental ends."[51-53]

The use of upper limbs and hands has developed into a very specialized adaptation, so that the unique movements, the sense of touch, the balance function, the reaching out, the gesturing, and fine manipulative capacities can be used separately or combined in infinitely varied ways to enable culturally derived occupations, unique to humans, to be carried out. Yet all humans are not able to use their upper limbs and hands with the grace of a Balinese dancer, the skill of an artist, or the strength of arm wrestler. Although the capacity to use hands is "one of the dominant aspects of our biological and cultural adaptation,"[54] there are differences between individuals, which is recognized in commonplace acceptance of particular attributes of individuals and which needs to be borne in mind when strategies for occupational justice are enacted.

Visual System

Upright posture and skilled hand use work in cooperation with vision. Because of humans' upright posture and height and eyes positioned at the front rather than the side of the head, they are able to see for relatively long distances. As well as enjoying the benefits of long sight, stereoscopic vision helps people to focus on objects that are close and to see these in three-dimensional form (Figure 3-4). This capacity has made it possible for humans to manipulate and appreciate the structure of materials, to become toolmakers, and, with practice, to produce objects of great variety and complexity that, in turn, have assisted human adaptation to different environments. Coupled with visual perception, humans are able to identify objects by color, hue, brightness, and form, in different orientations, and with sufficient clarity to pick out objects from their backgrounds whether they are still or moving. This range of visual capacity has been instrumental in the variety of occupations that can be undertaken and gives humans an evolutionary advantage over other animals despite them, perhaps, having better visual faculties of a particular kind.

Humans know about their world through their senses, and it is "the limitations of [human] senses [that] set the boundaries of...conscious existence."[55] To many, vision is the most important of our senses, and it has been estimated that between 75% and 90% of the information stored in the brain is derived from visual sources. Ninety-eight people of a group of 104 subjects surveyed by first-year occupational therapy students about their perceptions of sensory capacities identified vision as the sense they most used.[56] Despite this, loss of vision does not necessarily impair health or well-being, but the effects differ between people, perhaps according to how and to what extent they use it in valued occupations and how much they are able to compensate for the loss by using other senses.

"Since the world is constantly changing, the brain is flooded with information," even though "the eye [only] takes in a trillionth of the energy which reaches it."[6] In fact, the visual system and the brain selects, simplifies, and organizes so that what humans see "is not so much a replication of the real world as a calculated and very selective abstraction of it."[57] This capacity prevents people from being overwhelmed by extraneous information and helps them make sense of what they see and choose what it is necessary to attend to so that appropriate, or even fast, action can occur as necessary for survival and safety. For example, instead of seeing each color, shape, texture, and form of parts of a room as separate, people perceive the room as a whole coherent structure in which they can move and act, or a glimpse of part of an animal or another human who may threaten will be perceived and understood as a whole. To do this, "the brain constantly needs stimulation to develop, grow, and maintain its organization,"[6] and vision, like all other capacities, is dependent, to a large extent, upon use and upon what we learn through experience. Indeed, sensory systems are often especially tuned in to communication systems of the same species, because the activities of conspecifics often affect survival, health, and well-being.[58,59]

Language

This leads to consideration of language, which, because of the weight given to this capacity, its complexity, and its centrality in occupational evolution, merits an extended discourse.[60-62] Chomsky, along with many others, argues that complex human language is unique to humans as no other animal learns anything that resembles it.[63] Indeed, it is held by some that human language is so different from communication of other animals that comparison need not be made.[64,65] However, the more traditional view argues that language has evolved through a series of adaptive changes within mammalian communication systems[66] and "may rest on neural mechanisms that are present in reduced form in other living species and that were elaborated quite early during hominid evolution."[67]

Edelman argues that humans had the capacity to "produce and act on concepts" and to ascribe meaning prior to language acquisition. Then, at about the same time as the speech areas named after Broca and Wernicke emerged in the brain, changes occurred in the base of the skull as a result of bipedalism.

This provided a morphological basis for the evolution of...the supralaryngeal tract...As part of this evolutionary development, the vocal cords emerged and the tongue, palate, and teeth were selected to allow fuller control of air flow over the vocal cords, which in turn allowed for the production of coarticulated sounds, the phonemes.[1]

> *The comparative anatomy of living primates and of hominid fossils suggests that the evolution of the human supralaryngeal vocal tract probably...was not completed until the appearance of fully modern humans...complex patterns of human speech seem to have evolved only in the past 1.6 million years or so [and] there seems to be a link between the neural mechanisms involved in speech motor control and those responsible for syntax.*
> Lieberman P. Evolution of the speech apparatus. In: Jones S, Martin R, Pilbeam D, eds. *The Cambridge Encyclopedia of Human Evolution.* New York, NY: Cambridge University Press; 1992:136-137.

According to Edelman's theory of neuronal group selection and following the prior evolution of the specific brain structures mentioned above, the capacity for language was first linked by "learning with concepts and gestures," followed by semantics, and then syntax.[1]

Although early language was, undoubtedly, based on gesture, body signals, grunts, growls, cries, or even perhaps markers on trees for directional information in the hunt for food, speech is thought by some to have developed at the same time as people became tool users, because, among the more obvious social advantages, speech would have facilitated complex thinking abilities necessary for the manufacture of tools and the transfer of toolmaking skills as they occurred. Such claims are supported by the fact that the brain of *Homo habilis* was larger than other hominid species of the same period and a habilis skull, estimated to be 2 million years old, was found to possess a Broca's speech area, although not as prominent a feature as that of modern humans.[68] Earlier ancestors' remains have not revealed this feature, and there is considerable debate from studies of ape brain structure and behavior as to whether Broca or Wernicke areas, important for human speech, are present.[7] Even though chimpanzees are excellent communicators and "appear to have concepts and thought and...simple semantics,...they have no brain bases for the complex sequencing of articulated sounds [and]...lack an elaborated syntax."[1] The sounds produced by them mainly originate in the limbic system (as does the human scream) and are not commensurate with human spoken language, which originates in the cortex.[5] Their gestures, however, are generated in the cortex, and the greatest success in teaching primates to communicate has not been achieved through speech, but by sign language, such as "Ameslam," symbols, and using a computer keyboard.[69-72] In infancy, children rely on "the workings of the limbic system to call attention to their needs...They find temper tantrums, whimpering, or crying a much easier way...to express [emotions] than to explain." This is despite being able to use simple speech, such as two-word

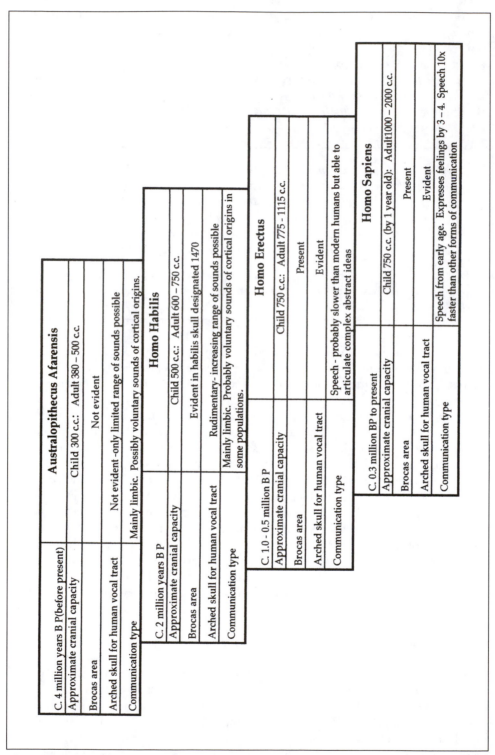

Figure 3-5. Overview of the evolution of language. Adapted from Campbell BG. *Humankind Emerging*. 5th ed. New York, NY: Harper Collins Publishers; 1988:367 and Lewin R. *In the Age of Mankind: A Smithsonian Book of Human Evolution*. Washington, DC: Smithsonian Books; 1988.

sentences, to communicate effectively about less emotional issues. Human speech is thought, by some, to have evolved in a similar fashion.[5] See Figure 3-5 for an overview of the evolution of language.

Most pre-historians seem to agree that some form of verbal language arose as long as 2.5 million years ago and that by about 30,000 years ago humans would have developed "modern language capacity, including the ability to articulate complex abstract ideas."[68] However, not all agree with the tool technology hypothesis, but a link between language and some type of occupational behavior is favored by many. Hewes emphasizes the role of gesture in the evolution of language and suggests that, as tool usage occupied hands, they became less available for communication, leading to increased use of facial gesture and sound.[73] Kimura agrees that speech is related to gesturing and tool usage and argues that it follows that evolution of speech occurred later than lateralization of brain function, which was instrumental in control of complex movement.[74] This theory is supported by observations that hand gestures still accompany speech, and when there are difficulties in verbal communication, such as people conversing in different languages, hand and facial gestures increase. Theories about lateralization flourished in the 1960s and 1970s, although much of the research was carried out with male subjects and often those with some abnormality of brain function. More recent evidence points to both hemispheres being involved in most activities (even though they may perform different parts of the task). It is also evident that the "complexity of neural networks involved are all highly dependent upon individual differences, talents, and learning, including one's sex and genetic endowment."[75]

Bruner hypothesizes that language is "virtually an outgrowth of the mastery of skilled action and perceptual discrimination," basing this claim on observations of ontogenetic development. From this beginning, he asserts language is progressively freed from its original dependence on action and experience.[51] Others name hunter-gatherer activities or complex social relationships as the driving force in the evolution of language, with de Laguna suggesting that the most likely explanation lies in the need for help associated with a sociotechnical way of life.[76] It would seem that as all these were occurring at about the same time, a combination of causes is probable, such as the theory that development of language followed similar stages to those apparent in ontogenesis. This seems to make sense of the evidence from archaeology and other primates. Simple tool usage and communication similar to that of chimpanzees increased in complexity as bipedalism freed the hands and led to structural anatomical and physiological change in the base of the skull and head, all of which facilitated more complex occupational behavior, social structures, speech, and language.

Spoken language is the foundation of culture, because, without language, complex technology and social structures would be impossible. Reminiscence, singing, and the telling of stories, myths, and legends is central in handing down to the next generation occupational "know how," culturally sanctioned behaviors, taboos, and spiritual beliefs, all of which are intimately related to survival, health, and well-being. (No material record or proof of these aspects of technical, cultural, and spiritual occupations are available as, before the fairly recent advent of writing, human discourse and song simply vanished.) Without language, individuals are peripheral to society and devalued, and as a consequence well-being would be hard to experience in cultures, such as our own, that value language-related occupations.

The capacity to communicate is not the only benefit of language. As Percy Bysshe Shelley observed in *Prometheus Unbound*, "He gave man speech, and speech created thought, which is a measure of the universe."[77] Although Piaget argues that "language is not enough to explain thought, because the structures that characterize thought have their roots in action and in sensorimotor mechanisms that are deeper than linguistics,"[78] language allows individuals to explore ideas, to think in abstract as well as concrete terms, and to bring to their occupational pursuits concepts based on their unique life experience and ways of thinking. Lewin suggests "mankind's exaggerated intellectual power focuses on the need to build a better mental construct of reality...It may have required a complex propositional language, not so much that we could converse with others, but so we could think better."[40]

Thinking about and searching for truths about life and its meaning must have developed along with language. It is probable that intellectual activities of the type now called philosophy first emerged as wonder at the natural world and that early belief systems were based on animals and environmental forces important in survival terms. This speculation is founded on the types of images humans left behind in cave drawings and in ornamentation and the fact that the earliest monumental buildings, such as those in Uruk and Ur in Mesopotamia, had religious significance frequently associated with natural phenomena. Early Greek philosophy, which emerged in Miletus, with Thales (c. 600 BC), also reflects this dual interest in matters natural and spiritual. Thales is reported as saying that "all things are full of gods."[79] It was not until the Sophists came into prominence, shortly before Socrates, that philosophy became interested in mankind apart from nature and in reasoning per se. This interest led to a recurring theme in philosophy and psychology—the debate about the nature of consciousness, which is the next human characteristic to be considered, but from the perspective of its role in the occupational nature of humans rather than in philosophical history.

Consciousness

Consciousness is an example of a "super-capacity," which is a combination of many other capacities and is integral to the use of other capacities. Capacities seldom work in isolation, but combine with others according to the environment and experience. They are multifunctional and the combining of specific capacities with others increases the potential variability that individuals will demonstrate through their occupations. Capacities can be used in an insular focused way or act as an integrated part of several capacities, being utilized in different ways at any one time. They are responsive to inner needs and external variables, as well as being capable of rapid reaction to emergency. Each capacity is "relatively independent of the others," but they may "work in concert. This means that the faculty itself, seen as a whole, is bound to vary from one person to another."[36] A similar theme in modern psychology is that a single mental capacity may represent a "family of competencies." Harvard psychologist Howard Gardner calls these "frames of mind."[80]

Consciousness is defined in the 1981 *Macquarie Dictionary* as "the state of being conscious; inward sensibility of something; knowledge of one's own existence, sensations, cognitions, etc.; and the thoughts and feelings, collectively, of an individual or of an aggregate of people."[81] It has been described as "the tool of the social animal"[40] and by Watson as "the capacity to see ourselves and to put ourselves in someone else's place. We are not only self-aware, but conscious of being so." It is "the key...[and]...the power which motivates and drives all human affairs."[57] Consciousness enables us to know what we know and to experience our own feelings and the outcomes of what we do. It "is a kind of continuous apprehension of an inner reality, the reality of one's mental states and activities,"[82] providing us with a model of the world, "based on sense and body information, expectations, fantasy and crazy hopes, and other cognitive processes."[83] Consciousness is deemed by many writers to demonstrate the difference between humans and other species, in that humans alone can "examine all options in advance...look inward upon themselves, and...observe the processes of their own minds."[5] There is, however, evidence that some other primates have some degree of consciousness and, for example, "can recognize themselves on television and even determine whether an image is taped or live."[72,84]

Edelman has proposed a biological model of the evolution of consciousness according to his theory of neuronal group selection. The processes of natural selection gave rise to form and tissue patterns, which are the basis of behavior. From this developed a "primary repertoire of variant neuronal groups in the brain" that are involved in selection. Selection "assumes that, during behavior, synaptic connections in the anatomy are selectively strengthened or weakened by specific biochemical processes," carving out a variety of functioning circuits. "Correlation and coordination of...selection events are achieved by 're-entrant' signalling and by strengthening of interconnections between the maps" in the brain. This selection process linked, during evolution, the older areas of the brain (brainstem and limbic system), which take care of bodily functions, internal states, and values, and the thalamo-cortical system, which perceives and categorizes world events. Together, through "value-category" memory, they enable perceptual categorization and the subsequent development of primary consciousness, which, in conjunction with changes to the structure of the brain, such as Broca and Wernicke areas (mentioned with regard to language), in quite a short time span evolved higher order consciousness.[1]

In considering the evolutionary purpose of consciousness, it would seem that awareness of the possible consequences of action is necessary for an organism with free will. Such a capacity can, but may not always, act as a guard to ensure continued well-being and survival. Without it, the organism can, more easily, use its other capacities in ways, and for occupations, that will be detrimental to itself, to the species, and the ecologies upon which it is dependent.

Complex occupational behavior would be impossible without consciousness and, apart from it being a prerequisite, consciousness plays an important part in choice and execution of occupation. Ornstein hypothesizes that, although individuals are generally unaware of it, consciousness vetoes or permits every action that is initiated at an unconscious level from the "many different kinds of minds" responsible for human responses to the world, talents, capacities, and characteristics within the brain organization.[83] Additionally, states of consciousness can be affected by the types of occupations in which individuals choose to engage. Csikszentmihalyi has found that "when challenges are high and personal skills are used to the utmost, we experience a rare state of consciousness," which he calls "flow." Flow is enjoyable, narrows attention to a clearly defined goal, provides a sense of control over actions although awareness of time disappears, and people are absorbed and involved. "The activity can be wildly different, but when people are deeply involved [in] meeting a manageable challenge, the state of mind they report is the same the world over."[85-87] Csikszentmihalyi, who embraces a "personal growth" view of health, recognizes that flow experiences resulting from "growth enhancing occupations" are an important aspect of positive health.[85]

In an argument similar to Edelman's argument that consciousness depends upon perceptual and conceptual categorization, semantics, syntax, and phonology, all of which allow learning to occur, Csikszentmihalyi proposes that consciousness depends particularly on three other capacities. He believes "attention, awareness, and memory...act as a buffer between genetic and cultural instructions on the one hand, and behavior on the other." His view that "consciousness frees the organism from its dependence on the forces that created it and provides a certain [if precarious] control over our behavior" is similar or complementary to that stated above. Consciousness, in fact, negates the need for a multitude of separate genetic programs to link stimuli and responses and "increases the possibilities" between "programmed instructions and adaptive behaviors." The "self-system" has a main goal to "ensure its own survival. To this effect, attention, awareness, and memory are directed to replicate those states of consciousness that are congenial to self and to eliminate those that threaten its existence." On the down side, consciousness has given humans enormous independence and power, with the potential to destroy the environment from which they evolved and on which they depend, and "it is by no means certain that [this] choice and control...will serve us better than the blind instructions of our genes."[37]

While consciousness is an essential capacity for the forward planning and execution of occupational behavior, it has the unenviable role of prompting humans to consider the consequences of their actions. It is central in the balancing act between occupational achievement, health, and well-being, in both the short- and long-term.[88-90] Its watchdog role is made complex by its susceptibility, just as other capacities, to enculturation. For example, raising the consciousness of people about lifestyle issues relating to ill health can be viewed as both a cause and effect of "health education" initiatives, and this important matter is discussed in some detail in the last chapter. It is an integral part of other agendas, such as those aimed at cultural awareness, social justice, or sustainable ecology. Consciousness raising also emerged in the 1960s as part of the feminist movement to enable women "to express and explore themselves," to understand the effects of patriarchal societies, and to validate "women's knowledge and experience" from a personal and political viewpoint. Similar groups are emerging for men.[91] This broader consciousness raising is important as part of a holistic view of health and well-being.[92-95] For example, advocates of transpersonal psychology recognize that an "optimal state of consciousness" is a central process in the achievement of positive health. Optimal states of consciousness, they believe, enable people "to achieve deep states of relaxation, [to experience] increased inner awareness, ...bodymind self-awareness and, [make] effective choices...more accessible."[96] They link psychological and physiological states, incorporating notions from many Asian religions including the Patanjali concept that "all the body is in the mind, though not all of the mind is in the body."[97] In a way similar to Ornstein's and Sobel's pragmatic view that the brain minds the body, the "psychophysiological principle" claims that every conscious or unconscious change in either physiologic or mental-emotional state is accompanied by an appropriate change in the other and that health can be facilitated by awareness and self-regulation of normally unconscious processes.[97]

Creativity

Consciousness is one of the most complex, poorly understood human mental capacities. Similarly complex and subject to many different interpretations is the last capacity to be discussed—creativity. This capacity is not a prerequisite of occupational behavior, but results from the amalgam of the rich variety of capacities available, and as such is important to an occupational perspective. It has, in the minds of many, been closely associated with occupational therapy, though often in a limited, craft-oriented way, rather than in the holistic way creativity is used here. Just as occupation is used to refer to all purposeful activity, so is creativity used in relation to all types of activities, products, or ideas, and just as consciousness is seen as combining other capacities so does creativity. Creativity is both a capacity in its own right and a super-capacity integrating or involving almost every other human capacity. Gordon suggests that "to create is one of man's most basic impulses."[98] Jung classified it as one of five major instinctive forces in humans,[99] and Sinnott argues that it is in "inherent creativeness" of the ordinary affairs of people that the "ultimate source" of creativeness is to be found.[100]

Creativity derives from the Greek word "krainein," meaning to fulfill, and the Latin word "creare," meaning to make.[101] Dictionaries describe it as the "ability to bring into existence or being, to originate, to beget, to shape, to bring about, to invest with new character, and to be inventive."[2,102] William Morris suggested that creativity is an integral part of the human contest with nature describing his perception thus:

> *But a man, making something which he feels will exist because he is working at it and wills it, is exercising the energies of his mind and soul as well as of his body. Memory and imagination help him as he works. Not only his own thoughts, but the thoughts of the men of past ages guide his hands; and, as a part of the human race, he creates.[103]*

Creativity requires the ability to conceptualize outcomes from actions. Some describe such abstract conceptualization as the ultimate human gift, and Lewin suggests that the creation of paintings, carvings, and engravings represents a true abstraction of thought and mind, and traces examples back perhaps 300,000 years.[40] However, John Halverson of the University of California argues that early creative images were "unmediated by cognitive reflection" but rather were clear, representational, and repeated for their own sake. The extent of early humans' creativity has been hard to assess because although they appeared to possess very little in the form of creative artifacts this may be a consequence of an "inescapable conflict between mobility and material culture."[68] For example, the !Kung carry only about 12 kilograms each when they travel, so most of their culture is carried in their heads. This is also true of the Australian Aboriginals following a traditional lifestyle and reminds us that creativity is much more than the manufacture of material artifacts. It includes those intellectual and abstract reasoning skills so dear to philosophers and academics and the evidences of culture that are carried in the minds and recreated regularly throughout history. Sinnott suggests that the biological basis for creativity is the "organizing, pattern forming, questing quality" of life itself, which, when applied to behavior and the complexity of the human brain, results in an almost infinite number of new mental patterns.[100]

Marx, as noted earlier, suggested that labor is the collective creative activity of mankind; certainly it was the creative abstract occupations that, integrated with tool technology, evolved eventually into high-technology activities through cultural evolution. High technology is the epitome of human creativity, yet the products of the industrial and technological age have had a serious effect on individual creativity. For example, although not true of all people, many no longer make products that they need, preferring to buy, and seldom create their own entertainment, preferring to watch and listen to prepackaged material. Similarly, the creative behavior of many children has changed with the advent of television as hours are spent in viewing images rather than experimenting, playing, or creating their own.

Creativity is a capacity that has excited much interest and discussion, yet sources seldom agree on a definition, with one paper written in 1953 offering no fewer than 25.[104] Many psychologists, from behaviorists to social psychologists, have offered theories about it.[98,105-109] For example, it has been suggested that psychoanalytic theorists, such as Freud and Adler, accepted the view of creativity held early this century, which limited the concept to the arts.[109,110] The arts were held to be socially acceptable activities that were an outlet for sublimation of libidal energy and other unconscious conflicts, drives, and needs. Creativity was seen as stemming from neurotic tendencies, offering the resolution of guilt feelings and compensation for feelings of inferiority.[111-113] Despite this, Freud recognized parallels between the creative nature of children's play and the creative artist and, along with others of the psychoanalytical school, suggested that creative people were subject to better health as well as more sickness than the average.[110,114]

It is not surprising that humanist and gestalt psychologists have linked creativity with the experience of health and with individual potential. They hold the view that creativity is much more than innate talent or genius exemplified by exceptional individuals in the arts and is evident in all aspects of life as the potential to self-actualize is given to all human beings at birth.[115] Humanists, such as Maslow and Rogers, have proposed that self-growth motivates creativity and that creativity and the achievement of individual potential are synonymous with health. Rogers describes "man's tendency to actualize himself, to become his potentialities" as the mainspring of creativity,[116] and Maslow observes "that the concept of creativeness and the concept of the healthy, self-actualizing, fully human person seem to be coming closer and closer together, and may perhaps turn out to be the same thing."[117]

Maslow reached this conclusion following a study of self-fulfilled people, whom he saw as mentally healthy, in order to discover how people are enabled toward growth and self-actualization and to determine the attributes and components of a basically healthy intrinsic nature. He described the healthiest and most effective people as transcenders. Such people are responsive to beauty, holistic in their perceptions of humanity, motivated by the satisfaction of being and service values, able to adjust well to conflict situations, and more likely to accept others with an unconditional positive regard. They are less attracted by the rewards of money and objects, and work whole-heartedly toward goals and purposes. They tend to fuse work and play and have more peak or creative experiences.

There are definite similarities between traits of Maslow's transcenders and traits believed to characterize creative people as identified by the Institute of Personality Assessment at the University of California. The latter are described as intuitive, open, spontaneous, expressive, independent, self-accepting, flexible not authoritarian, and autonomous, functioning best when working independently on their interests. They are relatively free from fear and are not interested in detail but in meaning and implications, with the ability to synthesize and integrate material and experiences. They have well-developed intrinsic values and are goal directed.[118] Indeed, the links between creativity (and, by inference, occupation) and mental health appear strong—

for example, high creativity has been found to correlate with a high degree of normal mature positive self-esteem.[119] This discussion should be kept in mind when mental well-being is discussed in Chapter 5.

Making the assumption that creativity is closely related to occupation, from low levels observed in solving the problems of daily life to significant levels in terms of contributions to advances in technology, intellectual, or sociocultural activity, there appear to be strong links between individuals and particular forms of creative occupation. This supports the notion of inherent capacities, which emerge or peak at different parts of the life cycle, as discussed earlier in the chapter.[107,120-123] It also appears that, for most people, potential requires incubation, education, diligence, nurturing, and opportunity, despite some evidence of particular individuals having the ability to overcome detrimental circumstances in order to actualize their occupational creativity.[107,108,120,124,125]

These examples from the range of capacities with which humans are endowed demonstrate how anatomical structures and physiology focus on occupational behavior. The incredible flexibility of specific parts of the body for different functions, such as those noted in the hands, bipedalism, and vision, coupled with the extensive range of higher cortical capacities, which are central to consciousness and creativity, for example, prompts, motivates, and enables an infinite variety of occupational exploration, experimentation, interest, choice, and skill, as well as imbuing people with the need for purpose and meaning. Additionally, every other physiological characteristic influences, promotes, or supports humans' occupational behavior. The next section considers sleep and homeostasis from this perspective.

Sleep

Most animals appear to need a balance between activity and rest, the two seeming to be opposites of the same system. Kleitman explored and then described the day/night sequence as the "basic rest activity cycle."[126] He saw sleep as complementary to wakefulness in that "the one related to the other as the trough of a wave is to the crest."[36]

Over the past 40 years, sleep patterns have been the subject of intense scrutiny, and sleep is recognized as an important aspect of health and well-being, relaxation and sleep providing the natural mechanism to prevent overuse and a time for repair. Additional understanding is now emerging about the complex relationship between it and occupation carried out during waking states. Theories about this relationship center around recuperation, information processing, energy conservation, and self-preservation.[59] As sleep deprivation results in symptoms such as decreased coordination and reaction times, irritability, and blurred vision,[127] which affect occupational performance, sleep can be viewed as necessary to engagement in occupation. Together they form part of the complex neural system aimed at maintenance of health.

Leger suggests that "just as musicians' pauses are a component of the performance, pauses from the stream of behavior are a component of the repertoire. The organism 'doing nothing' is doing something."[59] All sleep stages have a homeostatic function, although the system does not operate on feedback principles but on intrinsic timing mechanisms.[36] These mechanisms differ slightly for each individual and change throughout the lifespan. In evolutionary terms, the oldest form of sleep known as non rapid eye movement sleep, or slow wave sleep (SWS), shows different patterns of

EEGs for several different stages. SWS is responsible for replenishing the body and maintaining physiological and metabolic fitness. After a day of strenuous physical occupation, SWS increases, and it is only during SWS that growth hormone, essential for restoring damaged tissue, is released.[128] Following sleep deprivation, SWS takes priority in "catching up." For example, studies, such as those conducted by Shapiro and others, on ultra-marathon runners demonstrated an increase in SWS as well as total sleeping time over 4 nights following the run.[129] This effect appears most developed among people who are physically fit,[130] suggesting a close relationship between sleep patterns and regular occupations.

As the association areas of the neocortex expanded during evolution, additional "servicing" was required for the maintenance of structures specializing in mental and social functions. This is provided by rapid eye movement (REM) sleep when circuits are tested and neurotransmitters are replenished by being rested selectively.[36] During this stage, the brain is very active and "actually consumes more oxygen than it does during intense physical or mental activity when one is awake."[131] Speculations about other functions of REM sleep include the integration of knowledge acquired during the day, consolidation of information, assistance in dealing with emotionally charged material, and the laying down of long-term memory.[36,132,133] (However, some claim that SWS also assists memory formation and recall.[134]) Experiments using EEGs on rats, rabbits, and cats have demonstrated that theta rhythms exhibited during important species-specific occupations (i.e., exploring, burrowing, or pouncing) are also present during REM sleep. Fox speculates that "current information, blocked from the hippocampus and the limbic circuit during waking, is allowed in there during sleep to be 'matched' against those wired-in survival behaviors that are the species' ethogram." If the information is deemed relevant, it is processed "for at least 3 years in some form or other" during dreams before being "stamped in" to long-term memory and eventually stored in the neocortex.[135] This process enables the neocortex to assess experience toward future goal-directed action. Although REM sleep may serve a similar purpose in humans, Fox suggests that dreaming has been freed, to some extent, from phylogenetic ties and species-specific experience, allowing the "matching" to relate to prenatal and childhood experience.

There are "gating mechanisms" that facilitate passage between sleep and awake states.[136] REM sleep, which usually occurs four to five times a night, is seen as the easiest exit point from sleep and possibly evolved in part as a "sentinel device, a monitor in case of danger."[36] At rhythmical times during wakefulness, there are "sleepability gates" when it is easier to sleep. The most obvious of these is the biological slump occurring in the afternoon, which is taken as siesta time in many traditional cultures. (Winston Churchill is quoted as saying "You must sleep sometime between lunch and dinner, and no half measures. Take off your clothes and get into bed. That's what I always do." in *My Dear Mr. Churchill* by Graebner.) Biphasic activity peaks are part of our biological heritage, are evident in behaviors of other primates, and are probably an adaptation resulting from the need to reduce occupation during the hottest part of the day. However, duration of sleep is hard to change because need differs from person to person. Ultradian rhythms of arousal and non-arousal concerned with placement of sleep are easily overruled by sociocultural demands, such as social and family routines and obligatory and freely chosen occupations.[137] For example, in a study of 64 children, 10 to 14 years of age, weekly changes of sleep patterns during the school year disappeared during vacations when sleep increased considerably.[138]

Studies using EEGs have demonstrated differences in brainwaves throughout sleep and awake states. Particularly in the awake states, these seem to relate to when the organism is best fitted for different types of occupation or rest, although these are flexible and can be overridden, as happens in "post-industrial" working days and 24-hour working shifts, which enable humans to behave as nocturnal rather than diurnal animals. The sleep systems are therefore facilitatory to immense occupational flexibility, as well as servicing all systems so they can be used as required in occupational behavior.

Homeostasis

The last physiological characteristic to be explored is homeostasis, which is defined as "a tendency to stability in the normal body state's [internal environment] of the organism."[139] It "is an evolutionary strategy for preserving internal sameness by resisting and smoothing out the changes" and variations from the external environment.

> *Homeostasis is especially necessary for the proper functioning of the central nervous system of animals on the higher rungs of the evolutionary ladder. Before intelligent life could appear, and well before the culminating event of consciousness, the mechanism to ensure the sameness of the internal milieu had to be in place.*[36]

It was Claude Bernard, a 19th century French physiologist, who developed the concept that the internal environment—the milieu intérieur—of a living organism must maintain reasonable constancy despite external circumstances. He recognized that humans, despite their apparent indifference to the environment, are "on the contrary in a close and wise relationship with it, so that its equilibrium results from a continuous and delicate compensation established as if by the most sensitive balances" and that animals able to maintain "inner sameness" have greater freedom to live in many different environments and are less vulnerable to ecological change. This perhaps results in their apparent indifference to the environment.[140]

Bernard's first recorded use of the term "milieu intérieur" was in the first lecture of a series entitled "Lectures on the Physiological and the Pathological Alterations of the Liquids of the Organism," at the University of Paris on December 9, 1857. In this lecture, Bernard said that in living beings there is a spontaneous organic evolution which, although it needs the external environment to manifest itself, is nevertheless independent of that environment in its course because "in the living being, the tissues are, in reality, removed from direct external influences and protected by a true internal environment (milieu intérieur), mostly constituted by fluids circulating in the body."

Bernard C. Lectures on the phenomena of life common to animals and vegetables (1878-1879). In: Langley LL, ed. *Homeostasis, Origins of the Concept*. Straudsburg, Pa: Hutchinson and Ross, Inc; 129-147.

The term homeostasis was suggested by Walter Cannon, an American physiologist, in 1926.[141] He recognized that homeostasis is a system working cooperatively with brain and body and found that at "critical times" of environmental stress "economy is secondary to stability" in that important substances such as water, sugar, or salt are eliminated in order to maintain constancy.[142] Cannon researched and described the way a fluid matrix provides a stable context for highly specialized cells, which, by themselves, can only survive in specific conditions, to enact their part in complex, flexible, and versatile activities. He postulated that homeostasis leaves humans free to do new occupations, to be adventurous, and to seek beyond survival to the "unessentials" that are part and parcel of civilization.[142]

Homeostasis is a successful adaptation that is central to humans' occupational nature, because not only is the need for "sameness" used to maintain constancy in body physiology, but in mental processes as well. To make sense of the world, psychological mechanisms seek "sameness" in what is received and perceived. This is facilitated by an "internal milieu, [which] seems to be more constant for the cells of the brain than for other parts of the body."[36] In 1890, William James claimed in *The Principles of Psychology* that the capacity to recognize sameness is a prerequisite for the existence of a sense of self and "the very keel and backbone of our thinking" as it is central to recognition, of giving meaning, and of appreciating contrast and difference.[143] This capacity is also central to occupational behavior. Without it, every time engagement in occupation occurred, it would appear as a new experience, take longer, be in the nature of trial and error, and no ongoing learning could occur. The occupational evolution of the species would indeed be different.

Summary

In this chapter, it has been found that biological characteristics and capacities, which have been identified as important by evolutionary scientists, archaeologists, anthropologists, neuroscientists, and other disciplines, form the basis of the occupational nature of humans. Such characteristics have allowed humans to learn and to adapt culturally to many different natural and social environments. A superprimate brain capable of the whole range of sociocultural adaptations that have characterized occupational evolution is common to humankind but is also unique in each individual. During the exploration, the role of human capacities in survival, health, and well-being began to emerge, setting the scene for later consideration. Occupational behavior is a result of the processes of natural selection throughout evolution as organisms have adapted to their environment, genetic inheritance, individual biological structure and form, epigenetic processes, ontogenesis, and learning. The next chapter will explore the evolution of occupational behavior, which has resulted from this biological inheritance.

References

1. Edelman G. *Bright Air, Brilliant Fire: On the Matter of the Mind.* London, England: Penguin Books; 1992:7,16-19,23,25,48,51,57,64,83-85,117-119,126,129-130,134.
2. *The Standard English Desk Dictionary.* 2nd ed. Oxford, UK: Oxford University Press; 1975.
3. Roget PM. *Roget's Thesaurus of Synonyms and Antonyms.* London, England: The Number Nine Publishing Co; 1972.
4. *Word Finder: The Australian Thesaurus.* Sydney, Australia: Reader's Digest; 1983.
5. Campbell BG. *Humankind Emerging.* 5th ed. New York, NY: Harper Collins Publishers; 1988:47,52,86-87,360,364-365,374-378.
6. Ornstein R, Sobel D. *The Healing Brain: A Radical New Approach to Health Care.* London, England: Macmillan; 1988:36,39,57,105-106,218.
7. Kolb B, Whishaw IQ. *Fundamentals of Human Neuropsychology.* 3rd ed. San Franscico, Calif: WH Freeman and Co; 1990:4,123.
8. Sperry R. *Some Effects of Disconnecting the Cerebral Hemispheres.* Les Prix Nobel; 1981:209-219.

9. Snell GD. *Search for a Rational Ethic.* New York, NY: Springer Verlag; 1988:140,147,165.
10. Penfield W, Boldrey E. Somatic motor and sensory representation in the cerebral cortex as studied by electrical stimulation. *Brain.* 1958;60:389-443.
11. Brodmann K. *Vergleichended lokalisations lehre der Grosshirnrinde in prinzipien dargestellt auf grund des zellenbaues.* Liepzig: JA Barth; 1909.
12. Lassen NA, Ingvar DH, Skinhoj E. Brain function and blood flow. *Scientific American.* 1978;239:62-71.
13. Roland PE. Applications of brain blood flow imaging in behavioral neurophysiology: cortical field activation hypothesis. In: Sokoloff L, ed. *Brain Imaging and Brain Function.* New York, NY: Raven Press; 1985:87-104.
14. Kety SS. Disorders of the human brain. *Scientific American.* 1979;241:202-214.
15. Mazziotta JC, Phelps ME. Human neuropsychological imaging studies of local brain metabolism: strategies and results. In: Sokoloff L, ed. *Brain Imaging and Brain Function.* New York, NY: Raven Press; 1985.
16. Restak R. *The Brain.* New York, NY: Bantam Books; 1984.
17. Deacon TW. The human brain. In: Jones S, Martin R, Pilbeam D, eds. *The Cambridge Encyclopedia of Human Evolution.* New York, NY: Cambridge University Press; 1992:121.
18. Gagne F. Toward a differentiated model of giftedness and talent. In: Colabango N, Davis G, eds. *Handbook of Gifted Education.* Mass: Allyn and Bacon; 1991.
19. Haldane JBS. *The Causes of Evolution.* Ithaca, NY: Cornell University Press; 1966.
20. Jones S. Genetic diversity in humans. In: Jones S, Martin R, Pilbeam D, eds. *The Cambridge Encyclopedia of Human Evolution.* New York, NY: Cambridge University Press; 1992:264-267.
21. Plomin R, DeFries JC, McClearn. *Behavior Genetics. A Primer.* San Francisco, Calif: WH Freeman; 1980.
22. Loehlin JC, Nichols RC. *Heredity, Environment and Personality: A Study of 850 Sets of Twins.* Austin, Texas: Texas University Printers; 1976.
23. Vandenberg SG. Hereditary factors in psychological variables in man, with special emphasis on cognition. In: Spuhler JN, ed. *Genetic Diversity and Human Behavior.* Chicago, Ill: Aldine; 1967:99-133.
24. Coon CS. *Racial Adaptations: A Study of the Origins, Nature and Significance of Racial Variations in Humans.* Chicago, Ill: Nelson Hall; 1982.
25. Mellars P, Stringer C, eds. *The Human Revolution: Behavioural and Biological Perspectives on the Origins of Modern Humans.* Edinburgh: Edinburgh University Press; 1989.
26. Tobias PV. Race. In: Kuper A, Kuper J, eds. *The Social Science Encyclopedia.* London, England: Routledge; 1985:681-682.
27. Garn SM. *Human Races.* 3rd ed. Springfield, Ill: Thomas; 1971.
28. Garn SM, ed. *Readings on Race.* 2nd ed. Springfield, Ill: Thomas; 1968.
29. Lewontin RC. The apportionment of human diversity. *Evolutionary Biology.* 1972;6:381-398.
30. Littlefield A, Lieberman L, Reynolds LT. Redefining race: the potential demise of a concept in physical anthropology. *Current Anthropology.* 1982;23(6):641-647.
31. Scarr S. *Race, Social Class and Individual Differences.* NJ: Hillsdale; 1980.
32. Scarr-Salapatek S. Race, social class and IQ. *Science.* 1971;174.
33. Harris LJ. Sex differences in spatial ability: possible environmental, genetic and neurological factors. In: Kinsbourne M, ed. *Asymmetrical Function of the Brain.* New York, NY: Cambridge University Press; 1978.
34. Waber DP. Sex differences in cognition: a function of maturation rate? *Science.* 1976;192:572-573.
35. Campbell J. *Winston Churchill's Afternoon Nap.* London, England: Palladin Grafton Books; 1986:44-54,166,194,290.
36. Lieberman P. Evolution of the speech apparatus. In: Jones S, Martin R, Pilbeam D, eds. *The Cambridge Encyclopedia of Human Evolution.* New York, NY: Cambridge University Press; 1992:136-137.
37. Csikszentmihalyi M, Csikszentmihalyi IS, eds. *Optimal Experience: Psychological Studies of Flow in Consciousness.* New York, NY: Cambridge University Press; 1988:20-23.
38. Selye H, Monat A, Lazarus RS. *Stress and Coping: An Anthology.* 2nd ed. New York, NY: Columbia University Press; 1985:28.
39. Fleagle JG. Primate locomotion and posture. In: Jones S, Martin R, Pilbeam D, eds. *The Cambridge Encyclopedia of Human Evolution.* New York, NY: Cambridge University Press; 1992:79.
40. Lewin R. *In the Age of Mankind: A Smithsonian Book of Human Evolution.* Washington, DC: Smithsonian Books; 1988:174,179-180.
41. Jelinek J. *Primitive Hunters.* London, England: Hamlyn; 1989:24.
42. Watanabe H. Running, creeping and climbing: a new ecological and evolutionary perspective on human locomotion. *Mankind.* 1971;8(1):1-13.
43. Alexander RMcN. Walking and running. *American Scientist.* 1984;72:348-354.
44. Alexander RMcN. Characteristics and advantages of human bipedalism. In: Rayner JMV, Wootton R,

eds. *Biomechanics in Evolution*. New York, NY: Cambridge University Press; 1991.

45. Goodall J. *The Chimpanzees of Gombe*. Cambridge, Mass: Harvard/Belknap; 1986.

46. Brewer SM, McGrew WC. Chimpanzee use of a tool-set to get honey. *Folia Primatologica*. 1990;54:100-104.

47. Almquist EE. Evolution of the distal radioulnar joint. *Clinical Orthopedics*. 1992;Feb(275):5-13.

48. Brodmann K. *Vergleichended lokalisations lehre der Grosshirnrinde in prinzipien dargestellt auf grund des zellenbaues*. Liepzig: JA Barth; 1909.

49. Penfield W, Boldrey E. Somatic motor and sensory representation in the cerebral cortex as studied by eletrical stimulation. *Brain*. 1958;60:389-443.

50. Bell Sir Charles. *The Hand: Its Mechanism and Vital Endowments as Evincing Design*. Brentwood: The Pilgrims Press; 1979:108.

51. Bruner J. Nature and uses of immaturity. *American Psychologist*. 1972;August:687-708.

52. Birch HG. The relation of previous experience to insightful problem solving. *Journal of Comparative and Physiological Psychology*. 1945;38:367-383.

53. Schiller PH. Innate constituents of complex responses in primates. *Psychological View*. 1952;49:177-191.

54. Tinkaus E. Evolution of human manipulation. In: Jones S, Martin R, Pilbeam D, eds. *The Cambridge Encyclopedia of Human Evolution*. New York, NY: Cambridge University Press; 1992:349.

55. Coren S, Porac C, Ward LM. *Sensation and Perception*. 2nd ed. Orlando, Fla: Academic Press; 1984.

56. Wilcock AA. Research carried out as part of "occupation and health." University of South Australia, Adelaide, 1993.

57. Watson L. *Neophilia: The Tradition of the New*. Great Britain: Hodder and Stoughton Ltd; 1989:43,67.

58. Hopkins CD. Sensory mechanisms in animal communication. In: Dewsbury DA, Slater PJB, eds. *Animal Behavior, Vol. 2: Communication*. New York, NY: Freeman; 1983.

59. Leger DW. *Biological Foundations for Behavior: An Integrative Approach*. New York, NY: Harper Collins Publishers; 1992:374.

60. Chomsky N. *The Origin of Language: Its Nature Origin and Use*. New York, NY: Praeger; 1986.

61. Bickerton D. *Language and Species*. Chicago, Ill: University of Chicago Press; 1990.

62. Lieberman P. *Uniquely Human: The Evolution of Speech, Thought and Selfless Behavior*. Cambridge, Mass: Harvard University Press; 1991.

63. Chomsky N. *Language and Mind*. New York, NY: Harcourt Brace Jovanovich; 1972.

64. Lenneberg EH. *Biological Foundations of Language*. New York, NY: Wiley; 1967.

65. John-Steiner V, Panofsky CP. Human specificity in language: socio-genetic processes in verbal communication. In: Greenberg G, ed. *Cognition, Language and Consciousness: Integrative Levels*. Hillsdale, NJ: Erlbaum; 1987.

66. Lieberman P. *The Biology and Evolution of Language*. Cambridge, Mass: Harvard University Press; 1984.

67. Lieberman P. Human speech and language. In: Jones S, Martin R, Pilbeam D, eds. *The Cambridge Encyclopedia of Human Evolution*. New York, NY: Cambridge University Press; 1992:137.

68. Leakey R. *The Making of Mankind*. London, England: Michael Joseph Ltd; 1981:101-103,139.

69. Premack AJ, Premack D. Teaching language to an ape. *Scientific American*. 1972;227:92-99.

70. Gardner BT, Gardner RA. Two way communication with an infant chimpanzee. In: Schrier AM, Stolinitz F, eds. *Behavior of Nonhuman Primates*. Vol 4. New York, NY: Academic Press; 1971.

71. Rumbaugh DM, Gill TV. Lana's aquisition of language skills. In: Rumbaugh DM, ed. *Language Learning by a Chimpanzee*. New York, NY: Academic Press; 1977.

72. Savage-Rumbaugh ES. Language training of apes. In: Jones S, Martin R, Pilbeam D, eds. *The Cambridge Encyclopedia of Human Evolution*. New York, NY: Cambridge University Press; 1992:141.

73. Hewes GW. Language origin theories. In: Rumbaugh DM, ed. *Language Learning by a Chimpanzee*. New York, NY: Academic Press; 1977.

74. Kimura D. Neuromotor mechanisms in the evolution of human communications. In: Steklis HD, Raleigh MJ, eds. *Neurobiology of Social Communication in Primates: An Evolutionary Perspective*. New York, NY: Academic Press; 1979.

75. Moore JC. *Sexual Dimorphism and Brain Functions*. Material prepared for a 1996 conference paper. Personal communication, 1996.

76. de Laguna GA. *Speech: Its Function and Development*. Bloomington, Ind: Indiana University Press; 1963 (originally published 1927).

77. Percy Bysshe Shelley. *Prometheus Unbound*, II, IV. London, England: C and J Ollier; 1820.

78. Piaget J. *Six Psychological Studies*. New York, NY: Random House; 1967:98.

79. Hamlyn DW. *A History of Western Philosophy*. England: Viking; 1987:15.

80. Gardner H. *Frames of Mind. The Theory of Multiple Intelligences*. New York, NY: Basic Books; 1983:290.

81. *The Macquarie Dictionary*. NSW: Macquarie Library Pty, Ltd; 1981.

82. Churchland PM. *Matter and Consciousness*. Rev ed. Cambridge, Mass: Bradford Book; 1988:73.

83. Ornstein R. *The Evolution of Consciousness: The Origins of the Way We Think*. New York, NY: Touchstone; 1991:228.

84. Premack D, Woodruff G. Does the chimpanzee have a theory of mind? *Behavioral and Brain Sciences*. 1978;4:515.

85. Csikszentmihalyi M. Activity and happiness: toward a science of occupation. *Journal of Occupational Science: Australia*. 1993;1(1):38-42.

86. Sato I. Bosozuko: flow in Japanese motorcycle gangs. In: Csikszentmihalyi M, Csikszentmihalyi IS, eds. *Optimal Experience: Psychological Studies of Flow in Consciousness*. New York, NY: Cambridge University Press; 1988.

87. Delle Fave A, Massimini F. Modernization and the changing context of flow in work and leisure. In: Csikszentmihalyi M, Csikszentmihalyi IS, eds. *Optimal Experience: Psychological Studies of Flow in Consciousness*. New York, NY: Cambridge University Press; 1988.

88. Dossey L. Consciousness and health: what's it all about. *Topics in Clinical Nursing*. 1982;3(Jan):1-6.

89. Newman MA. Newman's theory of health as praxis. *Nursing Science Quarterly*. 1990;3(1):37-41.

90. Burch S. Consciousness: how does it relate to health? *Journal of Holistic Nursing*. 1994;12(1):101-116.

91. Grimshaw A. Consciousness raising. In: Bullock A, Stalleybrass O, Trombley S, eds. *The Fontana Dictionary of Modern Thought*. 2nd ed. London, England: Fontana Press; 1988:166.

92. Thomas B. Challenges for teachers of women's health. *Nurse Education*. 1992;17(5):10-14.

93. Ford-Gilboe MV. A comparison of two nursing models: Allen's developmental health model and Newman's theory of health as expanding consciousness. *Nursing Science Quarterly*. 1994;7(3):113-118.

94. Koerner JG, Bunkers SS. The healing web: an expansion of consciousness. *Journal of Holistic Nursing*. 1994;12(1):51-63.

95. Smith-Campbell B. Kansans' peceptions of health care reform: a qualitative study on coming to public judgement. *Public Health Nursing*. 1995;12(2):134-139.

96. Dossey BM. The transpersonal self and states of consciousness. In: Dossey BM, Keegan L, Kolkmier LG, Guzzetta CE, eds. *Holistic Health Promotion. A Guide for Practice*. Rockville, Md: Aspen Publications; 1989:32.

97. Green E, Green A. Biofeedback and transformation. In: Kunz D, ed. *Spiritual Aspects of the Healing Arts*. Wheaton, Ill: The Theosophical Publishing House; 1985:145-162.

98. Gordon R. The creative process. In: Jennings S, ed. *Creative Therapy*. London, England: Pitman Publishing; 1975:1.

99. Jung CG. *Collected Works*. Princeton, NJ: Princeton University Press; 1959.

100. Sinnott EW. The creativeness of life. In: Vernon PE, ed. *Creativity*. London, England: Penguin Books; 1970:115.

101. Young JG. What is creativity? *Journal of Creative Behaviour*. 1985;19(2):77-87.

102. *The Concise Oxford Dictionary of Current English*. Oxford, UK: Clarendon Press; 1911.

103. Morris W. 1884. In: Morton AL, ed. *Political Writings of William Morris*. London, England: Lawrence and Wishart; 1973.

104. Morgan DN. Creativity today. *Journal of Aesthetics*. 1953;12:1-24.

105. Skinner BF. *The Science of Behaviour*. New York, NY: Macmillan; 1953.

106. Maslow AH. *Toward a Psychology of Being*. 2nd ed. New York, NY: D Van Nostrand Co; 1968.

107. Amabile TM. *The Social Psychology of Creativity*. New York, NY: Springer Verlag; 1983.

108. Gardner H. *Creating Minds: An Anatomy of Creativity Seen Through the Lives of Freud, Einstein, Picasso, Stravinsky, Eliot, Graham, and Gandhi*. New York, NY: Basic Books; 1993.

109. Bruce MA, Borg B. *Frames of Reference in Psychosocial Occupational Therapy*. Thorofare, NJ: SLACK Inc; 1987.

110. Taylor IA, Getzels JW, eds. *Perspectives in Creativity*. Chicago, Ill: Aldine Publishing Co; 1975.

111. Freud S. *A General Introduction to Psychoanalysis*. Boni and Liveright; 1920:326-327.

112. Freud S. *Creativity and the Unconscious*. New York, NY: Harper and Row; 1958.

113. Freud S. Creative writers and daydreaming. In: Strachey J, ed. *The Standard Edition of the Complete Psychological Works of Sigmund Freud*. Vol 9. London, England: Hogarth Press; 1959:143-144.

114. Barron F. *Creative Person and Creative Process*. New York, NY: Holt, Rinehart and Winston; 1969.

115. Maslow AH. *Motivation and Personality*. New York, NY: Harper and Row; 1954.

116. Rogers CR. Towards a theory of creativity. In: Vernon PE, ed. *Creativity*. London, England: Penguin Books; 1970:140.

117. Maslow A. *The Further Reaches of Human Nature*. New York, NY: Viking Press; 1971.

118. Payne WA, Hahn DB. *Understanding Your Health*. 2nd ed. St. Louis, Mo: Times Mirror/Mosby College Publishing; 1989.

119. Solomon R. Creativity and normal narcissism. *Journal of Creative Behaviour*. 1985;19(1):47-55.

120. Feldman D. *Beyond Universals in Cognitive Development*. Norwood, NJ: Ablex; 1980.

121. Dennis W. Creative productivity between the ages of 20 and 80 years. *Journal of Gerontology.* 1966;21:106-114.
122. Lehman H. *Age and Achievement.* Princeton, NJ: Princeton University Press; 1953.
123. Simonton DK. Sociocultural context of individual creativity: a transhistorical time-series analysis. *Journal of Personality and Social Psychology.* 1975;32:1119-1133.
124. Stein MI. *Stimulating Creativity.* Vols 1 and 2. New York, NY: Academic Press; 1974 and 1975.
125. Golann SE. Psychological study of creativity. *Psychological Bulletin.* 1963;60:548-565.
126. Kleitman N. *Sleep and Wakefulness.* Chicago, Ill: University of Chicago Press; 1963:188.
127. Horne JA. A review of the biological effects of total sleep deprivation in man. *Biological Psychology.* 1978;(7):55-102.
128. Sassin JF, Parker DC, Mace JW, Gotlin RW, Johnson LC, Rossman LG. Human growth hormone release: relation to slow wave sleep and sleep waking cycles. *Science.* 1969;165:513-515.
129. Shapiro CM, Bortz R, Mitchell D, Bartel P, Jooste P. Slow wave sleep: a recovery period after exercise. *Science.* 1981;214:1253-1254.
130. Foret J. To what extent can sleep be influenced by diurnal activity? *Experientia.* 1984;40:422-424.
131. Moore JC. *The Lifespan in Relation to the Nervous System.* Melbourne, Australia: Australian Association of Occupational Therapists; June 1994:188.
132. Pearlman CA. R.E.M. sleep and information processing: evidence from animal studies. *Neuroscience and Neurobehavioural Reviews.* 1979;57-68.
133. Smith C. Sleep states and learning: a review of the animal literature. *Neuroscience and Neurobehavioural Reviews.* 1985;9:157-168.
134. Fowler MJ, Sullivan MJ, Ekstrand BR. Sleep and memory. *Science.* 1973;179:302-304.
135. Fox R. *The Search for Society.* New Brunswick, NJ: Rutgers University Press; 1989:179.
136. Winson J. *Brain and Psyche: The Biology of the Unconscious.* Garden City, NY: Anchor Press/Doubleday; 1985:Chapter 8.
137. Campbell SS. Duration and placement of sleep in a "disentrained environment." *Psychophysiology.* 1984;21(1):106-113.
138. Szymczak JT, Jasinska M, Pawlak E, Zwierzykowska M. Annual and weekly changes in the sleep-wake rhythm of school children. *Sleep.* 1993;16(5):433-435.
139. *Dorland's Illustrated Medical Dictionary.* 25th ed. Philadelphia, Pa: WB Saunders; 1974:720.
140. Bernard C. Lectures on the phenomena of life common to animals and vegetables (1878-1879). In: Langley LL, ed. *Homeostasis, Origins of the Concept.* Straudsburg, Pa: Hutchinson and Ross, Inc; 129-147.
141. Cannon W. *Physiological Regulation of Normal States: Some Tentative Postulations Concerning Biological Homeostatics.* Paris, France: Charles Richet; 1926:91-93.
142. Cannon W. *The Wisdom of the Body.* New York, NY: WW Norton and Co Inc; 1939:317,323.
143. James W. *The Principles of Psychology.* Vol 1. New York, NY: Dover Publications; 1890:239.

Suggested Reading

Campbell BG. *Humankind Emerging.* 5th ed. New York, NY: Harper Collins Publishers; 1988.
Campbell J. *Winston Churchill's Afternoon Nap.* London, England: Palladin Grafton Books; 1986.
Edelman G. *Bright Air, Brilliant Fire: On the Matter of the Mind.* London, England: Penguin Books; 1992.
Jones S, Martin R, Pilbeam D, eds. *The Cambridge Encyclopedia of Human Evolution.* New York, NY: Cambridge University Press; 1992.
Ornstein R. *The Evolution of Consciousness: The Origins of the Way We Think.* New York, NY: Touchstone; 1991.
Ornstein R, Sobel D. *The Healing Brain: A Radical New Approach to Health Care.* London, England: Macmillan; 1988.

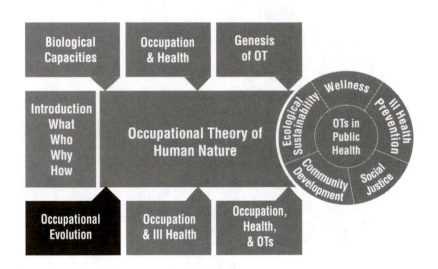

Chapter 4
Occupational Evolution

This chapter presents the reader with ideas about:
- Occupational evolution from the first of the *Homo* species
- The lifestyles of early and modern humans through the occupational eras of hunter-gathering, agriculture, industry, and the present turbulent times
- The function of engagement in occupation, basic occupational drives, diversification, and complexity

In the last chapter, it was established that humans have the biological capacity for occupation. The history of human engagement in occupation will be explored in this chapter, from the time of the earliest known hominids between 2 and 3 million years ago, in order to discover whether this, too, supports an evolutionary theory of human nature based on occupation. Proto humans, such as *Australopithecus*, are thought to have existed at least 5 million years ago, and *Homo sapiens*—modern humans—are believed to be little more than 100,000 years old.[1] Evidence of complex, cultural, and technological occupational behavior is increasingly apparent from this time on, but this is founded on behavior of earlier members of the species.

Archaeological and anthropological texts were used as the source for much of the material about early humans' occupations. Along with *The Cambridge Encyclopedia of Human Evolution*,[2] several texts have been particularly useful, such as Jacob Bronowski's *The Ascent of Man*,[3] Bernard Campbell's *Humankind Emerging*,[4] *The First Humans* edited by Goran Buranhult,[5] and a range of texts by Leakey and Lewin.[6-8] Richard Leakey's interest in pre-history grew from early exposure to archaeology via his famous parents, Mary and Louis Leakey, responsible for many important finds in Olduvai, Africa. Later, he became director of the Kenya National Museum. Roger Lewin, originally a biochemist, and then a writer for *Science* in Washington DC, was a consultant with Leakey to the BBC during the production of the television series "The Making of Mankind."

All take a common evolutionary view of human history in which occupational development is considered in conjunction with the biological and cultural development of the human species. Most debate similar topics that are apparently important in archaeological and anthropological research; yet, apart from detail, there appears to be remarkable agreement between them. The scholarship exhibited within the texts, and others of similar nature used throughout this chapter, rests upon a range of hypotheses founded on the study of archaeological finds and their context, the subjecting of these to scientific analysis and archaeological reconstruction, and from ethnographic studies of modern people still engaging in early lifestyles.

Throughout the book, the terms "developed" or "undeveloped," or "first world" or "third world" countries have been avoided, because these suggest superiority of one occupational form over another. To describe the differences these terms seek to define, the occupational form itself has been used, such as hunter-gatherer or post-industrial societies. This follows a trend in archaeology and anthropology in which the eras of mankind's history are frequently described in occupational terms, that is, hunter-gatherer, agricultural, and industrial eras.

Occupation is so central to the study of the origins and development of humans in society that much of the evolution of the human species, from pre-*Homo sapiens*, is traced by studying occupations, such as tool usage, food production, creativity, and domestic and communal activities.[9,10] In fact, Roland Fletcher uses occupational behaviors to define what is meant by "human." Along with bipedalism and toolmaking, he lists "the capacity to control fire, to interact socially with their dead, and to represent the universe in art" as marks of humanness in evolutionary terms.[11] Archaeologists and anthropologists recognize strong links between human occupation and biological evolution. These two avenues of study are interdependent because "the tangled triple influence of bipedalism, brain development, and the manipulation of objects cannot [easily] be separated."[4] Clearly, this chapter is built upon, and extends, the discussion of those matters in the previous chapter.

Hunting and Gathering

The first section explores the probable lifestyles and occupations of early humans until agriculture became the dominant economy. It considers, briefly, ideas held about occupations ranging from the practical matters of tool technology, food acquisition, division of labor, and education of the young to social occupations and those of an abstract nature.

Interest in differences between humans and other animals because of the tools they used for their various occupations has been central to the evolutionary debate, with some pre-historians arguing that tool technology was the driving force of the evolution of the human brain,[12,13] and others, such as Blumenberg, opposing the hypothesis that tool technology or any other activities were solely, or in combination, responsible for the advanced hominid brain, despite their importance in survival or social behavior.[14] Another recent controversial view based on temperature regulation of the brain following ecological change in the African Savannah, known as the "radiator theory," points to bipedalism preceding increased brain capacity and complex tool technology following it.[15,16] However, there is general agreement that changes in tools over the millenia reflect changes that affect culture as a whole, and Gowlett suggests that stone tools "provide a framework for mapping out human activities from the distant past to recent times."[17] The interactive nature of the evolution of toolmaking is shown in Figure 4-1. Throughout history, people have sought methods and tools to make tasks less arduous, which, in some instances, has made new occupations possible well into the future. Indeed, as Jelinek proposes, adaptation through experimentation is the driving force of technological evolution, just as adaptation per se is a central tenet of evolutionary theory, and "a new discovery [does] not have to find its relevance immediately" but can provide "a new solution" to some future need.[18]

Debate about the daily occupations of our early ancestors, however, is speculative, based as it is on skeletal remains, the environment in which they were found, and fossils and tools found adjacent. Like all large primates, hominids almost certainly subsisted principally on plant foods, and *Homo habilis* was probably an opportunistic

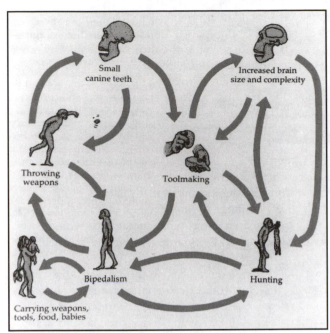

Figure 4-1. Interactive nature of the evolution of toolmaking. "Numerous feedback systems occur in nature and are often interlocking. Negative maintains stability, but positive feedback brings about major adaptive changes that constitute evolution. Shown here in simplified form is a positive feedback system that has been important in human evolution." *Humankind Emerging*. 5th ed. Campbell BG. Copyright 1988. Reprinted by permission of Addison-Wesley Educational Publishers Inc.

omnivore, occupied by scavenging, rather than hunting, with "...animal products such as birds' eggs, larvae, lizards, and small game [playing] a much more important role than big game" in the same way that they constitute "...an important part of the diet of present-day hunter-gatherers."[5]

"Scavenging requires no division of labor and does not imply sharing or any other social behavior approaching our own," although habilines probably lived in small groups with a structure similar to that of chimpanzees.[19] This very gradually developed into a systematic food-sharing economy based on cooperative foraging of meat and plant foods, and possibly some division of labor.[20-22] This led eventually to "some turning point in our history [when] the primitive *Homo* males began to take a serious interest in hunting as another way of providing meat."[6] It may well have started through self-protective behaviors, such as stone throwing, required because of human's physical vulnerability in comparison to many other animals. Barbara Isaac suggests that stone throwing, as observed in the Hottentots in South West Africa and the Australian Aboriginals in the Musgrave Ranges and the northern Kimberleys, was a possible early method of attacking prey for food.[23] Recent debate has suggested no clear-cut distinctions between hunting and herding[24] and between hunter-gatherers per se and horticulturalists who also hunt and gather,[25] but rather between "immediate return economies," characterized as "hand to mouth" existence, such as that lived by the Hadza, a hunter-gatherer people who live in Tanzania,[26] and "delayed return economies" in which a time investment for the future is part of daily life.[27]

How occupation was divided according to gender in the early days of human evolution has long been a point of debate in archaeology and anthropology. The extent of sexual dimorphism and the maturation rates of early humans set some parameters to the debate,[28] and others reflect concerns of the modern societies from which the ideas emanate, such as power relations, monogamy, and the nuclear family.[29] Most recent opinion seems to favor the idea that as hunting became an important aspect of subsistence, women, along with their child-bearing and care roles, engaged in the fabrication of household implements and clothing and continued with the foraging-gathering role, sharing their finds as the hunters shared their meat.[20] A recurring motif in rock paintings and engraving shows women with digging sticks weighted with per-forated round stones.[20] It has been estimated that women contributed more than half of the required subsistence calories and that diets were very diverse which increased the likelihood of balanced nutrition.[30,31] The necessity for women to assume respon-sibility for tasks in a sequential order of those closer to home to those farthest afield was due to the need for women to undertake occupations close to camp because of child-rearing restraints.[32] For men, the opposite is true.[33] Although by about 100,000 years ago dimorphism was similar to that found in modern humans,[29] evidence from primate ethology and ethnology of foragers demonstrates that male specialization in hunting and defense gives a "selective advantage to larger males" with resultant sex-ual dimorphism.[34] There may well have been a selective advantage for women who demonstrated child-rearing, food gathering and preparing, and fine manipulative skills.

Herskovits observes there would be no exemptions from some kind of labor except for the very young and that everyone would be primarily a hunter or gather-er and tool/household-implement-maker, even those with extracurricular activities, such as shamans, chiefs, or warriors.[35] In a similar vein, Coon, the Harvard anthro-pologist, infers from his study of modern hunter-gatherer societies that most individ-uals would be "jacks of all trades," living and working mostly outdoors, their senses acute and, like their bodies, well exercised. Their schedules and routines would be seldom monotonous and often adventurous.[36] Many anthropologists argue that this simple, but obviously effective, economy provided a very successful and persistent quality of life, with Marshall Sahlins of the University of Chicago naming it "the orig-inal affluent society...in which all the people's wants are easily satisfied."[8] Coon sug-gests there is a closeness of fit between hunter-gatherer people and their environ-ments. "Such people" he writes:

> *Have had the energy, hardihood, and ingenuity to live and live well in every climatic region of the world not covered by icecaps. They have done so with stone tools and no firearms. In every well-documented instance, cases of hardship may be traced to the intervention of modern intruders.*[36]

Hunter-gatherers, like most primates and modern humans, lived in social groups. In Ethiopia, Johanson found numerous bones ascertained to be more than 3 million years old and to have come from at least 13 individuals, perhaps killed together in some kind of natural catastrophe.[37] Social psychologists and sociobiologists offer var-ious reasons for humans having lived in social groups throughout their evolution, including the need to meet biological drives through group activity, dependency, affil-iation, dominance, sex, self-esteem,[38] nepotism,[39-41] coercion,[42] and reciprocity.[43] Jerome Bruner observes "there is no known human culture that is not marked by rec-iprocal help in times of danger and trouble, by food sharing, by communal nurtu-rance for the young or disabled, and by the sharing of knowledge and implements for expressing skill."[44] This as well as other theories, such as "the hunting band was an effective, adaptive solution to the survival and development of a partly carnivo-rous species"[45] and that social groups offered some protection against predators, implies occupational behavior of a social nature.

Because of the way evolution and natural selection work, it is argued by anthropologists that social structures are not only determined by what is best for individuals in terms of sexual success,[6] but that the kinds of social groups found in higher primates are facilitatory to "kin selection." As was noted in Chapter 2, this extends the Darwinian notion of individual "fitness" to include "social fitness," thereby increasing the survival, well-being, and reproductive success of all individuals in a social group who carry an individual's genes.[4] Within modern hunter-gatherer societies, such as those of Australian Aboriginals, Kalahari Bushmen, and the Birhhor of Northern India, survival needs and peaceful coexistence are major determinants of group size, which ethnographic studies demonstrate are usually made up of between 20 and 70 people.[46] "A lone individual rarely survives for more than a year, whereas a group of five can continue for up to a generation (about 30 years). A group of about 25 has a good chance of surviving for perhaps 500 years" and appears to be compatible with minimal conflict. To avoid inbreeding, these groups usually form part of larger tribes of about 500 to 800 people.[5] It is possible to argue from these studies of modern traditional societies that from early in human evolution there appears to have been a preference for small groups in everyday life, for the larger social get-togethers to be occasional, and for social gatherings to be purposive rather than accidental. Humans group together for the purposes of achieving large-scale occupations and for the enjoyment that can be experienced from being with and doing things with others. People with like occupational interests find pleasure and challenge in discussing and sharing their enthusiasm. Stimulation from social and group occupational interests will often lead to profound personal exploration of ideas and to individual occupations that lead toward self-growth and actualization.

The evolution of the role of societies in education of the young of the species is an important aspect in understanding how the occupational nature of humans can be developed or inhibited; after all, learning that occurs in the first formative years of life has significant lifelong effects. In fact, because what is best for the safety and development of offspring is of vital importance to the species, education of the young is one of the strongest arguments given for people living in social groups: it provides children with role models for their own future survival, as well as the protection and guidance of adults before being burdened with their responsibilities. Primate young have a lot to learn and, compared with other animals, a long childhood. Learning by observation and imitation combined with the imaginative creativity of play provides education for human young to learn about self-care, safety, and survival occupations. It also provides the experience of fun and the development of skills and self-worth, which are potential motivators for continued engagement in occupation. As humans evolved into more complex animals, the years of childhood, play, and education extended and changed. For example, until recent times, play and education were an integral part of the day-to-day occupations of adults and children, taking place in an environment relevant to the families' work and leisure activities. Today, in post-industrial societies, children, and often young infants, are separated from their families for much of their waking day, and education is provided according to socially and politically devised criteria. The effects of this change have not been assessed in terms of adult engagement in, or value given to, occupation.

There are some who challenge the present segregation of education from parents. Coon, for example, compares unfavorably the contact and guidance "through the puberty ordeals" of the young provided by parents in urban societies with that possible in hunting societies. He suggests that "the secrecy that once formed a part of puberty rites is transferred to the parents, to whom they (the adolescents) will not reveal what they are doing."[36] In contrast, Lorenz in *On Aggression* discusses etho- logical causes of what he describes as "war between the generations," which he asserts is part of a "species-preserving function to eliminate obsolete elements hin- dering new developments."[47] In puberty, young people go through a stage of "phys- iological neophilia" in which everything new is attractive. When somewhat older, they experience a revival of love of tradition or "late obedience." In occupational terms, Lorenz's explanation has some merit, in that physiological neophilia at an age when physical and mental capacities are acute will facilitate experimentation and explo- ration across a wide spectrum of activities, which may well provide survival and health advantages. Additionally, later development, growth, and adaptation may be based on successful experiences and individual interest, enhancing personal capaci- ties, health, and well-being.

Some authorities suggest that the demands of survival in harsh environments made the occupations of traditional societies necessarily very arduous and virtually contin- uous despite time spent in social activity.[48,49] Waechter and others argue that "the struggle for existence over nearly 4 million years by a creature with few weapons other than his developing brain allowed little time for activities not immediately con- cerned with survival."[48] However, others, basing their argument on evaluation of mod- ern hunter-gatherer lifestyles, have posited that the mixed economy of hunting and gathering brought with it time for leisure in the sense of occupation apart from labor concerned with survival.[6,7,20,50] Indeed, Marshall Sahlins in *Stone Age Economics* argued that more time is available for leisure in hunter-gatherer societies than in agrarian or industrial societies.[50] Providing evidence of this are the findings of Richard Lee and Patricia Draper[7] who, as part of a group of investigators mainly based at Harvard University, studied the hunter-gatherer lifestyle of the !Kung San who live on the northern fringe of the Kalahari Desert. (This lifestyle has been eroded, and now only a few continue in traditional ways.) Adults from 15 to 60 years of age only spend about 2.5 hours daily providing their necessities of life. These measurements were taken at a time of drought, and it may well be that in more plentiful times, the !Kung would have had even more time available for leisure.[6] The !Kung are not unique among hunter-gatherer societies in having time for leisure. In the 1840s, Edward John Eyre remarked on the few hours it took, "without fatigue or labor," for Australian Aboriginals to procure sufficient food to last the day.[51]

Labor, in the sense of procuring the physical needs of survival, is only one aspect of the occupational behavior necessary for the well-being of the organism, and other forms of occupation serve a built-in need to exercise, maintain, and develop the capacities inherent to each individual. In fact, as long as the second need is met by goal-directed, meaningful occupation, and it is possible for material needs to be pro- vided by other means, then the occupational nature of humans can be satisfied. Leisure, for example, frequently serves as a mechanism for children and adults to exercise their bodies, to be social, to develop their creativity, to fulfill "wishes at the fantasy level," and to sort out problems, as well as having a crucial role in teaching and maintaining "fluency with roles and conventions."[44] Its difference from work in meeting basic human needs is related directly to how it is valued by societies.

Hunter-gatherer societies left a legacy of more than stone tools to demonstrate the range of occupations valued by them. Deep in caves, they drew and colored images, usually depicting creatures and humans who were a part of their world. They carved throwing sticks and other implements, along with creating "new and stylistically more complex tools," and there is archaeological evidence of "a rich ceremonial life based on complex concepts and rituals."[5] However, it is difficult to determine if there existed any formal differentiation and value loading between labor, self-care, and leisure in the lives of early hominids. From study of hunter-gatherer people of recent times, it is possible to suggest that early in human history no distinction did exist between labor and leisure occupations. Wax observes "I do not believe that any Bushman could tell us—or would be interested in telling us—which part of [his] activity was work and which was play."[52] The separation of leisure from work appears to have occurred fairly recently; early societies seemed to have operated in such a way that a natural balance between work, leisure, self-care, and rest was an accepted part of their occupational lives. Their economic activities had built-in leisure components, such as "singing and telling stories at work."[53] Indeed, in hunter-gatherer societies, such as that of the Eskimos[54] or Australian Aboriginals,[49] there is no generic word for work or doing but many for specific occupations such as hunting. Such a lack of distinction is advantageous to health and well-being in that individuals would be able to develop their own traits and capacities according to need and opportunity, without subjugating their choice of activity to economic efficiencies or without regard to the kinds of sociocultural values imbued in work, self-care, or leisure that have made occupational choice so complex in present times.

This does not imply that sociocultural values did not exist or were not important to early humans. In fact, the simplistic notions held until recently that the hunter-gatherer lifestyle was essentially nomadic and that small bands of families would be unencumbered by material goods or social hierarchy are changing. Many of the complex features of our own way of life, such as social inequality, occupational specialization, long-distance exchange, and technological innovation, originated with hunter-gatherers.[8] These suggestions are supported by finds, such as "the remains of magnificently adorned children...buried with high honors before they are old enough to do anything outstanding raises the possibility of status by heredity rather than achievement"[5] and Mediterranean shells used as Paleolithic decoration as far inland as the Ukraine giving reason to suppose that trade was an occupation long before the establishment of agriculture or towns. King, anthropologist of the Historic Preservation Advisory Council, when discussing early Californian societies, observed they had "economic systems utilizing shell-bead currencies and validated by ritual exchange obligations," which "facilitated sharing of subsistence resources over broad areas."[8] The possibility of complex lifestyles is also supported by evidence in the Central Russian Plains of semi-permanent dwellings with vaults, arches, and buttresses, constructed of mammoth bones from about 30,000 years ago. Such constructions can be said to "represent the foundations of architecture."[18]

Such dwellings also indicate that fixed habitation and some domestication of crops probably occurred in some regions for thousands of years before the rapid spread of agriculture through most of the world from about 10,000 years ago, and, indeed, "many archaeological sequences also show that knowledge of agriculture and domesticated plants existed long before there was a real shift from hunting and gathering."[55]

Agriculture

The impact of the agrarian revolution on human occupation merits discussion, as it was the first major, rapid occupational change that we know of, is one that set the scene for increasing occupational complexity, and still impacts upon the daily life of many people.

Why agriculture occurred at all has been a topic of debate over decades, although it is generally accepted that the advent of permanent settlements was closely associated with environmental and climatic conditions that prevailed in different locations. Those that provided adequate food and shelter year-round probably supported resident populations, reducing to a great extent nomadic ways of life. Major theories about the rapid increase of permanent settlement range from ideas that hunter-gathering is not well adapted to support large numbers of people, and a rise in populations forced more intensive means of food production; that when the Pleistocene ice age ended, a major climate change occurred, which produced environments conducive to agriculture; and that increasing social complexity resulted in a need for more formalized food production because the food procuring system of small nomadic communities became inadequate. It is also possible that the developing occupational capacity of humans was instrumental in the change. That is, as humans experimented with material resources as their skills expanded, they began to challenge the environment and adapt it to meet their own needs and comfort, and they changed their social structures and behaviors to accommodate such change. This theory is supported by the fact that as agriculture developed so did the diversity of occupations in which humans engaged along with an expansion of goods and services regarded as necessary.[53]

When agriculture became the dominant economy, it was the men who changed their occupation from hunting to that previously done by women. However, the shift to male farming heralded a change in role for many women, who increasingly became engaged in household occupations.[56,57] For women, as for men, the roles they undertook differed according to the societies and cultures in which they lived. Ester Boserup found sexual division of labor in all the traditional societies she studied, but no common pattern; what was considered a natural occupation for women was seemingly determined by the fact that they had "undergone little or no change for generations."[58] Variability was particularly evident with regard to food production and care of domesticated animals.[34]

Agriculture did not necessarily mean the cessation of communal life. In many instances, it gave a focus for some combined activity for both individual and communal good, as well as time for celebration and fun. For example, Ashton reports that among the Basuto, working parties, which "are gay, sociable affairs comprising about 10 to 50 participants of both sexes" are a part of all aspects of agricultural activities.[59] Work structures that mix labor and leisure lessen drudgery and enable workers to meet their social and psychological needs, although, from a capitalist view in which labor is seen as separable from other types of occupation and as merely one aspect of the production process, in most instances, combining work and leisure is considered inefficient and uneconomical. In Western agricultural societies also, leisure, as well as work, was long associated with seasonal tasks, which included communal participation. When Christianity became the dominant religion, seasonal celebrations of an occupational and social nature were adapted to its religious observances.

Some peoples did not adopt an agrarian lifestyle. Coon argues that surviving hunters do not lack the intellectual capacity to progress, pointing, as evidence, to their ingenious methods of obtaining foodstuffs and to their complex social organizations.[36] The successful survival of Australian Aboriginals in a relatively inhospitable environment and their unusually complex structure of kinship relationships is a case in point.[18] Three possible reasons for the retention of a hunter-gatherer way of life are isolation, climatic conditions not conducive to profitable agriculture, and that they did not want to change.[36] Coon suggests that they had an eminently satisfactory way of living together in small groups, free from tedious routine, and all the food they needed, and he argues that adopting agriculture would have imposed a "whole new system of human relationships that offer no easily understood advantages, and disturbs an age-old balance between man and nature and among the people who live together."[36]

Coon's argument is supported by observations made of hunter-gatherer communities currently in the process of adopting a sedentary, agrarian lifestyle. For example, some of the !Kung are undergoing transition from a hunter-gatherer lifestyle to agriculture, under pressure from the government. A major source of apparent conflict and difficulty arises from differences between community life based on sharing, central to hunter-gatherers, and saving, that is, the husbandry of resources, central to agriculture. Another consequence for the !Kung is an apparent decrease in both social and sexual egalitarianism and a more rigid defining of male and female roles, obvious also in changed play behaviors of the children. There has been a tendency for individuals to accumulate material goods, as well as a marked rise in birth rate. The dispersion of shelters from villages clustered around a central, and publicly shared, space to more isolated shelters "owning" the land around them has changed the complex support mechanism of the older type of communities.[7] All of these changes are manifest in occupational behavior.

With the advent of agriculture, a more stable provision of food for those who adopted agrarian practices led to greater population density, an apparent need for territorial defense, and the ever-recurring occupation of war.[8] Leakey suggests that "man is not programmed to kill and make war, nor even to hunt: his ability to do so is learned from his elders and his peers when society demands it."[7] His argument is based on no evidence of inflicted death and warfare being found before the advent of temple towns making "this...too recent an event to have had any influence on the evolution of human nature." This cultural view of human aggression is one aspect of the ongoing debate about whether or not humans are innately aggressive and wars inevitable. In contrast, Lorenz argues that, in common with other animals, humans are innately aggressive in order to maintain sufficient space for existence, to ensure the strongest males father offspring, and to establish a pecking order.[47] Others propose that an inevitable consequence of tribal bonding is hostility to other tribes.[45] It is true that people have expended vast amounts of mental and physical effort as well as resources on the development and accumulation of weapons. These may be seen as an expression of a human need to feel safe, of innate aggression, or, as a consequence of either, an occupational need to develop tool technology without adequate consideration of the possible consequences of the technology so produced. The weapons of war are only one aspect of tool technology developing beyond and perhaps to the detriment of human well-being. This may be a reflection of the planlessness of evolution, that adaptation to one set of environmental conditions millions of years ago may prove to be a handicap in another type of environment.[60] In particular, the expression of capacities through ongoing experimentation and technological development is a strong force, especially when valued highly by society. The brain's ability to override biological needs with a highly developed cognitive capacity responsive to sociocultural influences has disadvantages as well as advantages.

Another disadvantage of the human capacity for occupational experimentation is that agriculture changed the earth as a result of deforestation, land clearing and ploughing, and irrigation schemes, such as blocking or moving river beds.[61] As part of the agricultural process, domestication of animals "involved an accelerating process of elimination of the great diversity of wild animals and plants to replace them with a few species that could be easily managed and manipulated." It has also resulted in the proliferation of some, such as the rabbit.[62] "Erosion and the alteration of the balance of species became inevitable."[61]

Towns and City States

With the fairly recent formation of cities, at least 6,000, and possibly 10,000, years ago, more elements of modern occupational behavior began. Lewin considers that it is possible from this time to trace occupational developments in architecture, art, writing, commerce, religion, increased technological innovation, and social administration. Administrative functions, organization, and control of cities in those early days, often combined with religious activity and monumental architecture, developed to help communities cope with socioenvironmental stress, uncertainty, and unpredictability.[8] The stressors arose from within communities living in much larger, specialized populations than they had been used to, and also in response to possible dangers to the community from outside. Neff observes that during this period occupation began to acquire distinctions and qualifications and an increasingly complicated infrastructure of evaluative meanings, including a distinction between labor and leisure.[49]

It is, perhaps, in early Greek culture that the greatest distinction between labor and leisure is made. The Greek city states were established by conquest during the third and second millenia BC, when the Greek citizen "managed to divest himself of all need to labor," leaving this to slaves, free peasants, artisans, and craftsmen who were usually the indigenous people of conquered domains.[49] Labor and work were regarded as "brutalizing the mind, making man unfit for thinking of truth or for practicing virtue; it was a necessary evil which the visionary elite should avoid."[53] In contrast, leisure, which was the domain of the elite, was concerned with occupations worthy of free men, such as those of an intellectual, political, and social nature, and war-like pursuits, along with "a conscious abstention from all activities connected with merely being alive."[53] Aristotle argued, in concurrence with the cultural norms of his day, that without labor it is not possible to provide all the necessities of life, but that to master slaves is the human way to master necessity and thus is not against nature.[63] He supposed that the supreme end for human endeavor is happiness, that the function of man is reasoning, and that happiness for man is the good performance of reasoning.[64] Hannah Arendt (1906-1975), who is considered an authority on concepts of work and labor in the Greco-Roman world, came to agree, in large part, with the classical views of which she wrote, regarding labor and work as degrading and less than human, and that the leisure pursuits of Athenian gentlemen demonstrated the true human condition.[65] (Arendt recognized the lack of modern day theory about *animal laborans* [the labor of the body] and *homo faber* [the work of our hands] which she found surprising because of the present-day glorification of labor and work as "the source of all values.") Her view is challenged by Neff who argues that although Arendt probably correctly reflected ideas held about occupation in Classical Greece and Rome, "it is not work itself that is degrading but the power relationships and social structure which surround it." Work, he believes, takes on a "servile" nature when subjugation of one people to another is part of the equation, and that to the dominant group it may appear "degrading to perform certain kinds of work, since to do so is to be akin to a slave or an alien."[49] Similarly, this occupational theory holds that no occupation of itself is degrading; that sociocultural structures and values that force people into restricted occupational choice is counter to our occupational nature and to "occupational justice"; that humans need to recognize and accept, as part of the human condition, their similarities with as well as their differences to other animals; and that if, in the future, other means are found to provide humans with the necessities of life without work or labor, humans will not suffer deleterious effects to their health and well-being so long as the whole range of each individual's physical, mental, and social capacities have the opportunity for exercise and growth in a sociocultural environment that values such activity (occupational justice).

The notion of the elite having a choice of occupational pursuits, to the extent that choice is equated to this day with leisure, continued in feudal and agricultural societies. However, the idea that leisure is superior to work was challenged in Christian societies partly by a reformed monastic rule, which saw occupation as one honorable way of serving God, as well as being necessary for the material well-being of monastic communities. For example, rule XLVIII of the Benedictine order ordained that "idleness is the enemy of the soul and therefore, at fixed times, the brothers ought to be occupied in manual labor, and again at fixed times, in sacred reading."[66] Such views were based, in part, on the Hebrew notion of God as one who works and the commandment of 6 days of labor followed by a day of rest on the Sabbath.[67] Although much earlier than the Reformation, some argue that such ideas can be considered precursors of what is usually called the "Protestant work ethic." The work ethic, a concept originating with Max Weber, who sought to understand the religious and idealistic roots of modern capitalism,[68] is usually reserved for reference to the Reformers' doctrine of salvation and is particularly relevant to Calvinism. Salvation was God's gift in response to faith, and work was a "fruit" of faith. A life of obedience that included hard work and thrift were deemed necessary for those elected to serve God and to be saved by God, and who He could favor with prosperity. Perhaps because the notion of predestination, central to Calvinist doctrine, was difficult to accept, worldly success following methodical labor gradually came to be equated with being of the chosen few.[69] Such Reformation ideas appealed to the masses who, by necessity, labored and benefited growing numbers of merchants and artisans, living in cities, who were able to mix their opportunities for prosperity on earth with hope for preferment in heaven, although Protestant creed did stress that it was the work rather than its fruits that were important.

The ennobling of one aspect of occupation over others may have done disservice to the occupational nature of humans. It has the potential to deprive individuals of a balanced use of their innate capacities, of using some and not others to the detriment of overall well-being. Closer to my view is the more holistic notion of occupation followed by the pre-industrial society of the Baluchi of Western Pakistan—that occupation can be divided into the sphere of obligatory duty and the sphere of one's own will, with the latter being the valued domain in which individuals choose to spend energy and creativity.[52] However, it was the work ethic rather than freely chosen occupation that continued in ascendance as agriculture gave way to industrialization, and discussion of ideas that grew from this time on will be the focus of the last part of the chapter.

Industry

From the turn of the 18th century in the Occident, the occupational nature of humans was subjected to perhaps its greatest challenge. With remarkable speed, occupation as a valued part of life became focused on paid employment, increasingly within capitalist forms of industry. Indeed, in England, which led the change to industry, there was a "steady assimilation of small professional and business families, diverse in point of both wealth and activity" on whom "primarily, depended the viability and growth of the national economy...social flexibility and stability..."[70,71] This new middle class, "frequently self-made and always dependent on aggressive use of their talents, ...were genuine 'capitalists' in terms of the investment of their labor and their profits in entrepreneurial activity, whether commercial or professional," dominated work, education, play, and diversion.[70] Their fascination with pragmatics and applied technology lingers today, along with one of the most influential forces on occupation in our own time, economics, which also developed at this time.

Adam Smith (1723-1790), whose *An Inquiry Into the Nature and Causes of the Wealth of Nations*[72] is considered the foundation of classical economics, proposed that the key to increasing a nation's wealth was by the accumulation of capital and the division of labor, both of which would increase with the freeing of trade. He held that the division of labor would enhance workers' specialist skills because "the difference of natural talents...is not...so much the cause, as the effect of labor. The difference...seems to arise not so much from nature, as from habit, custom, and education." However, he also recognized that the division of labor could decrease the quality of work.[73] In the broad sense, division of labor has led to modern exchange economy, that is, specialization followed by exchange between specialists, which is a fundamental aspect of all modern economies.[74] While it appears that the vast majority of the population have accepted that material wealth provided by occupational specialization is logical and acceptable, one could raise the basic question of whether division of labor and specialization is conducive to well-being, notwithstanding material wealth. This is not a straightforward question as there are many dimensions to specialization, from that resulting from the development of personal and professional skills to specialization that is imposed by a system. In the former, strengths and capacities can be developed but, in the latter, there may be a minimalizing of individual development except for minute and meaningless actions, as in some industrial processes, and for the majority of workers little opportunity to explore a wide range of occupations and discover their individual potential.

There has been a persistent stream of questioning of the ill effects that accompany the goods proclaimed by classical economics. For example, Frank Knight, professor of economics at Chicago University, argued that "the values of life are not, in the main, reducible to satisfactions obtained from the consumption of exchangeable goods and services."[75] John Kenneth Galbraith argued in *The Affluent Society*[76] that classical economics developed at a time when "wants" were chasing "goods" and is inappropriate when the opposite is true as in modern industrial nations where the "production machine has become an end in itself."[77] Even Lionel Robbins, an economist of the English neo-classical school, suggested that economists "have nothing to say on the true ends of life and that their propositions concerning what is or what can be involve in themselves no propositions concerning what ought to be."[78] Post-Ricardian economics have also been criticized for defending and rationalizing the interests of capitalism at the cost of impartiality, with Marxist writers describing as "vulgar economics" that which concentrates on "surface phenomena," such as "demand and supply to the neglect of structural value relationships" and the "class relationships underlying commodity transactions."[79] (David Ricardo [1772-1823] was an English political economist. In his work such as *Principles of Political Economy and Taxation*, the antagonism of class interests remains central.)

The extreme dichotomy, at the time of the industrial revolution, of economic conditions, social conditions, and the nature of occupations versus the values of employers and their employees led intellectuals as various as Karl Marx, John Ruskin, and William Morris to consider the effects of the industrial era on the occupational nature of mankind. Some of their ideas were similar to those expressed by Renaissance Utopians, that what people do can be a source of joy if it is creative and provides pleasure in the exercise of a range of skills.[80,81] A brief account of the views of Marx, Ruskin, and Morris follows.

Karl Marx,[82] in his early works, such as *Economic and Philosophical Manuscripts, The Holy Family,* and *The German Ideology,* formulated a "materialistic theory of history," arguing that it is social and economic conditions, rather than metaphysical or religious ideas, that drive human history and determine how people live.[83-86] (Marx had not intended these papers for publication, but from 1932 [Soviet translation] onward the work created enormous interest as it provided new insights on Marx's concepts of alienation and the self-creation of humanity through material labor.) Influenced by Hegel who saw "labor as man's act of self-creation,"[87] he founded much of his philosophy on the idea that "free conscious activity constitutes the species character of man."[82] Particularly in *Economic and Philosophical Manuscripts,* he discusses praxis as the free, universal, creative, and self-creative activity that differentiates humans from other animals and by which they make and change themselves and their world.[82] (Petrovic argues in *A Dictionary of Marxist Thought* that praxis is the central concept of Marxism.) This implies that it is natural for all people to be involved in productive activity to provide for their subsistence but that such occupation should also enable them to achieve fulfillment, dignity, and well-being. Marx argued that when labor is not a creative activity by which humans make and mold themselves, but is simply a process to earn a wage for subsistence, it is a contradiction of the nature of mankind, economic conditions having become more powerful than individuals. Fischer, in his comments on Marx's work, adds "the reduction of labor to empty wage earning is now accepted without question."[87] Additionally, Marx recognized that when work is destructive to people's physical and intellectual potential "the worker feels himself only when he is not working."[82] Marx criticized the capitalist industrial society of the time because it prevented individuals from being able to cultivate their unique talents and alienated them from their species' need to be an active, productive being, and, in fact, led to misery, exhaustion, and mental debasement. This idea of alienation, which will be considered in greater depth later, was a major theme of Marx's theories. These early humanist ideas of Marx are remarkably similar to the central focus of this text, that humans are occupational beings and that compulsion and subservience can act against the biological function of this species characteristic.

Ruskin and Morris differed from Marx in that they came to social criticism from the viewpoint of creative artists. Ruskin (1819-1900) as a well-known art critic challenged the traditional view of manual labor and intellect, and in 1860 turned to political economy, writing four essays that appeared in *Cornhill Magazine* and were published as *Unto this Last* in 1862.[88]

From this time, he added considerably to the challenge offered by Coleridge in *The Friend*[89] and Carlyle in *Sartor Resartus*[90] to classical political economists whom they characterized as ignoring the human factor in economics. Ruskin's central theme was that the quality of life that citizens enjoy is the true measure of a nation's prosperity, rather than the accumulation of wealth for its own sake. He attacked the boredom and monotony of the Victorian industrial system and the disconnection between leisure and work, and he advocated that training schools should be established at government expense for all children.[91] These schools should teach the laws of health, habits of gentleness and justice, and the "calling" by which each would live. In conjunction with these, he proposed that the government should establish factories and workshops, producing high standard goods, to run in competition with private business. Any person out of employment should be admitted immediately to a government school, trained, and given work for wages. For those unable to work, he proposed special training schemes or "tending" in the case of sickness. For those who objected to work, he suggested they be compelled to work in less desirable jobs, their wages retained until each learned to respect the laws of employment.

> *We want one man to be always thinking, and another to be always working, and we call one a gentleman, and the other an operative; whereas the workman ought often to be thinking, and the thinker often to be working, and both should be gentlemen, in the best sense.*
>
> Ruskin J. *The Stones of Venice*. Vol 2. London, England: Smith, Elder and Co; 1853.

William Morris (1834-1896), who was a member of the small Marxist Social Democratic Federation organized by Henry M. Hyndman, founded the Socialist League in England in 1884. He was the most notable of Ruskin's followers and, although abandoning Ruskin's elitism, among his many endeavors attempted to establish a working community on Ruskin's principles. Morris was a poet, architect, painter, printer, craftsman, and social reformer (known to some today for a revival in the popularity of his decorative fabrics and wallpapers).[92] As a craftsman, he too deplored the machine age and the fact that commerce had become a "sacred religion," turning work from a solace into a burden, and for the majority a mere drudgery:

> *The wonderful machines...have driven all men into mere frantic haste and hurry, thereby destroying pleasure...they have instead of lightening the labor of the workmen, intensified it, and thereby added more weariness yet to the burden which the poor have to carry.*[93]

He supported the destruction of social and economic inequalities, hoping that the manual arts could be restored as an integral part of people's lives. He accepted that "the race of man must either labor or perish [because] 'Nature' does not give us our livelihood gratis; we must win it by toil of some sort or degree" but he also believed that, under socialist conditions, the necessary work of society could be accomplished without overstrain or difficulty. Morris argued against the "stifling overorganization common to both capitalist and socialist versions of modern industrial society."[94] Additionally, he suggested that most work could be done with actual pleasure in the doing "since certainly in other matters ['Nature'] takes care to make the acts necessary for the continuance of life in the individual and race not only endurable but even pleasurable."[95] In *News from Nowhere,* he described a fictional communist utopia based on his ideas about the pleasures inherent in work when people are free and independent, and where poverty, exploitation, competition, and money all disappear.[96]

Marx, Ruskin, and Morris believed that purposeful, creative labor, which is close to what is being described here as occupation, is basic to human nature, but they saw that the industrial and commercial use of this innate characteristic was destructive both to individuals and to mankind in the long-term. The challenges aimed at changing the values of industry and commerce led by such socialist comment and mounted by the organized labor movement achieved some success, but social inequities and conditions of work have remained the major focus of debate and action. In contention over the exploitation of the workforce, the basic ideological arguments about the nature of occupation and the human need for purposeful creative activity were, on the whole, overlooked. Mainstream socialism "became enmeshed in the 'quasi-socialist machinery' of party politics" and followed the Fabian vision of a technocratic society with enlightened leadership, in preference to the anti-modern revolutionary stance of Ruskin and Morris.[94,97] Workers continued, in better conditions, to be servants of machines and, for many people, there was little opportunity for creativity or even the chance to be involved in a total process of production.

In early industrial society, even social and celebratory customs, as an integral part of work, diminished, and the division between work and leisure became clearer. This division was not absolute or the same for each individual,[98] and in many traditional workshops ritual patterns of fellowship and celebration continued.[99] However, the change was so evident that it encouraged entrepreneurs to recognize the commercial potential of separated entertainment, which has led to one of the most powerful industries of the present day.[100] The separation of work from leisure is also demonstrated in the way leisure was deplored by Victorian explorers, who perceived, in their encounters with hunter-gatherer peoples, that their "non-work ethic" was a major reason for lack of progress. This prejudice or bias remains today, with post-industrial nations encouraging more traditional peoples to change to an occupational way of life similar to their own without reference to the personal satisfaction, community well-being, or ecological sustainability of traditional occupational behavior.

Jenkins and Sherman argue in *The Leisure Shock* that because modern society is "work-oriented in a systematic, non-seasonal way, as it has been since the industrial revolution," it does not consider leisure seriously.[101] Leisure, they say, is often confused with pleasure, making it sound "vaguely sinful and hedonistic and frivolous enough to be frowned upon." Despite this, they observe that modern technology creates a situation in which all goods and services can be produced by fewer people, leading to a reduction in the availability of paid employment. This leaves many people with up to 100% leisure time, in a society that values technological progress and the material rewards of paid employment above all other forms of occupation, including those that are people or skills centered. Eventually, Jenkins and Sherman argue, societies are going to have to come to terms with the idea that the work ethic is fast becoming redundant and that the boundaries between work and leisure must be blurred. This need to blur work and leisure is a constant theme of writers concerned with their study.[53,102-106]

Throughout this century, the need for people to be seen to pass time usefully, to provide by one's own efforts for the necessities of life, sometimes despite unfulfilling, unsatisfying employment, has been a strongly held social value. Jahoda found, from study of the unemployed in the 1930s, that employment offered more than financial reward. It allowed purpose, a sense of achievement, a daily time structure, social contact outside the family, and social status, and its lack caused boredom, mental despair, apathy, and deterioration.[107] In the late 1980s, she remained convinced about these negative effects.[108] Similarly, Warr found that employment offers scope for developing new skills and decision-making, but that on the down side, the value given to employment causes the unemployed to suffer frequent humiliations and loss of social status.[109] Smith goes so far as to suggest that paid employment has become the central institution mattering more to individuals than "government, education, religion, defense, or health." He believes being unemployed may be worse than "being excommunicated, disenfranchised, illiterate, conquered, and diseased," with many people without paid employment feeling unwanted, as if they no longer belong to society, their impoverished days having neither structure nor purpose.[110]

Post-Industry

In the late 20th century, in post-industrial cultures, employment for remuneration still enjoys the greatest status among occupations for both men and women. People in the 1990s, though, have shifted their ideas from expecting to work to provide for their own needs toward an expectation that they have a right to work to provide themselves with status and material comforts. However, for many people, paid employment is not intrinsically satisfying.[111] For example, Winefield and his colleagues, in a prospective longitudinal study of more than 3,000 young Australians, found that people dissatisfied with their employment were no better off in terms of self-esteem, levels of depression, or lack of psychological well-being than the unemployed who were, as could be expected, significantly worse off than those satisfied with their employment.[112] The theme of the last two paragraphs, which begins to relate unemployment or unsatisfactory employment with ill health, will be developed in Chapter 6.

Because paid employment has assumed such high status, unless other forms of occupation assume a market status on par with it, they have become devalued. This has resulted in leisure activities becoming subject to high technological development and over-regulation. An example is the preoccupation with product development rather than sailing skill in the America's Cup. In this, we see the value once given solely to human occupational achievement taken over by the achievement of occupational technology. Effectively, this values material goods at the expense of people and process, and devalues skills as well as the goods people can produce by their own efforts.

Although not always linked with capitalist gain, technological experimentation and development have been strong characteristics of the occupational nature of humans throughout history because our "genetic constitution" is organized in such a way that all people experience the need to engage in exploratory, adaptive, and productive occupational behavior, seemingly for the purpose of reducing time spent on necessary occupations in favor of time for self-chosen occupations. The effort to save time in order to use it in some other way demonstrates how individuals unconsciously seek to use the range of their capacities. For some people, the range of obligatory activities concerned with their work may meet their biological needs for physical, mental, and social stimulation and exercise; for others, this may be far from the truth.

Industrial processes and capitalist structures narrowed the range of activity of many individuals to those that were economically efficient and viable, reducing many of the peripheral occupations, often of a social or problem-solving nature, that in earlier economies had given exercise to a wide range of capacities.

Industrialization certainly signaled an enormous change from a long period of human occupation based mainly on natural processes through either hunting and gathering or agriculture to occupations that were man-made and, in some cases, many steps removed from nature and natural needs or processes. As early as 1935, Carrel, a Nobel prize-winning medical scientist, in his call for the scientific study of man, suggested that "it is difficult...to know exactly how the substitution of an artificial mode of existence for the natural one and a complete modification of their environment have acted upon civilized human beings."[113]

This question remains as people seem to accept that technological change is necessarily an improvement and that the development of machines to reduce occupational effort is inevitable and desirable. Just as from the 1920s on, most people continue to joyfully welcome "modern civilization," adopting new modes of life and "ways of acting and thinking," laying aside "old habits," because these "demand a greater effort."[113] In this way, new technology leads to new cultural adaptations, which, in turn, lead to further technological change, and so on. This can be constructive or destructive and, depending on the viewpoint taken, can be either or both.

In technically advanced societies, the industrial era has evolved rapidly into a new electronic era. Arthur Penty, a follower of Morris, is credited with coining the phrase "post-industrial society" at the turn of the century,[114] but social commentators as diverse as Daniel Bell, Alain Touraine, and Barry Jones give us contemporary descriptions.[115-117] To them, post-industrial society is characterized by a change from production to service industries, from manual to professional and technical workers, and to decision-making based on information technology. Toffler observes that these economic changes are part of "a crisis that is simultaneously tearing up our energy base, our value systems, our sense of space and time, our epistemology as well as our economy," and will result in a "wholly new and drastically different social order."[118] In fact, the social forms and values that developed and prevailed during industrial domination of human choice in labor and leisure occupation remain. The tension between traditional social forms and modern post-industrial arrangements has been responsible for a period of unprecedented uncertainty and loss of direction for many people. Jones suggests that, despite "universal literacy, an omnipresent media, and a vast information industry," post-industrial society is threatened by its "preoccupation with materialism, a conviction that national and international salvation is to be found in economic growth alone, and emphasis on externalized (consumption-based) value systems."[117] Similarly, the American futurologist, Richard Louv, in *Working in America II*, commenting on the speed of change in the information age, observed that "even the post-industrials have a gnawing feeling that the transforming economy is like a blizzard or tornado: unpredictable, beyond control, or, more precisely controlling us."[119]

Both Jones' and Louv's concerns can be seen as a criticism of the complacent, confident predictions of the futurologists of the 1950s and 1960s in which "the fruits of applied science...were seen able to produce...an era of leisure and abundance."[120-123] Following the economic recessions of the late 1970s and 1980s, a more cautionary note has appeared in futurological speculation often in reference to social limits of growth[124] and frequently allied with ecological theory. However, many people do appear to experience the difficulties alluded to by Louv, such as feeling loss of control or that the world is changing too rapidly for comfort, despite these feelings, in some measure, being countered by excitement as technological development sweeps all before it.

The value given to technology has also caused a devaluation of older members of society. Many are confused by the rapid social and technical changes occurring around them; whereas in agricultural societies they were often viewed as wise counselors and spiritual leaders, in post-industrial societies they have been effectively displaced because their early life experiences are no longer seen as relevant, and they are viewed as being part of a "stagnant, marginal social category."[125] The same attitude is evident in dealings with non-modern technology-based societies. In large part, the lack of understanding and recognition of the human need for occupation has contributed to humans allowing technological development to drive them rather than the other way around and in accepting that the driving force of such development, at present, is based on economic theory rather than on human nature and needs.

Countering this could be possible if all people had a better understanding of the purpose and meaning of occupation in a generic sense. Such understanding demands:

A sociological imagination that reminds us of the real range of social behavior...necessary so that we can collectively decide which kinds of work and which kinds of leisure are appropriate to a good life and create the opportunities for these to be realized.[53]

In fact, from the industrial era on, occupation for its own sake seems to have lost its efficacy and value, perhaps because it is no longer obviously associated with nature. The major changes in ways in which people have met the physiological requirements of food, shelter, and safety, while nurturing their social and mental needs, have evolved from being an integral part of a self-sustaining ecological lifestyle to one that is superimposed on and destructive to natural resources. This can be seen to have obscured some biological needs that are germane to species' survival. Meeting the needs of long-term species' survival is not, for most people in post-industrial societies, a day-to-day concern, and, in fact, human occupation, its technology, and the social structure and values that surround it are now so complex that they are almost unrecognizable as developing from the simple survival occupations of our ancestors. The need to use human capacities in a creative, problem-solving, inventive, or adaptive way has led to the domination of occupational technology over the ecology, queries about the survival of the species in the long-term, and ironically to the detriment of present and future use of personal skills. I agree with Lorenz's viewpoint that such domination can be considered a "disorder(s) of certain special behavior mechanisms originally possessing survival value."[126]

Some commentators argue that when humans become sufficiently focused on these culturally created problems, the same drive that created them will be able to counteract the ill effects. This could already be in train. Indeed, Toynbee suggested in the 1960s that even though "in making...tools progressively more effective" and the "misuse of them progressively more dangerous" the "World's most powerful nations and governments have shown an uncustomary self-restraint on some critical occasions" demonstrating an "advance in social justice" and an increase in humanitarianism.[127] In present times, there is widespread questioning of the wisdom of continuing with economic policies that place technological development and the expansion of trade before human well-being and diminishing natural resources. Robertson, in

Future Work, calls for people to reject a future of technological determinism in which technology rather than value systems dictate choice; and Jones suggests that "the most appropriate analogies for economic processes are to be found in biology—with growth, maturation, nourishment, excretion, and decline—rather than physics."[105,117] Despite this, at a recent United Nations Conference on Environment and Development, the government delegates appeared to support maintaining the status quo and transnational corporations by arguing for "promoting sustainable development through trade liberalization."[128] A reluctance by industrialists and world leaders to pay more than lip service to ecological or pre-industrial society's issues points to a bias toward maintaining the first, or possibly the second, of three possible scenarios for the future—"business as usual," in which development continues similar to the present; "hyper-expansionism" based on super-industrial development of science and technology; or a "sane, humane, ecological" vision that focuses on human development and ecological sustainability.[105] Future health and well-being depends on the latter vision, with all human beings using their occupational nature through activities that sustain the ecological balance and that enable personal growth and potential. This issue will be picked up in the final chapter.

Functions of Occupation

The exploration of biological and cultural occupational evolution in Chapters 3 and 4 has established the force of the idea that the biological need to engage in occupation is a major characteristic of humans aimed at enabling species' survival and individual health. Four major functions of occupation have been identified:

1. To provide for immediate bodily needs of sustenance, self-care, and shelter
2. To develop skills, social structures, and technology aimed at safety and superiority over predators and the environment
3. To maintain health by balanced exercise of personal capacities
4. To enable individual and social development so that each person and the species will flourish

However, because of the strength of the occupational needs that are prerequisite to meeting those four functions, imbalance is possible, and the needs may be counter to survival, particularly if they are not recognized for what they are.

While it is relatively easy to see that there is a correlation between obvious survival occupations and health, because what people do has direct bearing on their type of shelter, their access to food, clean air, and water, which have been well researched, the correlation between health and the innate need of humans to engage in other types of occupations is obscure, complex, and poorly researched. Because of the complexity of occupation, teasing out its positive or negative attributes is difficult. Engagement in occupation cannot easily be separated from the other basic requirements of life, and the complexities of these interactions need much more inquiry. The interaction of mind, body, and spirit; obligatory and choice issues; differences in genetic capacities; the nature of and need for occupational mastery, risk taking, and challenge; optimum levels of personal satisfaction; or the relationship to sociocultural values of any occupation are just a few of the variables that may make a difference in how occupation affects health.

In conclusion, it may seem that, in comparing early and present forms of occupations that have continued throughout evolution, this chapter has condemned current practices. To some extent, the comment may be justified as, in exploring the differences between natural and culturally acquired occupational behaviors, it would seem that people living in post-industrial countries do not appear happy or satisfied. Despite many apparent material and social welfare advantages, people cannot be described as experiencing well-being, but rather a "drifting dissatisfaction" that, according to anthropological studies, does not occur in the "more primitive social groupings nor, indeed, in the less developed countries."[101] Some of the probable causes alluded to in the chapter include the division of occupation for gender, economic, and age reasons; limitations, restrictions, and impositions due to dominant philosophies and policies of societies; conflict between technological development, individual need, and the ecology; and the problem of achieving balance between occupations of choice and necessity. The literature reviewed in this chapter also suggests that the basic occupational needs of people have been obscured by the current complexity of occupational technology and economy, and the sociopolitical structures, divisions, and values that have been established progressively. This leads to the notion that cultural views of occupation dominate biological needs for occupation and that this may be a cause for less than healthy survival. Because the origins and nature of occupations have become obscure, we have failed to recognize them as a basic need, accepting instead the materialistic, value-loaded results of occupation as the central focus of modern life and occupation's purpose. This poses many questions for the future, not least, from the perspective of this theory, is the question of what these changes mean to the occupational nature of people and to their health. The next chapter will explore ideas about health and well-being from this occupational view of human nature.

References

1. Pilbeam D. What makes us human? In: Jones S, Martin R, Pilbeam D, eds. *The Cambridge Encyclopedia of Human Evolution.* New York, NY: Cambridge University Press; 1992.
2. Jones S, Martin R, Pilbeam D, eds. *The Cambridge Encyclopedia of Human Evolution.* New York, NY: Cambridge University Press; 1992.
3. Bronowski J. *The Ascent of Man.* London, England: British Broadcasting Corp; 1973.
4. Campbell BG. *Humankind Emerging.* 5th ed. New York, NY: Harper Collins Publishers; 1988:230.
5. Buranhult G, ed. *The First Humans: Human Origins and History to 10,000BC.* Australia: University of Queensland Press; 1993:59,93,95,98-99.
6. Leakey R, Lewin R. *People of the Lake: Man: His Origins, Nature, and Future.* New York, NY: Penguin Books; 1978:32-33,88,120.
7. Leakey R. *The Making of Mankind.* London, England: Michael Joseph Ltd; 1981:226-229,242.
8. Lewin R. *In the Age of Mankind: A Smithsonian Book of Human Evolution.* Washington, DC: Smithsonian Books; 1988:190,195,204,224.
9. Foley R, ed. *Hominid Evolution and Community Ecology.* London, England: Academic Press; 1984.
10. Klein RG. *The Human Career: Human Biological and Cultural Origins.* Chicago, Ill: University of Chicago Press; 1989.
11. Fletcher R. The evolution of human behaviour. In: Buranhult G, ed. *The First Humans: Human Origins and History to 10,000BC.* Australia: University of Queensland Press; 1993:17.
12. Lancaster J. The dynamics of tool using behaviour. *American Anthropologist.* 1967;70:56-66.
13. Tobias PV. The emergence of man in Africa and beyond. *Philosophical Transactions of the Royal Society.* 1981;292:43-56.
14. Blumenberg B. The evolution of the advanced hominid brain. *Current Anthropology.* 1983;24(5):589-623.
15. Falk D. *As It Happened: Some Liked It Hot.* Television documentary. SBS (Adelaide), UK, March 21, 1996.
16. Falk D. Cerebral cortices of East Afrian early hominids. *Science.* 1983;221:1072-1074.
17. Gowlett JAJ. Tools—the Palaeolithic record. In: Jones S, Martin R, Pilbeam D, eds. *The Cambridge Encyclopedia of Human Evolution.* New York, NY: Cambridge University Press; 1992:350.
18. Jelinek J. *Primitive Hunters.* London, England: Hamlyn; 1989:42,66.

19. Rowley-Conway P. Mighty hunter or marginal scavenger? In: Buranhult G, ed. *The First Humans: Human Origins and History to 10,000BC*. Australia: University of Queensland Press; 1993:61-62.

20. van der Merve NJ. Reconstructing prehistoric diet. In: Jones S, Martin R, Pilbeam D, eds. *The Cambridge Encyclopedia of Human Evolution*. New York, NY: Cambridge University Press; 1992:369-372.

21. Wing ES, Brown AG. *Paleonutrition: Method and Theory in Prehistoric Foodways*. New York, NY: Academic Press; 1978.

22. Isaac GLI. The food sharing behaviour of protohuman hominids. *Scientific American*. 1978;238(April):90-106.

23. Isaac B. Throwing. In: Jones S, Martin R, Pilbeam D, eds. *The Cambridge Encyclopedia of Human Evolution*. New York, NY: Cambridge University Press; 1992:358.

24. Ingold T. *Hunters, Pasturalists and Ranchers*. New York, NY: Cambridge University Press; 1980.

25. Ellen RF. *Environment, Subsistence and System*. New York, NY: Cambridge University Press; 1982.

26. Foley R. Studying human evolution by analogy. In: Jones S, Martin R, Pilbeam D, eds. *The Cambridge Encyclopedia of Human Evolution*. New York, NY: Cambridge University Press; 1992:336.

27. Woodburn J. Hunters and gatherers today and reconstruction of the past. In: Gellner E, ed. *Soviet and Western Anthropology*. London, England: Duckworth; 1980.

28. Potts R. The hominid way of life. In: Jones S, Martin R, Pilbeam D, eds. *The Cambridge Encyclopedia of Human Evolution*. New York, NY: Cambridge University Press; 1992.

29. Lampl M. Sex roles in prehistory. In: Buranhult G, ed. *The First Humans: Human Origins and History to 10,000BC*. Australia: University of Queensland Press; 1993:30-31.

30. Lee RB, DeVore I. *Man the Hunter*. Chicago, Ill: Aldine Publishing Co; 1968.

31. Dalberg F, ed. *Woman the Gatherer*. New Haven, Conn: Yale University Press; 1981.

32. Brown JK. A note on the division of labor by sex. *American Anthropologist*. 1970;72(5):1073-1078.

33. Burton ML, Brudner LA, White DR. A model of the sexual division of labor. *American Ethnologist*. 1977;4(2):227-251.

34. Burton ML, White DR. Division of labour by sex. In: Kuper A, Kuper J, eds. *The Social Science Encyclopedia*. London, England: Routledge; 1985:206.

35. Herskovits MJ. *Economic Anthropology*. New York, NY: Knopf; 1952.

36. Coon CS. *The Hunting Peoples*. London, England: Jonathan Cape Ltd; 1972:3,388-389,392.

37. Johanson D, Edey M. *Lucy: The Beginnings of Humankind*. New York, NY: Simon and Schuster; 1981.

38. Argyle M. *The Psychology of Interpersonal Behaviour*. Harmondsworth: Penguin Books; 1967.

39. Alexander RD. *Darwinism and Human Affairs*. Seattle, Wash: University of Washington Press; 1979.

40. Chagnon N, Irons W, eds. *Evolutionary Biology and Human Social Behaviour*. North Scituate, Mass: Duxbury Press; 1979.

41. Symons D. *The Evolution of Human Sexuality*. New York, NY: Oxford University Press; 1979.

42. van den Berghe PL. Sociobiology. In: Kuper A, Kuper J, eds. *The Social Science Encyclopedia*. London, England: Routledge; 1985.

43. Trivers RL. The evolution of reciprocal altruism. *Quarterly Review of Biology*. 1971;46(1):35-57.

44. Bruner JS. Nature and uses of immaturity. *American Psychologist*. 1972;August:687-708.

45. Morris D, Marsh P. *Tribes*. London, England: Pyramid Books; 1988:9.

46. Liljegren R. Animals of ice age Europe. In: Buranhult G, ed. *The First Humans: Human Origins and History to 10,000BC*. Australia: University of Queensland Press; 1993.

47. Lorenz K. *On Aggression*. London, England: Methuen; 1966:52.

48. Waechter J. *Man Before History*. Oxford, UK: Elsevier-Phaidon; 1976.

49. Neff WS. *Work and Human Behaviour*. 3rd ed. New York, NY: Aldine Publishing Co; 1985:33,35.

50. Sahlins M. *Stone Age Economics*. Chicago, Ill: Aldine-Atherton; 1972.

51. Eyre JE. *Journals of Expeditions of Discovery Into Central Australia and Overland*. London, England: T and W Boone; 1845.

52. Wax RH. Free time in other cultures. In: Donahue W, et al, eds. *Free Time: Challenge to Later Maturity*. Ann Arbor, Mich: University of Michigan Press; 1958:3-16.

53. Parker S. *Leisure and Work*. London, England: George Allen and Unwin; 1983:14,17,19,119.

54. Boas F. *The Mind of Primitive Man*. New York, NY: Macmillan; 1911.

55. Binford LR. Subsistence—a key to the past. In: Jones S, Martin R, Pilbeam D, eds. *The Cambridge Encyclopedia of Human Evolution*. New York, NY: Cambridge University Press; 1992:365-368.

56. Ember CR. The relative decline in women's contribution to agriculture with intensification. *American Anthropologist*. 1983;85(2):285-304.

57. Burton ML, White DR. Sexual division of work in agriculture. *American Anthropologist*. 1984;86(3):568-583.

58. Boserup E. *Women's Role in Economic Development*. New York, NY: St. Martin's Press; 1970:15.

59. Ashton H. The Basuto. In: Parker S. *Leisure and Work*. London, England: George Allen and Unwin; 1983:131.
60. Lorenz K. *The Waning of Humaneness*. London, England: Unwin Paperbacks; 1983.
61. Hole F. Origins of agriculture. In: Jones S, Martin R, Pilbeam D, eds. *The Cambridge Encyclopedia of Human Evolution*. New York, NY: Cambridge University Press; 1992:373-379.
62. Clutton-Brock J. Domestication of animals. In: Jones S, Martin R, Pilbeam D, eds. *The Cambridge Encyclopedia of Human Evolution*. New York, NY: Cambridge University Press; 1992:380-385.
63. Aristotle. Politics. In: Barnes J, ed. *The Complete Works of Aristotle*. Rev Oxford trans. UK: Princeton University Press; 1984.
64. Aristotle. Nicomachean ethics. In: Barnes J, ed. *The Complete Works of Aristotle*. Rev Oxford trans. UK: Princeton University Press; 1984.
65. Arendt H. *The Human Condition*. Chicago, Ill: University of Chicago Press; 1958:83-85.
66. Bettenson HS, ed. *Documents of the Christian Church*. New York, NY: Springer; 1963.
67. Exodus 20: verses 9-11. *The Holy Bible*. Authorized King James version. London, England: Oxford University Press; 1972.
68. Weber M. *The Protestant Ethic and the Spirit of Capitalism*. Parsons T, trans. London, England: George Allen and Unwin Ltd; 1930.
69. Kalberg S, Weber M. In: Kuper A, Kuper J, eds. *The Social Science Encyclopedia*. London, England: Routledge; 1985:892-896.
70. Langford P, Harvie C. The eighteenth century and the age of industry. In: Morgan KO, ed. *The Oxford History of Britain*. Vol IV. Oxford, UK: Oxford University Press; 1992:42,44-45.
71. Morgan KO, ed. *The Oxford History of Britain*. Vol V. Oxford, UK: Oxford University Press; 1992.
72. Smith A. (1776). In: Campbell RH, Skinner AS, Todd WB, eds. *An Inquiry Into the Nature and Causes of the Wealth of Nations*. Chicago, Ill: University of Chicago Press; 1976.
73. Raphael DD. *Adam Smith*. Vol 1. Oxford, UK: Oxford University Press; 1985:17.
74. Bannock G, Baxter RE, Rees R. *The Penguin Dictionary of Economics*. 2nd ed. New York, NY: Penguin Books; 1978.
75. Knight FH. Some fallacies in the interpretation of social cost. 1924. Reprinted in Arrow KJ, Scitovsky T. *Readings in Welfare Economics*. London, England: George Allen and Unwin; 1969:226-227.
76. Galbraith JK. *The Affluent Society*. London, England: Hamish; 1958.
77. Roll E. *A History of Economic Thought*. 4th ed. London, England: Faber and Faber; 1973:600.
78. Robbins L. *Politics and Economics, Papers in Political Economy*, London, England: Macmillan; 1963:7.
79. Desai M. Vulgar economics. In: Bottomore T, ed. *A Dictionary of Marxist Thought*. 2nd ed. Oxford, UK: Blackwell Ltd; 1991:574.
80. More T. *Utopia*. Turner P, trans. Harmondsworth: Penguin Books; 1965.
81. Campanella T. *City of the Sun*. Donno DJ, trans. Berkeley, Calif: University of California Press; 1981.
82. Marx K. *Early Writings*. New York, NY: Penguin Classics; 1992:326,328.
83. Marx K. Economic and philosophical manuscripts. In: *Early Writings*. New York, NY: Penguin Classics; 1992.
84. Bottomore T. *A Dictionary of Marxist Thought*. 2nd ed. Oxford, UK: Blackwell Ltd; 1991.
85. Marx K, Engels F. *The German Ideology*. 1845-46. London, England: Lawrence and Wishart, 1964.
86. Marx K. *The Holy Family. 1844*. London, England: Lawrence and Wishart, 1957.
87. Fischer E. *Marx in His Own Words*. London, England: Allen Lane, The Penguin Press; 1970:31,49.
88. Ruskin J. Preface. In: Yarker PM, ed. *Unto This Last*. London, England: Collins Publishers; 1970.
89. Coleridge ST. *The Friend*. New York, NY: Freeport; 1971.
90. Carlyle T. Sartor Resartus 1833-1834. In: *Sartor Resartus, and On Heroes and Hero Worship*. London, England: Dent; 1908. Reprinted New York, NY: Dutton; 1973.
91. MacCarthy F. *William Morris: A Life for Our Time*. London, England: Faber and Faber; 1994:70-71.
92. Cole GDH. In: Selgman ERA, ed. *Encyclopaedia of Social Science*. New York, NY: Macmillan; 1933.
93. Morris W. Art and socialism. In: Morton AL, ed. *Political Writings of William Morris*. London, England: Lawrence and Wishart; 1973:110-111.
94. Jackson Lears TJ. *No Place of Grace: Antimodernism and the Transformation of American Culture 1880-1920*. New York, NY: Pantheon Books; 1981:63-64.
95. Morris W. Useful work versus useless toil. In: Morton AL, ed. *Political Writings of William Morris*. London, England: Lawrence and Wishart; 1973.
96. Morris W. News from nowhere. In: Morton AL, ed. *Three Works by William Morris: News from Nowhere, The Pilgrims of Hope, A Dream of John Ball*. London, England: Lawrence and Wishart; 1968.
97. Mackenzie N, Mackenzie J. *The Fabians*. New York, NY: Weidenfeld and Nicolson; 1977.
98. Lowerson J, Myerscough J. *Time to Spare in Victorian England*. Hassocks: Harvester Press; 1977.
99. Bailey P. *Leisure and Class in Victorian England*. London, England: Routledge; 1978.

100. Cunningham H. *Leisure in the Industrial Revolution*. London, England: Croom Helm; 1980.
101. Jenkins C, Sherman B. *The Leisure Shock*. London, England: Eyre Methuen Ltd; 1981:1,5.
102. Keniston K. Social change and youth in America. *Daedalus*. 1962;Winter:145-171.
103. Friedlander F. Importance of work versus non-work among socially and occupationally stratified groups. *Journal of Applied Psychology*. 1966;December:437-441.
104. Hollander P. Leisure as an American and Soviet value. *Social Problems*. 1966;3:179-188.
105. Robertson J. *Future Work*. England: Gower Publishing Co; 1985.
106. Pettifer S. Leisure as compensation for unemployment and unfulfilling work. Reality or pipe dream? *Journal of Occupational Science: Australia*. 1993;1(2):20-26.
107. Jahoda M. *Employment and Unemployment*. New York, NY: Cambridge University Press; 1982.
108. Jahoda M. Economic recession and mental health: some conceptual issues. *Journal of Social Issues*. 1988;44(4):13-23.
109. Warr P. Twelve questions about unemployment and health. In: Roberts R, Finnegan R, Gallie D, eds. *New Approaches to Economic Life*. Manchester: Manchester University Press; 1985.
110. Smith R. *Unemployment and Health; A Disaster and a Challenge*. Oxford, UK: Oxford University Press; 1987.
111. Aungles SB, Parker SR. *Work, Organisations and Change: Themes and Perspectives in Australia*. Sydney, Australia: George Allen and Unwin; 1988.
112. Winefield AH, Tiggerman M, Goldney RD. Psychological concomitants of satisfactory employment and unemployment in young people. *Social Psychiatry and Psychiatric Epidemiology*. 1988;23:149-157.
113. Carrel A. *Man the Unknown*. London, England: Burns and Oates; 1935:24-25.
114. Bullock ALC. Post industrial society. In: Bullock A, Stalleybrass O, Trombley S, eds. *The Fontana Dictionary of Modern Thought*. 2nd ed. London, England: Fontana Press; 1988:670.
115. Bell D. *The Coming of Post Industrial Society. A Venture in Social Forecasting*. New York, NY: Basic Books; 1973.
116. Touraine A. *Post Industrial Society*. London, England: Wildwood House; 1974.
117. Jones B. *Sleepers, Wake! Technology and the Future of Work*. Melbourne, Australia: Oxford University Press; 1982:44-45.
118. Toffler A. *The Eco-Spasm Report*. New York, NY: Bantam Book Inc; 1975:3.
119. Louv R. *Working in America II*. New York, NY: Penguin Books; 1983.
120. Jungk R, Galtung J, eds. *Mankind 2000*. London, England: George Allen and Unwin; 1969.
121. Jantsch E. *Technological Forecasting in Perspective*. Paris, France: OECD; 1967.
122. International Future Research Conference, Oslo. In: Bell D, ed. *Towards the Year 2000*. London, England: George Allen and Unwin; 1968.
123. Kumar K. Futurology. In: Kuper A, Kuper J, eds. *The Social Science Encyclopedia*. London, England: Routledge; 1985:325.
124. Hirsch F. *Social Limits to Growth*. London, England: Routledge; 1977.
125. Hazan H. Gerontology, social. In: Kuper A, Kuper J, eds. *The Social Science Encyclopedia*. London, England: Routledge; 1985:337.
126. Lorenz K. *Civilized Man's Eight Deady Sins*. Latzke M, trans. London, England: Methuen and Co Ltd; 1974:2.
127. Toynbee AJ. A study of history. Vol XII. Reconsiderations. In: Kohn H, ed. *The Modern World*. New York, NY: Macmillan; 1963:303-304.
128. Korten D, ed. *Economy, Ecology and Spirituality*. The Asian NGO Coalition, Manila, IRED Asia, Columbo, The People-Centred Development Forum, New York, NY, 1993:2.

Suggested Reading

Boserup E. *Women's Role in Economic Development*. New York, NY: St. Martin's Press; 1970.
Bronowski J. *The Ascent of Man*. London, England: British Broadcasting Corp; 1973.
Buranhult G, ed. *The First Humans: Human Origins and History to 10,000BC*. Australia: University of Queensland Press; 1993.
Campbell BG. *Humankind Emerging*. 5th ed. New York, NY: Harper Collins Publishers; 1988.
Dalberg F, ed. *Woman the Gatherer*. New Haven, Conn: Yale University Press; 1981.
Jackson Lears TJ. *No Place of Grace: Antimodernism and the Transformation of American Culture 1880-1920*. New York, NY: Pantheon Books; 1981.
Jones B. *Sleepers, Wake! Technology and the Future of Work*. Melbourne, Australia: Oxford University Press; 1982.
Jones S, Martin R, Pilbeam D, eds. *The Cambridge Encyclopedia of Human Evolution*. New York, NY: Cambridge University Press; 1992.

Korten D, ed. *Economy, Ecology and Spirituality.* The Asian NGO Coalition, Manila, IRED Asia, Columbo, The People-Centred Development Forum, New York, NY, 1993.

MacCarthy F. *William Morris: A Life for Our Time.* London, England: Faber and Faber; 1994.

Marx K. *Early Writings.* New York, NY: Penguin Classics; 1992.

Neff WS. *Work and Human Behaviour.* 3rd ed. New York, NY: Aldine Publishing Co; 1985.

Parker S. *Leisure and Work.* London, England: George Allen and Unwin; 1983.

Pettifer S. Leisure as compensation for unemployment and unfulfilling work. Reality or pipe dream? *Journal of Occupational Science: Australia.* 1993;1(2):20-26.

Sahlins M. *Stone Age Economics.* Chicago, Ill: Aldine-Atherton; 1972.

Smith R. *Unemployment and Health; A Disaster and a Challenge.* Oxford, UK: Oxford University Press; 1987.

Winefield AH, Tiggerman M, Goldney RD. Psychological concomitants of satisfactory employment and unemployment in young people. *Social Psychiatry and Psychiatric Epidemiology.* 1988;23:149-157.

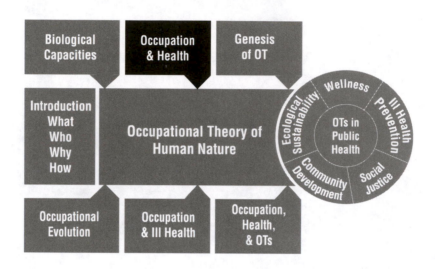

Chapter 5
Health: An Occupational Perspective

This chapter presents the reader with ideas about:
- Positive health and well-being, holism, and health promotion from an occupational perspective
- A view of "natural" health based on the "natural" lifestyles and health experiences of hunter-gatherer peoples
- Biological needs as a mechanism for health, and engagement in occupation as a "biological need"
- Occupational determinants of health and well-being

Ideas about what is health differ according to cultural and spiritual philosophies, socially dominant and individual views, the type of economy, and the health technology available. In this chapter, a particular view of health from the perspective of humans as occupational beings will be discussed, focusing on what makes and keeps people well, rather than what causes or prevents them from being ill. It starts by exploring definitions and concepts held about health, well-being, holism, and World Health Organization (WHO) directives to promote health. From this exploration, and building upon the ideas about occupation that have emerged in earlier chapters, the view of health held in this text is described. This relates to survival of the species, to how individuals and communities flourish, and to ecological sustainability. To support the central notion that engagement in occupation is a biological mechanism for health, the chapter goes on to explore how the "natural" occupational behaviors of early hunter-gatherers related to their health status.

Defining Health

There are many definitions of health, but the WHO definition that it is "a state of complete physical, mental, and social well-being not merely the absence of disease or infirmity" has survived 50 years of rapid social change and is one that a significant body of health writers have kept in mind,[1] despite some criticism about the definition from medical scientists that it is "idealistic, unattainable, largely irrelevant," and difficult to measure.[2,3] The focus of Western medical efforts on illness rather than health might also appear to gainsay the broader intent of the definition. This focus is not surprising as, on the whole, in countries with advanced medical technology, people have been socialized to think about health and illness in terms of medical and physical sciences and their commodities, to the extent that Newman, a nursing theorist, observes that the view of health as the absence of disease has pervaded most of our thinking from very early in life.[4]

Health as "more than the absence of illness" is particularly difficult to explicate, although there have been many attempts. For example, Blaxter discusses in *Health and Lifestyles* some of the many ways health may be conceptualized.[5] Her monograph, based on a survey undertaken in the United Kingdom with a sample of 9,000 adults, found that, as well as the absence of disease and illness, people described health as having a reserve to combat problems, behavior aimed at healthy lifestyle, physical fitness, energy and vitality, social relationships, being able to function, and psychosocial well-being. The survey outcomes support the belief that views of health differ over the life course, have clear gender differences, and are, for most, a multi-dimensional concept. The view of health presented in this chapter accepts these conclusions, and some of Blaxter's results are used to illustrate particular points. Blaxter's findings also appear to link health and well-being in accord with the WHO definition. Understanding what is meant by well-being appears to be a key issue, so this will be explored in some depth in the next pages.

Defining Well-Being

As early as 490 BC to 429 BC, Pericles made the connection between health and a feeling of well-being. More recently, well-being has been defined within the health promotion fraternity as "a subjective assessment of health which is less concerned with biological function than with feelings such as self-esteem and a sense of belonging through social integration."[2]

In the thesaurus, "well-being" stands with words like happiness and prosperity, as well as health.[6] While happiness and health have an intuitive fit, prosperity may be linked with well-being, insofar as people with no monetary concerns are able to make most use of health promoting opportunities. They are more easily able to meet the basic requirements for health than poorer people, as well as having none of the stress or worries attributed to poverty. In addition, the high social value accorded to money in the present day increases its potential effect on health status. Standardized mortality and morbidity statistics support the association of people with limited resources experiencing poorer health (and, it can be argued, less well-being).[7] For example, it has been found that children of unskilled workers in Britain are twice as likely to die in their first year of life as are those of professional people,[8] and numerous other studies support the notion that well-being is related to income, financial status, and employment.[9-15]

Despite these acknowledged "material" associations, the feeling of well-being is as intangible and amorphous a concept as charm or style. Subjectively, well-being can be described as a pleasant and desirable physiological sensation, which can differ from person to person. Some people describe well-being as "being on top of the world" or in conjunction with "being in love." Others describe it as when they indulge in a favorite hobby or relax in a special place, and some even experience it in pursuit of their paid occupation or vocation. John Hersey, for example, admitted to "feeling nourished and transformed" as a result of his literary work.[16] Other feelings include happiness, contentment, peace, joy in simple aspects of the environment or being with others, energy and anticipation, confidence and concentration, satisfaction with ongoing achievement, or a sense of timelessness and "flow."[17] Csikszentmihalyi found that "the typical working adult in the United States" experiences "flow" at work "three times (54%) as often as in free time (17%)" and during the experience of flow feels "very significantly more happy, strong, satisfied, creative, and concentrated."[18,19] Blaxter's study found that for women who defined health in terms of energy they

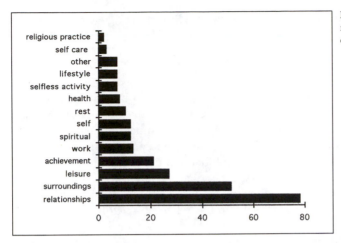

Figure 5-1. Situations or environments with which respondents associated well-being.

described it in similar ways as "feeling like conquering the world, being keen and interested, lots of get-up-and-go, and properly alive."[5] At times of absorbing interest, when physical, social, and mental capacities are able to meet the challenge, people are said to be able to resist disease and seem impervious to many problems and difficulties that beset them.

Fragments of other empirical research point in the same direction. When Pybus and Thomson asked 444 New Zealanders in 1979 what, in their experience, was being well, the answers included replies like being "able to do what I want to and enjoy it" and "energy and interest," as well as "being full of life" and "feeling alive and vital," with "energy for things extra."[20,20a] In order to explore these ideas about well-being, an Adelaide survey asked subjects to define their concept of well-being, how it felt to them, and how often they experienced the feeling. Seven convenience cluster samples were selected from high school students, an elderly citizens' village, family units, a suburban neighborhood, the city shopping center, churchgoers, and fourth-year occupational therapy students. The three most common responses related to having a sound mind, a healthy body, and being happy. Ninety-five percent of 138 respondents agreed they had experienced a feeling they would describe as well-being, with 50% admitting they experienced this feeling frequently. Fifty-two percent described the feeling associated with well-being as happiness, 35% with peace, and 22% with confidence. Subjects were asked with what situation or environment they associated a feeling of well-being, and of the two most common responses, 56% concerned relationships and 37% concerned surroundings. Interesting are the number of occupational categories such as work, leisure, rest, religious practices, self-less activity, self-care, and achievement, which when added together total 83 responses (60%). This total does not take into account any occupations carried out in conjunction with social relationship or spiritual (as opposed to religious) situations, so it could well be that most of the sample identified some form of occupational situation or environment as one of the circumstances associated with their experience of well-being (Figure 5-1). The majority of subjects were women, single, fit, and young, which may well have given a particular cast to the responses. In other studies, well-being has been related to social supports, community cohesion, marital state, education, and religious attitudes, beliefs, and activities.[9-12,21,22]

To explore positive health and well-being in more depth, physical, mental, and social well-being need to be considered separately and linked to engagement in occupation.

Physical Well-Being

Physical well-being is, perhaps, the aspect of health that has received the most attention and is the easiest to understand. The experience of physical well-being is often recognized when body function is challenged beyond the norm and the challenge is met, such as the relaxing after-effects of exercise. Indeed, Maslow suggests that muscular people have to use their muscles to "feel good and to achieve the subjective feeling of harmonious, successful, uninhibited functioning."[23] According to Blaxter, young people, and men in particular, associate health with physical fitness, with strength, energy, and athletic prowess and, in line with this, identify sports figures as their idea of health in others. Women tend to relate physical fitness and energy in terms of outward appearance and work-related activity rather than sports or particular leisure pursuits.[5] Small-scale studies carried out with students tend to confirm that young people view physical fitness and well-being as synonymous but that there are differences in how men or women perceive physical fitness, often in accord with how health and well-being are reported in the media.[24]

Popular media regularly encourage people to experience well-being and health by physical means, such as exercise and diet. The results of medical research, aimed mainly at physical well-being, are reported in abbreviated form in popular magazines, in medical columns of newspapers, on radio and television, and form much of the foundation for the current interest in the pursuit of health. The number of joggers or aerobic devotees are testament to the effectiveness of this type of promotion to the extent that health, in this popularized sense, has become a marketable product during recent years, with health farms, foods, centers, and shops springing up throughout metropolitan areas. For example, listings of health and fitness centers in the Adelaide *Yellow Pages* increased by 50% in a decade, from 81 in 1983 to 120 in the 1993 directory. In 1983, there were only 103 health food manufacturers/wholesalers/retailers listings, compared with 189 in 1993. The apparent rise of interest in feeling well along with defeating disease has also been associated with a growth of alternative health services for those unhappy with the solutions provided by conventional medicine. No "alternative health services" (so described) were listed in the 1983 directory compared with 59 in 1993, and the listings of a group of different services including acupuncture, herbalism, homeopathy, naturopathy, massage, and relaxation therapy grew in the 10 years from 379 to 600.

In some ways, such interest could be seen as resurgent rather than novel, as earlier societies have also perceived benefits of physical fitness. For example, in the first half of the 20th century, initiatives were taken in several countries to encourage and almost glorify health and fitness. These initiatives in the most part had patriotic national flavors and are most typified by the Nazi youth movement in Germany. In Australia, less fervent programs toward a healthy and strong white race were advocated by progressives such as Cumpston, Elkington, and Cilento.[25,26] Powles describes those early decades of this century as the "national" period in the public hygiene movement when physical fitness, eugenics, efficiency, vitality, and race purity were focal values.[27]

In contrast to those "national" and "physical" themes, present views are based to some extent on more holistic notions influenced by traditional Asian philosophies and associated with increasing acknowledgment that physical well-being is related to spiritual, social, and behavioral factors, such as where and how people live and what they believe, their self-care practices, the amounts and types of activity they pursue, and a balance between rest and work, "being" and "doing."[28] Subsequently, it is being recognized that physical well-being, achieved through use of physical capacities, has an effect on general well-being, for example, mental functioning benefits through increased blood supply to the brain and aerobic power and social interactions benefit through shared activity.[29,30] Examples of such recognition are provided by a review of the relationship between physical training and mental health in which Folkins and Syme found evidence of a positive relationship between exercise, well-being, self-concept, and work ability[31]; by Chamove's study, which found that moderate physical exercise by people with psychiatric disorders decreased their depression, anxiety, disruptive and psychotic behavior, increased self-concept and social well-being, and aided sleep and relaxation[32]; by Morgan's suggestion that non-specific aspects of exercise such as social contact may be instrumental in improved mental health and well-being[33]; and by Oliver's report that improved play and social interaction are benefits of physical education activity along with growth, fitness, agility, and coordination.[34]

The theory of human nature developed in this text leads to the proposition that people need to make use of their physical capacities to enjoy physical well-being and that this can be through engagement in individually motivating and ongoing occupations. If they are able or encouraged to pursue self-chosen occupations, as well as those that are obligatory, to enhance their physical capabilities, they will enhance their health, apart from supplying sustenance for survival and safety: "the best sort of exercise in terms of retaining one's powers is the kind you don't call 'exercise'...the best exercise is work."[35] Indeed, studies have demonstrated that older people who lead active lives following a wide range of occupations tend to feel better and to require less medical attention than isolated and sedentary elderly people.[36] The total range of an individual's purposeful and fulfilling occupations can provide sufficient exercise to maintain homeostasis and to keep body parts functioning at peak efficiency. For example, occupations can maintain and enhance joint stability and range, muscle tone, cardiovascular fitness, and respiratory capacity. A range of occupations can provide balance between physical challenges and relaxation, which prevent overuse and allow time for repair. When people are able to experience occupational well-being, in a physical sense, they will be able to carry out activities they need or wish to do without undue consideration of body functioning, and their physical status will enable effective use of mental and social capacities.

Mental Well-Being

This leads to consideration of mental well-being, which, in this theory, alludes to spiritual as well as cognitive and affective factors. Blaxter found that psychological fitness (well-being) was a popular concept of health across all the age groups and for both men and women when they described health for themselves rather than for others. While it tended to be used more by women and those with better education, "'health is a state of mind' or 'health is a mental thing more than physical' were common statements."[5] For a comparison between responses of subjects from her study concerning physical fitness and psychological fitness, see Table 5-1.

The National Mental Health Association of America describes mentally healthy people as those who:

	Males			**Females**		
Age	18-39	40-59	60+	18-39	40-59	60+
Physical fitness, energy	39%	27%	12%	41%	32%	16%
Psychological fitness	31%	40%	36%	48%	52%	44%

Table 5-1. Comparison of Concepts of "Physical Fitness" and "Psychological Fitness" for Describing What it Is to Be Healthy Oneself (N=9,000=100%). Compiled from data contained in Blaxter M. *Health and Lifestyles.* London, England: Tavistock/Routledge; 1990.

> *Feel comfortable about themselves, ...are not overwhelmed by their own emotions, ...can accept many of life's disappointments in their stride, ...experience all of the human emotions (e.g., fear, anger, love, jealousy, guilt, joy) but are not incapacitated by them. Feel right about other people, ...are comfortable with others, ...are able to give and receive love, ...are concerned about the interests of other people and have relationships that are satisfying and lasting, are able to meet the demands of life, ...respond to their problems, accept responsibility, plan ahead without fear of the future, and are able to establish realistic goals.*[37]

Mental health is described in these or similar terms in many popular texts addressing healthy living, including *The Good Health Guide*,[38] *Health Through Discovery*,[39] and *Understanding Your Health*.[37] The popular texts usually refer to the well-working and coping ability of both emotional and intellectual capacities and sometimes include spiritual capacities, all of which, in combination, enable individuals to find meaning in their lives, interact effectively with others, be reflective, process and act on information, solve problems, develop skills for making decisions, clarify values and beliefs, cope with stress, and be flexible and adaptable to changes in life circumstances and demands. According to this conception, while these varied capacities may not amount to well-being in themselves and the need to use them differs between people and at different life stages, they are seen as prerequisites to the experience of well-being.[40] They are also capacities, integral to engagement in occupation. If individuals are under- or overstressed in the use of emotional, intellectual, or spiritual capacities because of physiological, environmental, or social factors, or because of occupational deprivation, alienation, or imbalance, health and well-being may be undermined.[41-43] From Antonovsky's theory linking health with a "sense of coherence" comes the idea that one difference between who stays well and who does not is an individual's level of coping within his or her "own boundaries." These boundaries, which enclose what is most important to each individual, may be narrow for some and broad for others. That is, "one need not necessarily feel that all of life is highly comprehensible, manageable, and meaningful in order to have a strong 'sense of coherence,'" but those with this sense will be better able to cope and to experience "behavioral immunology," and to experience mental well-being.[44-47]

Some psychologists have pursued the study of mental well-being, particularly focusing on specific attributes and measuring satisfaction in various aspects of life.[48-50] Social psychologists—Strack, Argyle, and Schartz, for example—equate the concept of mental well-being with happiness.[51] Maslow, whose work based on the study of

Antonovsky defines a "sense of coherence" as:

A global orientation that expresses the extent to which one has a pervasive, enduring though dynamic feeling of confidence that (1) the stimuli deriving from one's internal and external environments in the course of living are structured, predictable, and explicit; (2) the resourses are available to meet the demands posed by these stimuli; and (3) these demands are challenges, worthy of investment and engagement.

Antonovsky A. The sense of coherence as a determinant of health. In: Matarazzo JD, Weiss SM, Herd JA, et al, eds. *Behavioral Health. A Handbook of Health Enhancement and Disease Prevention.* New York, NY: John Wiley and Sons; 1990.

people he considered mentally healthy has already been noted, is discussed in most books addressing the subject of mental well-being. He regards it as "full humanness," which he describes as the highest level of personal development enabling individuals to recognize their potentials and life roles and to fully use their personal strengths, without selfishness.[52] Maslow stands in a tradition of humanist psychology, based on existentialism,[53] which extends from Burnham's "wholesome personality"[54] through Fromm's "productive character"[55] to Rogers' descriptions of the "fully functioning person."[56] This humanist tradition can be said to stem from the "mental hygiene movement," founded in America in 1909, which was influential in the growth and development of mental health services of the first half of the century, including the birth of occupational therapy. The rhetoric of this approach became "equated with productiveness, social adjustment, and contentment—'the good life' itself."[57] In turn, the "mental hygiene movement" can be seen to uphold the Renaissance tradition of human achievement and the ideals of the "age of enlightenment." However, humanists have not, in a real sense, sought to integrate their perspective of mental well-being with physical and social well-being. Taken to extremes, that is, considering "achievement of one's goals" as the criterion for health is as focused and narrow as a biomechanical approach to health, which only considers physical factors. Despite this criticism, Boddy, a nurse educator, commends the approach as being "one of the few models that acknowledges the individuality of people and their creativity in defining their goals."[58] The central concept of these approaches, that well-being depends upon the meeting of individual potential, is also central to the theory of humans as occupational beings.

Occupationally, mental well-being embraces the belief that the potential range of individuals' occupations will allow each of them to be creative and adventurous as they experience all human emotions, explore and adapt appropriately, and without undue disruption meet their life needs. If mental well-being is to be attained, occupations need to provide self-esteem, motivation, socialization, meaning, and purpose as well as sufficient intellectual challenge to stimulate neuronal physiology and encourage efficient or enhanced problem-solving, sensory integration, perception, attention, concentration, reflection, language, and memory.[59,60] Additionally, a balance of occupations between intellectual challenges, spiritual experiences, emotional highs and lows, and relaxation is required. This does not imply constant high-powered mental "doing" or "feeling," rather that this should be interwoven with time for simply "being" or "becoming."[61] Mental well-being will be enhanced if people choose their occupations so that they are able to develop spiritual, cognitive, and emotive capacities; to experience timelessness and "higher-order meaning"[62]; and to adjust their activities to achieve a balanced combination of mental, physical, and social use.

Social Well-Being

Many of the characteristics of mental well-being include aspects of social interactions and relationships, which leads naturally to the consideration of social well-being. Nutbeam suggests that well-being in its entirety belongs within the broad context of the social model of health, as he considers its focus is on "social integration," "social support," and "social coherence for belonging."[2] This suggests that physical and mental well-being are dependent on the co-existence of social well-being.[63] Social well-being is usually described as resulting from satisfying interpersonal relationships, which depend on the ability to interact happily and effectively with people, within cultural and social parameters, without fear to challenge or develop ideas deemed of benefit to society. Social ease is acquired and often associated with socially sanctioned (moral) and respected occupational behavior.

The previous chapter showed that throughout time, people have displayed a need to be part of a cooperative social group. Some theorists even argue that there is a correlation between the size of the neocortex and the size of social groups among primates, humans having the largest brain relative to size and the largest and most complex societies.[64] It is, therefore, hardly surprising that reports of well-being are often associated with social interactions, as was found in the study reported earlier in the chapter. Some other empirical research supports this association. Argyle's study of the psychology of happiness reports several social factors that have been linked with health. He found that relationships, such as marriage and other close, confiding, and supportive relationships, enhance health by both preserving the immune system and encouraging good health habits.[10] He also reports that socially valued activities, including paid employment (if it is satisfying) and religion, appear to have a positive correlation with both health and happiness. Blaxter's findings also support this view, in that "not only socioeconomic circumstances and the external environment, but also the individual's psychosocial environment carry rather more weight, as determinants of health, than healthy or unhealthy behaviors."[5]

From the occupational perspective held here, social well-being occurs when the range of each individual's occupations and roles enables maintenance and development of satisfying and stimulating social relationships between family members, with associates, and within the community in which they live, and when engagement in occupation is balanced between social situations and time for quiet and reflection. Occupations that will have most obvious effects on health are those that are socially sanctioned, approved, and valued, even if only by a subculture with which people choose to associate and that endows individuals with social status enabling them freedom to effectively use physical and mental capacities in combination with social activity.[65] Doyal and Gough go so far as to suggest that "to be denied the capacity for potentially successful social participation is to be denied one's humanity."[66] Social well-being will be enhanced if people are able to develop their potential through practice in a range of socially valued occupations and to balance their social health needs because of increased awareness of the relationship of social activity and health.

Well-Being and Incapacity

With these ideas in mind, it becomes necessary to ask if health and well-being are possible despite some incapacity. One obvious answer is that, because no two individuals will possess the same range of capacities nor have the same experiences that impact upon their growth, in a sense, anyone can be seen as incapacitated to some extent. Some people can sing, others are tone deaf; some are athletic, others are clumsy. Such capacities endowed from birth, or the lack of them, are generally accepted as within the normal range of human differences, yet when these relate to a fundamental capacity, such as bipedalism, vision, intellect, or fluid movement, or when such capacity is lost in later life, individuals so afflicted are described by others as incapacitated or disabled and are frequently classified as unhealthy.

In this theory, it is argued that people can experience health and well-being without use of all possible capacities, and that this is the norm. The arguments already cited concerning individual differences provide empirical evidence of the truth of this claim. At a 1991 seminar on stroke held in New Zealand, opinions about the potential for people to experience health and well-being following stroke were canvassed. Most of those who had had a stroke, and their relatives and caregivers, agreed it is possible for people following stroke, with subsequent loss of capacity, to experience health and well-being, but not all health workers agreed. In fact, during the seminar, one physician expressed very vehemently his opinion that any person with hemiplegia could not be considered healthy.[67]

Well-Being, Occupation, Brain, and Mind

Physical, mental, and social well-being cannot easily be separated. They are part of an integrated system that warns, maintains, and rewards through people's awareness of how they feel. This will be discussed in greater detail later in the chapter. Yet, much of our health care system focuses on one or other aspects of these, usually according to which one is seen as dysfunctional, which one is diseased. This has led to recent health and wellness initiatives concentrating on particular aspects of fitness for their own sake and failing to make use of the potential health-giving properties to be found in everyday engagement in life's occupations. Contrasting markedly with initiatives of that type, occupational therapists have focused to a great extent on the integration of physiological, psychological, and social well-being, "doing" and brain/body functioning. For example, 15 occupational therapists who were the total population of attendees at a seminar were each asked to record eight immediate responses to the question "What is the relationship between health and occupation?" The responses were categorized and eight definite themes emerged that demonstrate their viewpoint. They are mental, physical, social, function, brain/body, quality of life, nature of the relationship, and environment (Table 5-2).

Similar integrative notions of health have been the subject of study from a variety of perspectives, but despite popular and scientific interest, neither these nor occupational therapists' concepts have been well-integrated into mainstream health care practices.[68-72]

One of the similar concepts, proposed by Ornstein and Sobel, that the principal function of the human brain is to maintain health, was introduced in Chapter 2. They claim that their view, which appears more logical than some of the lofty purposes attributed to the brain by those seeking to differentiate humans from their animal heritage, has largely "escaped the attention of the mainstream of medical practice and

Category	Frequency	Key Words (Common Responses)
Mental	28.5%	Self-esteem, motivation, meaning, satisfaction, purpose, concentration
Function	16.0%	Goal-directed, skills, talents, opportunities, competence
Physical	13.5%	Energy, strength, exercise, tone, cardiovascular fitness
Social	12.5%	Role, status, relationships, value
Brain/Body	10.0%	Balance, growth, unity, capacity
Quality of Life	7.0%	Quality of life, well-being, positive
Nature of Relationship	6.0%	Direct, inseparable, complementary, interdependent
Environment	2.5%	Adaptation, ecological, global
Other	4.0%	Hard to define, occupational therapy

Table 5-2. Occupational Therapists' View of Relationship Between Occupation and Health.

psychological thought." Medicine, they suggest, has largely regarded "the body as a mindless machine," and psychology has been restricted by "a view that the main purpose of the human brain was to produce rational thought. Never mind that the...neuron [does] not for the most part, serve thought or reason."[73] This idea is a recent contribution to the study of the mind, which has occupied the attention of philosophers, psychologists, medical scientists, and many others, probably for as long as humans have had the capacity for abstract thought. A brief diversion to review the changing concepts held about the mind is warranted to illustrate how concepts of health and well-being can change according to dominant views of societies and how occupational development influences concept formation.

"Mind" is derived from the old German word "gamundi" meaning to think, remember, intend, but in Classical Greece, the concept of mind was interwoven with concepts about the soul and spirit[74] with Plato proposing that the "mind is the attribute of the gods and of very few men" and that it is "separate and independent of the body."[75] Aristotle, however, viewed the soul as inseparable from the body and "the mind...(the thinking soul)...an independent substance implanted within the soul...incapable of being destroyed."[76] The evolution of the ideas about the relationship between body, brain, soul, and mind tends to reflect the occupational contexts of the age in which they were made. It is possible to speculate that a holistic view of the relationship was held by early humans who, because of their close relationship with the land and other living things, did not seek to distinguish special characteristics of the species. Rose argues that in medieval times in a world in which it was believed "the stars and planets were fixed to revolving glass spheres drawn by angel power, the body was the natural home of the soul and there was no incompatibility between them." Following discoveries that demystified the universe, such as those of Copernicus, Galileo, and Newton, Descartes reconciled his own mechanistic view with Catholic rhetoric. He separated the soul or mind (which he placed in the pineal gland) from the body and brain (which he viewed as operating as a "sort of hydraulic system") proposing that, theoretically, minds and souls can exist apart from the body and can withstand its corruption and death.[77] This Cartesian dualism has dominated ideas throughout the recent evolution of explanations of the relationships between body, brain, soul, and mind.[78] These explanations have been progressively expressed in terms of clockwork models, electrical and magnetic models, phrenology, telephone and factory management models to cybernetic and computer-based models.[77] Although integrated systems theories predominate today, the effects of dualism remain with disorders of mind and body being treated by different medical specialists in different locations, and the alleviation of social and ecological disorders being the province of totally separate agencies. Dualism is contrary to the holistic notion of health and occupation resulting from all parts of brain and body working in harmony with the environment.

Community and Ecological Well-Being

From the holistic point of view of the theory discussed in this book, the previous division of physical, mental, and social well-being was for the purpose of discussion only. So, too, is the fact that well-being was considered only from an individualistic perspective. Within capitalist societies, it is easy to disregard broader concepts of health that relate to families, communities, and to the ecology. Some other societies, such as the Australian Aboriginals, place more value on kin and community than individuality. This value is reflected in the way in which the Australian Aboriginal Health Organization defines health as referring to:

> *The social, emotional, spiritual, and cultural well-being of the whole community. Health services should strive to achieve that state where every individual can achieve their full potential as human beings (Aboriginals) and thus bring about total well-being of their community as a whole.*[79]

This might remind people from cultures dominated by individualistic values that such values are closely associated with materialism and are fairly recent.[80] Communities were originally a source of protection and succor to individuals and were small enough to reflect their basic needs but, because of their protective function, the good of "tribe" was seen as of more importance than individual survival. In societies in which individual goals and needs have assumed dominance over communal need, people commonly talk, with some degree of regret, about loss of community spirit, yet still seek to influence the way of life of other existing cultures who hold to community and extended family values much more in tune with the ecology. Indeed, people from post-industrial societies are so imbued with the values of material, technological, and economic growth and have given such "prominence to our separate nature that we have become alienated from the most fundamental truth of our nature, our spiritual oneness with the living universe," and our dependence on maintaining its physical health.[81,82]

My occupational view of health encompasses the relationship between all life from cellular to global factors, from biological to sociocultural, and microscopic to macroscopic levels. For example, human occupational behavior affects health and well-being on an individual basis through the integrative systems of the organism; on a social level through shared activity, the continuous growth of occupational technology and sociopolitical activity; and on a global level through occupational development affecting the natural resources and ecosystems. Any or all of these can have negative or positive effects on health, and all are inextricably linked. This implies that practitioners focusing on promoting the health-giving relationship of occupation cannot do so only at an individual level. All levels have to be considered or explored by focusing on education, behavioral, social, and environmental issues.

Holism

Widening the idea of health to include individual, community, and ecological well-being brings theories such as "holism" and "general systems theory" into consideration. Holism, from the Greek "holos" meaning whole, was first used by Smuts in 1928 to describe philosophies that considered whole systems rather than parts of systems (reductionism).[83,84]

Jan Christiaan Smuts (1870-1950) was a South African politician and military leader with anti-republican, anti-racist ideals, who helped found the United Nations. Between 1924 and 1933 when he was out of office he elaborated on his philosophy of holism and published *Holism and Evolution* in 1928.

Smuts observed "a basic tendency of nature and evolution to produce novel, irreducible wholes," and that living systems are more than the sum of their parts.[85] Also subscribing to this view, von Bertalanffy, who sought to discover general patterns, trends, and structures in natural, social, and technological systems, developed "general systems theory,"[86] which proved to be "a major source of impetus toward a more holistic approach" in the biological sciences and health care, including occupational therapy.[87] The view that people are more than a collection of cells, tissues, and organ systems encourages the study of health based on the integrated nature of human beings as part of their sociocultural and natural environment and draws on systems theory for its explanations.[88] In some ways, this may be considered a return to older values when it is appreciated that the word "health" is derived from the old English "haelth" from "hal" meaning whole.[89] Current dictionaries give wholeness as one of the synonyms of health,[90] so that the need to talk about holistic health is perhaps evidence of the term health having come to mean "something less than wholeness."[58] The concentration on reductionist research in the 20th century has, however, provided evidence that has enabled people to recognize the holistic nature of living systems.

Although holism was first mooted, in this century, in the 1920s, it did not gain prominence in the health debate until interest in alternative lifestyles and approaches to improve health and quality of life escalated from the early 1960s in many parts of the world. Many of those adopting alternative lifestyles rejected, to some extent, Western cultures in favor of Eastern philosophies and religions, particularly those such as Hinduism, which embodies "oneness with the universe."[58] However, holistic health labels have been applied to many approaches and disciplines, from which Kopelman and Moskop have identified five major common characteristics[85]:

1. Health being viewed from a positive perspective
2. The use of natural rather than invasive or high-technology solutions in the management of ill health
3. Self-responsibility for health, rather than professional responsibility
4. Professional responsibility should focus on health education
5. Change of emphasis within health services toward behavioral, social, and environmental issues

These characteristics do not appear to differ in any great degree from ideas central in the Ottawa Charter for Health Promotion. This states that "health is a positive concept," that "health promotion supports personal and social development through providing information, education for health and enhancing life skills" to enable people to "keep themselves, their families, and friends healthy," and that health services should be reoriented "toward the promotion of health."[91] Perhaps the similarities are merely figures of speech, as it can be argued that few health services or resource allocations for health purposes have been shifted in a holistic direction. The rhetoric may, in fact, be being used by health authorities to counter the criticisms leveled at the pragmatic technological approach of medical scientists. Lack of action in reorienting services toward holistic approaches may be due, in part, to the lack of empirical research supporting their benefits or because of the impossibility of comprehending the whole of the biological mechanism, even if all its elements were known.[82] Boddy suggests that exponents of holism have failed to justify much of its logic and need to take a more critical approach, similar to that expected of Western medical science. Within the holistic health movement, there is a common, unwritten assumption that health defined in holistic terms is good per se. She argues that if health is regarded as a "sufficient goal in its own right, (and as) the highest good rather than a means to achievement of some other higher good," then the active pursuit of health should be the primary goal of us all. Such a direction could be as limiting as a "biomechanical" or an "achievement of goals" model of health.[58]

Ottawa Charter for Health Promotion

It is important to consider further the Ottawa Charter for Health Promotion because this document is a primary source of contemporary health promotion directions. The Charter was developed and adopted by delegates from, mainly, post-industrial societies, representing 38 countries at the first international conference on health promotion jointly organized by Canadian and World Health Organizations. It proposes that action is required in five major directions:

1. Building healthy public policy
2. Creating supportive environments
3. Strengthening community action
4. Developing personal skills
5. Reorienting health services beyond the provision of clinical and curative services toward the pursuit of health

The Charter, which can be seen as developing the WHO definition and the ideas embodied in the Declaration of Alma Ata,[92] has been influenced by the concepts and views propounded by social health activists of the past 20 years. The Charter is holistic in its intent as it recognizes "the inextricable links between people and their environment [which] constitute the basis for a socioecological approach to health." It argues for:

> *The conservation of natural resources throughout the world, ...the need to encourage reciprocal maintenance, to take care of each other, our communities, and our natural environment...[so] that the society one lives in creates conditions that allow the attainment of health by all its members.*

It also calls for a commitment to "address the overall ecological issue of our way of living" and to "counteract the pressures toward harmful products, resource depletion, unhealthy living conditions, and environments." In acknowledging that urgent consideration needs to be given to factors detrimental to the natural and social environment, the Charter can be seen to recognize the adverse results of many current occupational structures and technology. However, it also recognizes the benefits of occupation. Although not formally acknowledged within the document, its "occupational" emphasis recognizes that what people do affects their health. Health, it is stated, "cannot be separated from other goals" because it "is created and lived by people within the settings of their everyday life; where they learn, work, play, and love." The Charter encourages communities and individuals to participate actively in life by the prescription that "to reach a state of complete physical, mental, and social well-being, an individual or group must be able to identify and to realize aspirations, to satisfy needs, and to change or cope with the environment."[93]

This encapsulates a theme central to the argument of this chapter, that there are primary links between health and occupation; that occupation is the fundamental mechanism by which people realize aspirations, satisfy needs, and cope with the environment; and that engagement in occupation to meet needs and aspirations provides the mechanism for the maintenance and growth of physical, mental, and social capacities. These are central to health. To utilize this mechanism effectively, humans need to develop or maintain natural and social environments in which the species will be able to sustain life and that provide sufficient challenge to exercise individuals' capacities and community potential. By this means, individuals and the species will flourish as an integrated part of the ecology.

Defining Health from an Occupational Perspective

Following this review of ideas about health and well-being, holism, and WHO directives toward health promotion from an occupational point of view, it is possible to summarize what is meant by health in this theory as:

- The absence of illness, but not necessarily disability
- A balance of physical, mental, and social well-being attained through socially valued and individually meaningful occupation
- Enhancement of capacities and opportunity to strive for individual potential
- Community cohesion and opportunity
- Social integration, support, and justice, all within and as part of a sustainable ecology

Health and Occupation for Hunter-Gatherers

Having established what I mean by health, the next section of this chapter explores, from this conception, the occupational behaviors of hunter-gatherers and views about the health-enhancing consequences of natural lifestyles. It does so in the belief that the basic biological health mechanisms of early humans will have been largely unaffected by culturally acquired knowledge, values, and behavior and that examination of their health will sustain the view that engagement in naturally driven occupation can be health promoting. This will be considered along with early hunter-gatherers' likely experience of morbidity and mortality.

In previous chapters, it has been argued that within hunter-gatherer cultures provision to meet the needs of sustenance, self-care, shelter, safety, self-esteem, and life satisfaction was similar for the total population. All able-bodied people were involved first-hand in occupations concerned with the getting and preparing of food and water, with finding or devising adequate shelter for safety and temperature control, and with the care and education of offspring. Few would have suffered the fate, or enjoyed the privilege, of not being able or eligible (for whatever reason) to participate in providing for themselves and others. Occupations were communal with on-the-job training and only limited division of labor. Such simple occupational structures did not obscure innate physiological needs, but catered for them.

Unlike many other animals, humans "exploit almost every link in the food chain," a characteristic that supported flexibility of habitat and provided motivation for hunter-gatherer peoples to move from "one resource to another."[94] Such a nomadic lifestyle assisted physical fitness, reduced the probability of illness due to unhygienic waste disposal, provided adventure, prevented boredom, and promoted bonding with fellow nomads. In common with other nomadic peoples, the Australian Aboriginals' "practice of moving camp as they journeyed throughout the tribal land ensured that many of the health problems associated with permanent settlement sites could not develop" is a case in point.[95] Indeed, the daily occupations of hunter-gatherers provided them with the type of exercise now being rediscovered as advantageous to cardiovascular fitness and tacked on to today's occupations, as well as providing opportunity to think ahead, plan, and use ingenuity and creativity to furnish their personal, kin, and community requirements. Communities were small enough not to require restrictive rules and regulations and probably, more so than in later occupational eras, the groups who lived together on a regular basis were stable and supportive. Survival would often have depended on the strength created by a cohesive group in combined activity. In fact, because of the constraints imposed by a nomadic way of life, the people making up each social "band" constituted the movable assets of the group, that is, the people rather than material assets were valued as central to survival. This would have influenced the development of a communal rather than an individual view of the world and of health.

Obligatory occupations, and many others of a creative, spiritual, or playful kind, were carried out as an integral part of the day-to-day business of wresting a living from nature. Hunter-gatherers were constrained to balance physical exertion with sedentary and rest occupations because, at least until they learned to create and control fire to their advantage, they would have been diurnal, so following basic circadian patterns of sleeping and waking. Additionally, and as noted in an earlier chapter, contrary to popular belief, the obligatory occupations of providing for immediate needs was not as time-consuming as the modern 8-hour day.

The development of individual potential by participation in occupations, many of which were directly related to maintenance of the organism and survival of individuals, their communities, and the species, was ensured by the development of a technology that was in tune with the natural world. Many consider that the occupational pursuits of the hunter-gatherer era generally would not have disturbed the environmental balance. At least, as Lorenz suggests, human hunter-gatherer cultures "influence their biotope in a way no different from that of animal populations."[96] Further, despite his suspicion that prehistoric people had the same characteristic need as modern humans to "overexploit every resource they can lay their hands on," Bill Stephenson, professor of zoology at Queensland University, observes that the Australian Aboriginals do not appear to have done so, perhaps because their long, isolated occupancy of Australia produced "a stable relationship between man and his resources."[94] King-Boyes agrees that "in full tribal life, the Aborigines presented an excellent example of a society working in rhythm with its environment."[95] This type of lifestyle, which was followed for probably at least 2 million years, provided a real test of the effectiveness of engagement in occupations to sustain health and well-being of people and the ecology.

There have been many speculations and comments about the health status of early humans from a rich variety of sources. Stephenson in *The Ecological Development of Man* observes "we know that people living a culturally primitive life (with less medical care) are generally more physically perfect than those from affluent societies,"[94] and McNeill in *Plagues and People* supposes that "ancient hunters of the temperate zone were most probably healthy folk" despite short lifespans compared with modern humans.[97] Such views are supported by reports from explorers in their initial contacts with people of primitive cultures, which suggest that they appeared both happy and healthy. For example, Nicholas Tunnes observed in 1656 that Eskimos in West Greenland who directed "all their efforts...toward acquiring, without too much trouble, what is absolutely necessary in the way of clothing and food" believed themselves "happy" and "favored,"[98,99] and Captain James Cook recorded in his journal (1768-1771) that he found the natives of the Pacific Islands he visited, happy, healthy, and full of vigor. Of the Australian Aboriginals, he wrote "they are far happier than we Europeans, ...they live in tranquility," and "they think themselves provided with all the necessarys of life, and that they have no superfluities."[100] It was, of course, a popular opinion at the time of Cook's voyages that "a state of nature" was the ideal state to create health and happiness, based on Rousseau's 1755 theories of man as a noble savage corrupted by civilization.[101] These theories were so popular, Dubos observes, that they "fostered an intellectual climate" that influenced philosophers of the "age of reason" and "practical sanitarians," contributing eventually to social reforms and improvement in health.[102] For example, Thomas Beddoes, British poet-physician, hypothesized that the blessed original state of health could only be recaptured by abiding by the simple order and purity of nature.[103] Julien Joseph Virey, the 19th century French physician-philosopher, asserted in *L'Hygiene Philosophique* that humans in a state of nature are endowed with an instinct for health that permits biological adaptation and that civilized humans have lost,[104] and Edward Jenner observed that "the deviation of Man from the state in which he was originally placed by Nature seems to have proved to him a prolific source of disease."[105]

Earlier Oriental examples demonstrate that Rousseau's theory was not original. In *The Yellow Emperor's Classic of Internal Medicine*, published in China in the 4th century BC, it was supposed that in the remote past "people lived to 100 years, and yet remained active and did not become decrepit in their activities."[106] Similarly Lao-tzu and Chuang-tzu eulogize about a golden age, the latter suggesting that when "the ancient men lived in a world of primitive simplicity...was a time when the yin and the yang worked harmoniously, ...all creation was unharmed, and the people did not die young."[107] Pao Ching-yen, at a later date, observed "Man in the morning went forth to his labor on his own accord and rested in the evening. People were free and uninhibited and at peace...Contagious diseases did not spread, and long life was followed by natural death."[108]

Despite these supposed advantages of the lifestyle, a high level of mortality at all ages is believed to have been the common experience containing the human population at the level at which their interaction with ecology could be maintained. Those who survived and procreated were those most able to live and adapt effectively to life's demands and, in fact, could be designated healthy. In this way, Coon observed

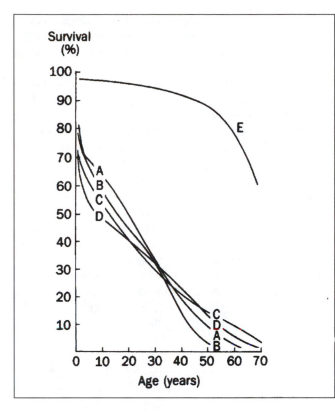

Figure 5-2. Mortality patterns of hunter-gatherer populations. A) Cariston-Annis, Kentucky [4000-2500 BC], 22.4 years; B) Libben, Ohio [750-1000 AD], 19.9 years; C) Yanomami, males only, 21.5 years; and D) "Maghreb"-Afaslou-bou-Rhummel and Taforalt, North Africa [10,000 years ago], 21.1 years. Curve E shows the survival profile of a modern post-industrial population—the United States in 1960. The average life expectancy of the recent US population of nearly 70 years contrasts sharply with the values for the other populations. From Meindel RS. Human populations before agriculture. In: Jones S, Martin R, Pilbeam D, eds. *The Cambridge Encyclopedia of Human Evolution.* New York, NY: Cambridge University Press; 1992:408. Reprinted with the permission of Cambridge University Press.

"natural selection is not thwarted, and in their breeding populations they do not build up increasing loads of disabling genes."[109] See Figure 5-2 for an illustration of mortality patterns of hunter-gatherer populations.

Early mortality and morbidity resulted from ecological forces acting on the population, for example, "parasites with high transmission rates and little or no induced immunity," such as worms, lice, and ticks, pathogens such as salmonella and trypanosoma (sleeping sickness), climate ("older people suffer gradual loss of the ability to buffer temperature extremes"[110]), and availability of food and water. "Occupational" accidents, aggression, and infanticide are also suggested causes.[111]

Such demographic and epidemiologic deductions do not contradict the claims that hunter-gatherers experienced general well-being, but rather, in common with modern humans they experienced ill health and accidents, the different nature of which, coupled with lack of specialist knowledge, led to early death for many of the population. Also, these deductions do not negate the notion that occupation, survival, and health are inextricably linked. In fact, they support this notion. Because of their occupational nature and potential, humans were able to strive to improve these survival odds and decrease the experience of ill health. Their technology, in the main, addressed the potential risk factors of a world in which people are not the fastest, strongest, largest, or best camouflaged of animals. Much has been written about "fight or flight" behavior and its appropriateness for the natural dangers facing early humans since Walter Cannon's description in the 1920s of the single automatic pattern of response of the organism to any challenge to equilibrium.[112] However appropriate, the response would have been unpleasant to experience and provided strong motivation to develop artifacts and social structures to overcome fear-producing situations. Social cohesion and education were used by hunter-gatherers, along with tool technology, as vehicles to improve superiority over prey and predators in the long-term. Survival pressures provided meaning, motivation, and opportunity for engagement in a variety of individual and community occupations that addressed the obvious health risks of the day. In pursuit of this, hunter-gatherers developed capacities, talents, and potentials and a satisfying balance of physical, mental, and social exercise with rest in tune with nature that, at the same time, promoted their health and well-being.

It is not known whether early humans made any conscious efforts to maintain health and prevent illness apart from shelter, sustenance, and the seeking out of substances they instinctively craved when sick, in a way similar to other animals.[113] Stephenson has suggested that the "animal" ability of primitive humans developed into a common sense approach to health and illness and "that with his omnivorous feeding habits and experimental frame of mind, primitive man established the curative values of a wide range of plant products, many of which are still in medicinal use."[94] King-Boyes notes of Australian Aboriginals that "many records exist of the remarkable healing capacity exhibited by their bodies subsequent to injury; and the knowledge of homeopathic medicine held by the women was considerable." These practices co-existed with the use of shamans at times of ill health, but without the expectation that "good health" was "an inalienable right of life."[95]

Views of Health and Healing

At least from the time of recorded history, humans appear to have valued healing science more than naturally healthy living. Dubos cites the history of the Greek gods Hygeia and Asclepius as symbolizing the never-ending oscillation between these different points of view. Hygeia was the goddess who once watched over the health of Athens. She symbolized the "virtues of a sane life in a pleasant environment" and probably personified reason. She was not involved in the treatment of the sick, but was closely associated with mental health. For followers of Hygeia, health was the natural order of things: they saw the most important function of medicine as the discovery and teaching of natural laws, which ensured health of mind and body. From the 5th century BC on, her cult progressively gave way to the god of healing, Asclepius, who before his creation as a deity lived as a physician in the 12th century BC. Followers of Asclepius believe that the chief role of medicine is to treat disease. In mythology, Hygeia became relegated to being either a member of his retinue, or his daughter, along with Panakeia. In most histories of medicine, she is mentioned briefly as subservient to Asclepius. Hippocrates attempted to marry the approaches of Asclepius and Hygeia, providing students of public health with a classical philosophy about the relationship between external and internal determinants of health. He observed that a physician "was to be skilled in Nature and must strive to know what man is in relation to food, drink, occupation, and which effect each of these has on the other."[102]

Medical science is dominant in current thinking about health, and it is medical experts who, on the whole, define for the general public what health is. Yet, it could be said that the meeting of biological needs, "with the weapons of Hygeia," seems to have little in common with modern medicine. Medicine's interest in healing may account for the large number of people who do equate health with the absence of illness. In fact, whether people can achieve health through meeting "natural laws which ensure health of mind and body" is, in many respects, socioculturally determined. Cultures and societies provide the occupational structure and value systems that determine which, how, and why particular needs can be met.

Yet, from "ancient times, the theory that most of the ills of mankind arise from failure to follow the laws of nature" has been reasserted time and time again.[102] Ideas and health practices purported to be based on natural lifestyles have resurfaced in this century with the countercultural movements of the 1960s, the growth of holistic and natural health approaches, the ecological "greenies" of the present time, and in this theory. While it is beyond the bounds of practicability to suggest that post-industrial societies should return to a "natural" lifestyle based on hunter-gatherer occupations in the cause of health and happiness, the repeated interest in the topic suggests that keeping in touch with humans' innate needs as evidenced by their early behaviors is important in refocusing attention on matters relating to healthy survival of the species.

Biological Needs: A Mechanism for Health

Biological mechanisms aimed at ensuring survival and health are basic to all animals, and adaptation occurs in response to long-term environmental conditions during a period of change. Such adaptations are not necessarily fitted to healthy living in future environments and, as some basic biological needs of humans are now obscured by millions of years of acquired values, present-day health awareness may not reflect needs that were, and probably still are, fundamental to healthy survival.

Health and well-being will now be considered by exploring the biologically based needs responsible for their maintenance through occupation. But, first, it is necessary to discuss the concept of biological needs, because, on the whole, and in a way similar to "instincts," the study of biological needs has been neglected of late. Perhaps the human quest for the new and different is partly to blame for this. As Allport remarked on fashion in scientific inquiry, "we never seem to solve our problems or exhaust our concepts; we only grow tired of them."[114] Alternatively, the false dichotomy between disciplines concerned with the long-running nature versus nurture debate and the recent emphasis on nurture may have resulted in need being more commonly explored from a sociocultural perspective.

The Concept of Needs and Drives

There are, however, numerous need theories that attempt to identify from a "natural" perspective what motivates human behavior.[115-122] Doyal and Gough, in *A Theory of Human Need*, recently called in question fashionable subjective and relativist approaches, arguing that health and autonomy are basic needs, the meeting of which are essential preconditions for participation in social life.[66] (There are some similarities between the model Doyal and Gough propose and my own. One basic difference is that while I conceptualize a needs theory in terms of positive health and well-being, they argue from a negative health perspective.) Doyal and Gough recognize biologi-

> *[We] define and measure physical health negatively as the minimalization of death, disability, and disease...and...autonomy negatively as the minimalization of mental disorder, cognitive deprivation, and restricted opportunities [considering] that these two negatives make a positive.*
> Doyal L, Gough I. *A Theory of Human Need*. Houndmills, Hampshire: Macmillan; 1991.

cal motivations or drives, but they separate from these their discourse of "universal needs" founded on human reason. Part of their stated reason for this separation is that physiological drives and needs can result from external sources, as in the case of someone who takes drugs "needing" a fix. In such cases this is obviously not a universal need, but an abnormal one.[66]

Maslow's "needs hierarchy theory" is probably the best known and most widely used needs theory, particularly in health texts. It is founded on the premise that individuals have innate needs that act as motivating forces.[122] He identified five basic need levels related to one another in a prepotent hierarchy. At the first level are needs, such as for food, which relate to the physiological function of the human organism, followed progressively by needs for safety and security, then belonging, love, and social activity, with the need for esteem and respect at the fourth level, and at the top of the hierarchy, self-actualization. The process of self-actualizing he saw as the "development of the biologically based nature of man, [empirically] normative of the whole species conforming to biological destiny, rather than to historically arbitrary, culturally local value models as the terms 'health' and 'illness' often do."[23] His theory is that more basic needs must be largely, but not necessarily completely, satisfied before higher level needs are activated and motivating. A similar three-level hierarchy proposed by Alderfer identifies existence, relatedness, and growth (ERG) as the need levels.[121]

Both Maslow's and Alderfer's theories are compatible with notions about innate "drives" common in psychology for the greater part of the century, but in disuse at present. Based on physiological discoveries, such as those pertaining to homeostasis, "drives" were seen as persistent motivations, organic in origin, which "arouse, sustain, and regulate human and animal behavior" and are distinct from external determinants of behavior, such as "social goals, interests, values, attitudes, and personality traits."[123] Dashiell, in *Fundamentals of Objective Psychology,* illustrated this view:

> *The primary drives to persistent forms of animal and human conduct are tissue conditions within the organism giving rise to stimulations exciting the organism to overt activity. A man's interest and desires may become ever so elaborate, refined, socialized, sublimated, idealistic, but the raw basis from which they are developed is found in the phenomena of living matter.[124]*

Eysenck, Arnold, and Meili, in the *Encyclopedia of Psychology,* report that the word "need," meaning a "central motivating variable," made its debut into academic psychology in the early 1930s. The concept of need, they say, eventually replaced the notion of instinct but, unlike instinct, an innate need, though undeniably goal-oriented, does not have a "repertoire of inherited, unlearned action patterns."[125] Snell bemoans the fact that "the term instinct has gone out of fashion," but thinks it "tempting to revive the term and to say we can now relate instinct to detailed brain structure."[126] In accord with this, Lorenz observes that although humans lack "long, self-contained chains of innate behavior patterns," they have more "genuinely instinctive impulses than any other animal."[96] These "instinctive impulses" are close to what I am terming the experience of "biological need."

Need is described in the *Dictionary of Behavioral Science* as "the condition of lacking, wanting, or requiring something which if present would benefit the organism by facilitating behavior or satisfying a tension" and also as "a construct representing a force in the brain which directs and organizes the individual's perception, thinking, and action, so as to change an existing, unsatisfying situation."[127] (It is interesting to note that almost all of the material about biological needs is found in psychological

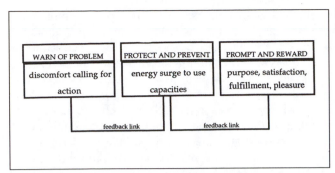

Figure 5-3. Needs: three-way role in health.

and social science texts before 1980. This is reflected in the references used here.)

The word "need," despite diverse common, conceptual usage, is employed in this section of the text to describe the mechanism by which unconscious biological requirements are communicated to neuronal systems concerned in engagement with the external world or that alerts the conscious state to the existence of some kind of disequilibrium. This view conforms with the suggestion made by Anscombe that needs, which are a matter of objective fact, relate to what is required for living organisms—plants, animals, or humans—to fulfill potential and flourish.[128,129] Anscombe's ideas are infused with new life some 30 years later by Ornstein's and Sobel's account of how the brain makes "countless adjustments" to maintain stability between "social worlds, our mental and emotional lives, and our internal physiology," each neuron producing "hundreds of chemicals" that "for the most part" are responsible for "keeping the body out of trouble, from commonplace problems like not falling over or walking into a wall to the myriad of tasks involved in maintaining the stability and health of the organism."[73] From my viewpoint, biological needs are activated by this process, and positive health and well-being is experienced when conditions allow humans to flourish because they are able to meet their needs and potential, usually through occupation.

According to this view, biological needs are homeostatically valuable—inborn health agents that recognize the organism as a "whole in interaction with the environment" as part of an open system. They do not differentiate between physical, mental, or social issues in the way in which modern society and medical or psychological practice do, but work as part of "a flow of processes" within biological systems relating structures and function.[130] They are integral to the collaboration between biological rhythms and homeostasis.

Three-Way Role in Health

Needs, from a homeostatic perspective, have a three-way role in maintaining the stability and health of the organism through occupation prompted by a specific feeling experienced.[131] They serve to warn when a problem occurs, to protect and prevent potential disorder, and to prompt and reward use of capacities so that the organism will flourish and reach potential. These three categories of needs provide both motivation and feedback (Figure 5-3). Each of these categories will now be discussed briefly.

First, to warn and protect, needs are experienced as a form of discomfort that calls for some kind of action to satisfy or assuage the need. Examples of these experiences are pain, fatigue, hunger, cold, fear, boredom, tension, depression, anxiety, anger, or loneliness. Many studies have researched these experiences as separate emotions.[132-134] Csikszentmihalyi, who has spent much of his professional life using a variety of methods such as questionnaires, diaries, interviews, and an "experience sampling method" to research the effects of occupation on individuals,[135] uses the term "psychic entropy" to describe these states.[18] He sees them as an "integrated response to the self system," with a main goal to "ensure its own survival," a view also held in this theory. There is debate about whether actions provoked by such experiences can be considered purposive; indeed, not all occupational therapists concede that activity that has unconscious, rather than socially valued, purpose can be described as occupation. In psychology literature, it is in texts contemporary with those discussing "biological needs" and "drives" that we find general acceptance of the notion of innate, biologically driven activity. Rex and Margaret Knight's *A Modern Introduction to Psychology* is a case in point, which suggests that activities that do not involve purposive "foresight, distant ends" or even, in some cases, "ideas or images" should be described as "conative," after the work of McDougall.[136] McDougall, the most famous advocate of the Hormic school of psychology, argued that the conative and emotional aspects of innate tendencies incline humans to act or to experience an impulse toward action that is conducive to biological well-being.[116]

In the second category, which involves preventing disorder and prompting the use of capacities, needs are experienced in a positive sense, such as a need to spend extra energy, walk, explore, create, understand or make sense of, use ideas, express thoughts, talk, listen or look, meditate or worship, spend time alone or with others, and so on. This mechanism, in interaction with the first, acts to balance over- or underuse. If capacities are overused, people feel fatigue, stress, and burnout, which can lead to increased susceptibility to accident and illness. If capacities are underused, they will atrophy, cause disturbance to equilibrium, and produce a decline in health. The balanced exercise of personal capacities to enable maintenance and development of the organism is perhaps the most primary and least appreciated function of human occupation, although it has been commented on from time to time by well-respected authorities from health science disciplines. Notable examples from throughout this century, some authors of which have already been mentioned, are listed below in order to demonstrate the striking similarities of their ideas. In 1922, the psychiatrist Adolph Meyer proposed "It is the use that we make of ourselves that gives the ultimate stamp to our every organ."[137] In 1935, Carrel, in analogous comment, observed:

> It is a primary datum of observation that physiological and mental functions are improved by work. Also, that effort is indispensable to the optimum development of the individual. Like muscles and organs, intelligence and moral sense become atrophied for want of exercise...the physiological and mental progress of the individual depends on his functional activity and on all his efforts. We become adapted to the lack of use of our organic and mental systems by degenerating...In order to reach his optimum state, the human being must actualize all his potentialities.[138]

In 1955, Sigerist, the medical historian, commented:

> Work in itself is not harmful to health; it is, on the contrary, essential to its maintenance, because it determines the chief rhythm of our life, balances it, and gives meaning and significance. An organ that does not work atrophies and the mind that does not work becomes dumb.[113]

In 1968, the psychologist Maslow echoed these earlier thoughts in his observation that:

Capacities clamor to be used, and cease their clamor only when they are well used. That is capacities are also needs. Not only is it fun to use our capacities, but it is also necessary for growth. The unused skill or capacity or organ can become a disease center or else atrophy or disappear, thus diminishing the person.[23]

The third category of needs considered to be integral to the occupational nature of humans and their healthy survival are those that reward use of capacities, such as the need for meaning, purpose, satisfaction, fulfillment, happiness, and pleasure. Pleasure and happiness, including laughter, have been recognized as powerful human needs by many writers, from Aristotle 2,300 years ago to current writers, whose work is particularly relevant to an occupational perspective, such as Argyle, Ornstein and Sobel, and Csikszentmihalyi. They maintain that pleasure is biologically related to health promoting activity.[10,17,139-144] This does not mean that pleasure is the ultimate drive of humans, but rather that it forms an integral part of health maintenance. Also, picking up on some of Doyal's and Gough's concerns about needs and drives, Csikszentmihalyi notes that:

A self originally organized around the pleasure principle might end up by working against the genetic teleonomy whose cause it had originally espoused...When a physiological need (such as hunger or sexual indulgence) becomes a goal, it ceases to be under the exclusive control of its original genetic instructions and begins to follow the teleonomy of the self.[135]

That pleasure is indeed innate is supported by experiments carried out in the 1950s in which rats could self-deliver a stimulus to the hypothalamus and from which James Olds and Peter Milner discovered what has subsequently been called the "pleasure center." Since then, other areas of the limbic system have also been found to elicit a pleasure response. Similar experiments on humans from the 1960s have been reported from America, mostly on inmates of mental hospitals. The subjects' descriptions of the experiences were vague, but included terms such as "feeling good," which they apparently did experience, to the extent that they were prepared to self-stimulate several hundred shocks an hour.[77]

Together, the second and the third categories of needs serve to establish a sense of individual identity and autonomy, the latter being identified by Doyal and Gough as one of two universal needs, the other being physical health. In the negative terms of their concept, autonomy includes minimization of "mental illness, cognitive deprivation, and restricted opportunities."[66]

To test the proposal about biological needs having a three-way role in maintaining stability and health, first-year occupational therapy students, as part of a survey about health, occupation, and capacities, each administered a questionnaire to three acquaintances to ascertain whether they had experienced such needs. Approximately 150 subjects with ages ranging from 6 to 98 years (mean: 35 years) were questioned. Ninety-nine percent admitted they had experienced discomfort that called for action, and almost all of these had acted in some way to alleviate the discomfort. Ninety-nine percent admitted to experiencing a need to use their capacities in various ways. Of these, nearly all had responded to such needs. If they did not respond to this type of need, approximately 87% admitted to experiencing the type of discomfort described in the first category. Ninety-nine percent also agreed they had experienced a need for purpose, satisfaction, fulfillment, and pleasure, with 95% usually taking action in response to these needs. When subjects did not respond to these needs, approximately 87% agreed that this lack of response resulted in discomfort. Additionally, the majority of those surveyed reported that they consider the satisfaction of these three categories of needs affects their mental, physical, and social health in a positive way.

Non-Omnipotence

This brings us to discussion of how sociocultural influences fit into this scheme. Needs are not omnipotent, and even ultradian rhythms of sleepability or wakeability can be overridden by the cortex. (Ultradian rhythms are those with a frequency of less than 20 hours. The term was coined by Franz Halberg, a chronobiologist at the University of Minnesota.) That is, needs are subject to scrutiny of, and adaptation by, the highly developed cognitive and intellectual capacities of humans, so that "primitive instinctive energy can be directed from its natural goal toward alternative ends that are a greater value." It is this process of redirection that enables the "highest achievements of humanity."[136]

This capacity for redirection and adaptation differentiates between biological and non-biological needs and allows individuals to make choices according to the particular circumstances in which they find themselves, with the future in mind. In this way, all impulses concerned with state of mind or action, whether deriving from "phylogenic or from cultural sources...[are] a link in a well-ordered, harmonious working system and, as such, [are] indispensable."[96] Even political theorists such as Fromm, Marcuse, Bay, and Macpherson recognize that needs and wants differ, that needs are not dependent upon wants, and that cognitive and intellectual capacities not only formulate wants, they interpret needs.[145-151] The two work in partnership, needs identifying biological requirements, and wants, in many instances, formulating ways that individual biological requirements can be achieved.

Our intellectual and cognitive capacity, freed by the mechanism of choice, has enabled humans, despite diverse challenges, to satisfy, in large measure, the biological needs described earlier. In post-industrial countries, action to satisfy or assuage discomfort, such as food production, the regulation of temperature, and measures to reduce pain, have reached a level of sophistication far beyond the simple methods used by all other animals living in natural habitats. To prevent disorder, humans have developed ways of using their capacities in adaptive, inventive, and exploratory fashions to the extent that they can provide purpose, reward, and the pursuit of happiness. In fact, the biological mechanism of needs has focused human energies toward developing both occupations and sociocultural structures to meet those needs. Because of this, humans have been successful survivors—to the point of overpopulation—although the occupations and sociocultural structures, in some instances, while answering one need may defeat another. There are downsides to the mechanism of choice in that humans can "act in ways that [go] against the millenial wisdom that natural selection had built into the biological fabric of the species," as was discussed in the section on consciousness in Chapter 3.[135] Because of the capacity to ignore biological needs, people may develop sociopolitical structures or make lifestyle choices that result in detrimental health consequences. Clear examples of this are starvation diets aimed early in this century at women's suffrage or currently at a fashionable appearance, which may lead to conditions such as anorexia nervosa or to untimely death.

Unless asked to consider such factors, or some process or part of the mechanism goes amiss, people are not usually conscious of survival and health-maintaining functions. These, rather like the autonomic nervous system, are built into the organism to just go on working. Because of this, we are able to use our capacities for our own purposes, to explain the purpose of life in abstract rather than biological ways, and to attribute meaning to our activity based on sociocultural influences. It follows that, in present circumstances, many individuals are not able to distinguish their biological needs, which ultimately impact on their health, from wants or preferences.[152] This is held to be partly because the complexity of sociocultural evolution makes differentiation difficult, so that "even phylogenetically evolved programs of...behavior are adjusted to the presence of a culture," which alters the significance of biological needs.[153]

The Underlying Influences on Health Through Occupation

These latter points lead naturally to the final items to be proffered in this chapter: the factors underlying the experience of positive health and well-being through occupation and the link between these and biologically based influences. These provide what can be regarded as a paradigm of the complex relationship between occupation, health, and well-being.

The ideas about occupation and health that have been explored in this chapter sustain the view that there are not only "occupational indicators of health and wellness," but also underlying factors that can positively influence occupational behavior and, subsequently, health. Figure 5-4, which was prompted by the Better Health Commission's graphic of the Social Determinants of Health, encapsulates the concept. There are three distinct categories of underlying factors:

1. The type of economy, such as nomadic, agrarian, industrial, post-industrial, capitalist, or socialist
2. National policies and priorities, such as toward war or peace, economic growth, sustainable ecology, wealth and power of multinational organizations, or self-generated community development
3. Dominant cultural values about such ideas as social justice and equity as they relate to occupation, how different aspects of occupation are perceived, the work ethic, individualistic or communal conventions, and respect for health or healing

These underlying factors give rise to particular occupational institutions and activities in any given society. For example, the type of economy has direct influence on the amount and type of technology in daily living; how labor is divided between classes, genders, and age groups; and employment opportunities. National priorities have direct influence on legislative and fiscal institutions that provide rules by which people live, commercial and material activities, and management of the environment and the ecology. Cultural values will impact upon the media, local regulations, social services, job creation schemes, education, and health care systems.

These activities and institutions can be positive influences upon community, family, or individual health by providing equitable opportunity to develop potential, creativity, and balanced use of capacities; to experience satisfaction, meaning and purpose, stability and support, belonging and sharing; and being able to contribute in a way that is socially valued, yet maintains natural resources and recognizes the rights of all living organisms. The effects of the underlying factors may not be the same for all communities or for all individuals. For example, although peace is advocated as a

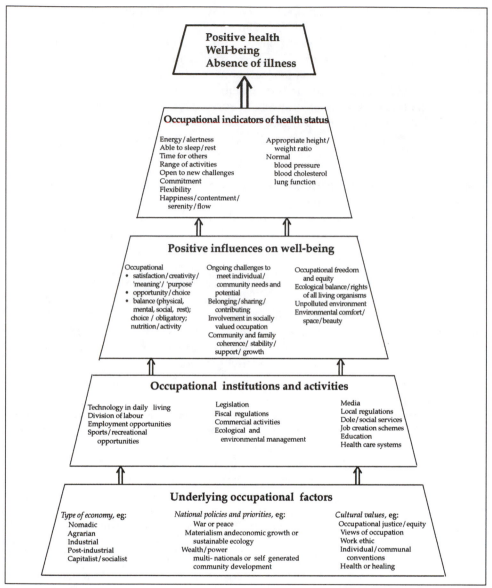

Figure 5-4. Occupational factors leading to health and well-being. Adapted from Better Health Commission. *Looking Forward to Better Health*. **Vol 1. Canberra: Australian Government Publishing Service; 1986:5.**

necessity for health by the Ottawa Charter, a view that is currently supported by many people, it may be that some communities and individuals find war to be a health-enhancing occupation. Although to the "green lobby," ecological sustainability appears to be the healthy way for all to survive, to power-broking economists and politicians the opposite may be conducive to their well-being. (Both war-mongers and power-brokers may pay lip service to opposite values.) What the more mature perceive as dangerous risk-taking behaviors by the young may produce happiness, exhilaration, and physical fitness.

Occupational indicators of health status include energy and alertness, a range of

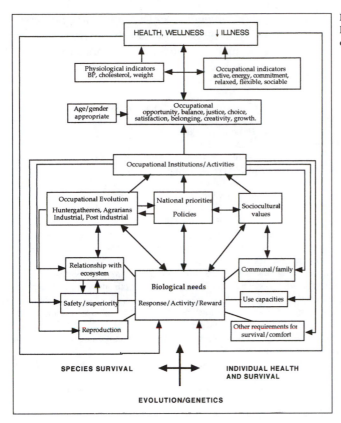

Figure 5-5. Factors underlying health and well-being from an occupational perspective.

activities, flexibility, interest, contentment, commitment, the ability to relax and sleep, time for others, openness to new challenges, and minimal absenteeism from obligatory tasks. These are likely to be compatible with more conventional health status indicators, such as appropriate height:weight ratio and normal blood pressure, cholesterol, and lung function. Figure 5-5 displays the interactive links between biological needs and sociocultural factors discussed throughout the chapter, as occupational determinants of health and well-being. Only the most direct links are shown in the figure in the interest of clarity, and it is especially important to note the link from the "health and well-being outcome" back to the underlying determinants, as the process is not linear, but interactive at all levels.

In summary, health and well-being result from being in tune with our "occupational" species' nature. Being responsive to biologically driven needs and using capacities has, in the past, been central to maintaining homeostasis and promoting physical, mental, and social well-being. Because physiological and innate biological mechanisms are informed, stimulated, influenced, and adapted by conscious social processes, these too become very influential determinants of human occupation and of health. For health and well-being to be experienced by individuals and communities, engagement in occupation needs to have meaning and be balanced between capacities, provide optimal opportunity for desired growth in individuals or groups, be flexible enough to develop and change according to context and choice, and be compatible with sustaining the ecology. Such engagement, if it is in accord with sociocultural values, will enable individuals, families, and communities to flourish and the species to survive. The complexity of the interaction of sociocultural processes with biological needs, along with lack of awareness about health's dependence on engagement in balanced and satisfying occupation, can lead to unhealthy consequences. These are discussed in the next chapter.

References

1. World Health Organization. *Constitution of the World Health Organisation*. International Health Conference, New York, NY, 1946.
2. Nutbeam D. Health promotion glossary. *Health Promotion*. 1986;1(1):113,126.
3. Caplan A, et al. *Concepts of Health and Disease*. Reading, Mass: Addison-Wesley; 1981:parts 1, 5.
4. Newman MA. *Health as Expanding Consciousness*. St. Louis, Mo: The CV Mosby Co; 1986.
5. Blaxter M. *Health and Lifestyles*. London, England: Tavistock/Routledge; 1990:24-26,29,233.
6. American Heritage Dictionary. *Roget's New Thesaurus*. Boston, Mass: Houghton Mifflin Co; 1980.
7. *Enough to Make You Sick: How Income and Environment Affect Health*. Australian National Health Strategy Research Paper, No 1, Sept 1992.
8. Whitehead M. *The Health Divide*. New York, NY: Penguin; 1988:229.
9. Cohen P, Struening EL, Genevie LE, Kaplan SR, Muhlin GL, Peck HB. Community stressors, mediating conditions and wellbeing in urban neighborhoods. *Journal of Community Psychology*. 1982;10:377-390.
10. Argyle M. *The Psychology of Happiness*. New York, NY: Methuen and Co; 1987.
11. Koenig H, Kvale J, Ferrel C. Religion and well-being in later life. *The Gerontologist*. 1988;28(1):19-27.
12. Burckardt C, Woods S, Schultz A, Ziebarth D. Quality of life of adults with chronic illness: a psychometric study. *Research in Nursing and Health*. 1989;12:347-354.
13. Ullah P. The association between income, financial strain and psychological well-being among unemployed youths. *The British Psychological Society*. 1990;63:319-330.
14. Isaksson K. A longitudinal study of the relationship between frequent job change and psychological well-being. *Journal of Occupational Psychology*. 1990;63:297-308.
15. Warr P. The measurement of well-being and other aspects of mental health. *Journal of Occupational Psychology*. 1990;63(4):193-210.
16. Hersey J. Time's winged chariot. In: Fadiman C, ed. *Living Philosophies: The Reflections of Some Eminent Men and Women of Our Time*. New York, NY: Doubleday; 1990.
17. Csikszentmihalyi M. *Flow: The Psychology of Optimal Experience*. New York, NY: Harper and Row; 1990.
18. Csikszentmihalyi M. Activity and happiness: towards a science of occupation. *Journal of Occupational Science: Australia*. 1993;1(1):38-42.
19. Csikszentmihalyi M, LeFevre J. Optimal experience in work and leisure. *Journal of Personality and Social Psychology*. 1989;56(58):5-22.
20. Pybus MW, Thomson MC. Health awareness and health actions of parents. ANZERCH/APHA Conference 1979. In: Boddy J, ed. *Health: Perspectives and Practices*. New Zealand: The Dunmore Press; 1985.
20a. Wilcock AA, van der Arend H, Darling K, et al. An exploratory study of people's perceptions and experiences of well-being. *British Journal of Occupational Therapy*. 1998;61(2):75-82.
21. McConatha JT, McConatha D. An instrument to measure self-responsibility for wellness in older adults. *Educational Gerontology*. 1985;11:295-308.
22. Homel R, Burns A. Environmental quality and the well-being of children. *Social Indicators Research*. 1989;21:133-158.
23. Maslow AH. *Toward a Psychology of Being*. 2nd ed. New York, NY: D Van Nostrand Co; 1968:vi,201.
24. Wilcock AA. Research carried out as part of student learning about the relationship between occupation and health. University of South Australia, 1991-1995.
25. Roe M. *Nine Australian Progressives: Vitalism in Bourgeois Social Thought 1890-1960*. Australia: University of Queensland Press; 1984.
26. Cilento R. *Blueprint for the Health of a Nation*. Sydney, Australia: Scotow Press; 1944.
27. Powles J. Professional hygienists and the health of the nation. In: Macleod J, ed. *The Commonwealth of Science*. Melbourne, Australia: Oxford University Press; 1988.
28. Hetzel BS, McMichael T. *L S Factor: Lifesyle and Health*. Ringwood, Victoria: Penguin; 1987.
29. Sydney KH, Shephard RJ. Activity patterns of elderly men and women. *Journal of Gerontology*. 1977;32(1):25-32.
30. Kirchman MM. The preventive role of activity: myth or reality—a review of the literature. *Physical and Occupational Therapy in Geriatrics*. 1983;2(4):39-47.
31. Folkins CH, Syme WE. Physical fitness training and mental health. *American Psychologist*. 1981;36:373-

389.

32. Chamove A. Exercise improves behaviour: a rationale for occupational therapy. *British Journal of Occupational Therapy.* 1986;49:83-86.

33. Morgan WP. Psychological effects of exercise. *Behavioral Medicine Update.* 1982;4:25-30.

34. Oliver J. Physical activity and the psychological development of the handicapped. In: Kane J, ed. *Psychological Aspects of Physical Education and Sport.* London, England: Routledge; 1972:187-204.

35. Comfort A. *A Good Age.* Melbourne, Australia: Macmillan Co Pty Ltd; 1977:82.

36. Corbin HD. Brighter vistas for senior citizens: salient thoughts. *Journal of Physical Education and Recreation.* 1977;October:52-53.

37. Payne WA, Hahn DB. *Understanding Your Health.* 4th ed. St. Louis, Mo: Mosby; 1995:26.

38. The Open University in association with the Health Education Council and the Scottish Health Education Unit. *The Good Health Guide.* London, England: Pan Books; 1980.

39. Dintiman GB, Greenberg JS. *Health Through Discovery.* 3rd ed. New York, NY: Random House; 1986.

40. Kanner AD, Coyne JC, Schaefer C, Lazarus RS. Comparison of two modes of stress management: daily hassles and uplifts versus life events. *Journal of Behavioral Medicine.* 1981;4:1-39.

41. Holmes T, Rahe R. Schedule of recent events and social readjustment rating scales. In: Pervin LA, Lewis M, eds. *Perspectives in Interactional Psychology.* New York, NY: Plenum; 1978.

42. Lazarus RS, Launier R. Stress related transactions between person and environment. In: Pervin LA, Lewis M, eds. *Perspectives in Interactional Psychology.* New York, NY: Plenum; 1978.

43. Pervin LA, Lewis M, ed. Perspectives in Interactional Psychology. New York, NY: Plenum: 1978.

44. Antonovsky A. The sense of coherence as a determinant of health. In: Matarazzo JD, Weiss SM, Herd JA, Miller NE, Weiss SM, eds. *Behavioral Health. A Handbook of Health Enhancement and Disease Prevention.* New York, NY: John Wiley and Sons; 1990:117,119.

45. White RW. Sense of interpersonal competence: two case studies and some reflections on origins. In: White RW, ed. *The Study of Lives.* Chicago, Ill: Aldine; 1963.

46. Bandura A. Self efficacy: toward a unifying theory of behavioral change. *Psychological Review.* 1977;84:191-215.

47. Kobasa SC, Maddi SR, Courington S. Personality and constitution as mediators in the stress-illness relationship. *Journal of Health and Social Behavior.* 1981;22:368-378.

48. Bradburn NM. *The Structure of Psychological Well-Being.* Chicago, Ill: Aldine; 1969.

49. Andrews FM, Withey SB. *Social Indicators of Well-Being.* New York, NY: Plenum Press; 1976.

50. Diener E. Subjective well-being. *Psychological Bulletin.* 1984;95:542-575.

51. Strack F, Argyle M, Schartz N, eds. *Subjective Well-Being: An Interdisciplinary Perspective.* Oxford, UK: Pergamon Press; 1991.

52. Maslow A. *The Farther Reaches of Human Nature.* Viking Press; 1971.

53. Bullock A. *The Humanist Tradition in the West.* London, England: Norton; 1985.

54. Burnham WH. *The Wholesome Personality.* New York, NY: Appleton-Century; 1932.

55. Fromm E. *Man for Himself.* New York, NY: Holt, Rinehart and Winston; 1947.

56. Rogers C. *On Becoming a Person.* Boston, Mass: Houghton Mifflin; 1961.

57. Ingleby D. Mental health. In: Kuper A, Kuper J, eds. *The Social Science Encyclopedia.* London, England: Routledge; 1985.

58. Boddy J, ed. *Health: Perspectives and Practices.* New Zealand: The Dunmore Press; 1985:48,113,116.

59. Lilley J, Jackson L. The value of activities: establishing a foundation for cost effectiveness. A review of the literature. *Activities, Adaptation and Aging.* 1990;14(4):12-13.

60. Foster P. Activities: a necessity for total health care of the long term care resident. *Activities, Adaptation and Aging.* 1983;3(3):17-23.

61. do Rozario L. Ritual, meaning and transcendence: the role of occupation in modern life. *Journal of Occupational Science: Australia.* 1994;1(3):46-53.

62. Rappaport R. *Ecology, Meaning, and Religion.* Richmond, Va: North Atlantic Books; 1979.

63. Kirkpatrick R, Trew K. Lifestyle and psychological well-being among unemployed men in Northern Ireland. *Journal of Occupational Psychology.* 1985;58:207-216.

64. Dunbar R. Why gossip is good for you. *New Scientist.* 1992;136(1848):28-31.

65. Maguire G. An exploratory study of the relationship of valued activities to the life satisfaction of elderly persons. *Occupational Therapy Journal of Research.* 1983;3:164-171.

66. Doyal L, Gough I. *A Theory of Human Need.* Houndmills, Hampshire: Macmillan; 1991:36-37,172,184.

67. Wilcock AA. Workshop: *Holistic Health Care, Occupational Therapy and Stroke.* Seminar on Stroke, National Heart Foundation, Auckland, New Zealand, November 1991.

68. Rosi EL. *The Psychobiology of Mind-Body Healing.* New York, NY: WW Norton and Co, Inc; 1986.

69. Pert C. The wisdom of receptors: neuropeptides, the emotions, and bodymind. *Advances.* 1986;3(3):8-16.

70. Dossey B. The psychophysiology of bodymind healing. In: Dossey B, et al. *Holistic Health Promotion: A Guide for Practice*. Rockville, Md: Aspen Publishers; 1989.
71. Emeth EV, Greenhut JH. *The Wholeness Handbook: Care of Body, Mind and Spirit for Optimal Health*. New York, NY: The Continuum Publishing Co; 1991.
72. Pelletier KR. *Sound Mind, Sound Body*. New York, NY: Simon and Schuster; 1994.
73. Ornstein R, Sobel D. *The Healing Brain: A Radical New Approach to Health Care*. London, England: Macmillan; 1988:11-12.
74. Valentine ER. Mind. In: Kuper A, Kuper J, eds. *The Social Science Encyclopedia*. London, England: Routledge; 1985.
75. Plato. "Timaeus" (51d) and "Phaedrus" (67a). In: Hamilton E, Cairns H, eds. *The Collected Dialogues of Plato*. New York, NY: Pantheon Books; 1961.
76. Aristotle (413 a 4) and (408 b 18). In: Barnes J, ed. *The Complete Works of Aristotle*. Rev trans. Oxford, UK: Princeton University Press; 1984:651,658.
77. Rose S. *The Conscious Brain*. Rev ed. Harmondsworth, England: Penguin Books; 1976:39,292-293.
78. Descartes R. *Discourse on the Method of Rightly Conducting the Reason, IV*. Translated with Introduction by Lafleur LJ. New York, NY: The Liberal Arts Press; 1954.
79. Agius T. Aboriginal health in Aboriginal hands. In: Fuller J, Barclay J, Zollo J, eds. *Multicultural Health Care in South Australia*. Conference proceedings. Adelaide: Painters Prints; 1993:23.
80. Lukes S. *Individualism*. Oxford, UK: Basil Blackwell; 1973.
81. The Asian NGO Coalition, IRED Asia, The people centred development forum. *Economy, Ecology and Spirituality: Toward a Theory and Practice of Sustainablity*. 1993.
82. Potter VR. Bioethics, the science of survival. *Biology and Medicine*. 1970;14:127-153.
83. Smuts JC. *Holism and Evolution*. London, England: Macmillan and Co Ltd; 1926.
84. Golley FB. *A History of the Ecosystem Concept in Ecology: More Than the Sum of the Parts*. New Haven, Conn: Yale University Press; 1993.
85. Kopelman L, Moskop J. The holistic health movement: a survey and critique. *Journal of Medicine and Philosophy*. 1981;6(2):209-235.
86. von Bertalanffy L. *Problems of Life*. New York, NY: Wiley; 1952.
87. Wilkinson P. General systems theory. In: Bullock A, Stalleybrass O, Trombley S, eds. *The Fontana Dictionary of Modern Thought*. 2nd ed. London, England: Fontana Press; 1988.
88. Pietroni PC. Holistic medicine. In: Bullock A, Stalleybrass O, Trombley S, eds. *The Fontana Dictionary of Modern Thought*. 2nd ed. London, England: Fontana Press; 1988.
89. *Funk & Wagnall's Standard Desk Dictionary*. Vol 1. New York, NY: Harper and Row; 1984:296.
90. *The Australian Concise Oxford Dictionary of Current English*; 1987.
91. World Health Organization, Health and Welfare Canada, Canadian Public Health Association. *Ottawa Charter for Health Promotion*. Ottawa, Canada, 1986.
92. World Health Organisation. *Primary Health Care*. Report of the International Conference on Primary Health Care, Alma Ata, USSR, 1978.
93. World Health Organization, Health and Welfare Canada, Canadian Public Health Association. *Ottawa Charter for Health Promotion*. Ottawa, Canada, 1986.
94. Stephenson W. *The Ecological Development of Man*. Sydney, Australia: Angus and Robertson; 1972:26,94,136,217.
95. King-Boyes MJE. *Patterns of Aboriginal Culture: Then and Now*. Sydney, Australia: McGraw-Hill Book Co; 1977:154-155.
96. Lorenz K. *Civilized Man's Eight Deadly Sins*. Latzke M, trans. London, England: Methuen and Co Ltd; 1974:3-5,12-13.
97. McNeill WH. *Plagues and People*. London, England: Penguin Books; 1979:39.
98. Tunnes N. 1656. Cited in: Dubos R, ed. *Mirage of Health: Utopias, Progress and Biological Change*. New York, NY: Harper and Row; 1959:11.
99. Fortuine R. The health of the Eskimos as portrayed in the earliest written accounts. *Bulletin of the History of Medicine*. 1971;45:97-114.
100. Wharton WJL, ed. *Captain Cook's Journal During His First Voyage Around the World Made in HM Bark Endeavour, 1768-1771*. London, England: Eliot Stock; 1893:323.
101. Rousseau JJ. Discourse on the origin and foundations of inequity amongst men. 1754. In: Mason JH, ed. *The Indispensable Rousseau*. London, England: Quartet Books; 1979.
102. Dubos R, ed. *Mirage of Health: Utopias, Progress and Biological Change*. New York, NY: Harper and Row; 1959:9,139,144.
103. Beddoes T. *Hygeia, or Essays Moral and Medical on the Causes Affecting the Personal State of Our Middling and Affluent Classes*. 3 vols. Bristol: R Phillips; 1802-1803.
104. Virey, JJ. *L'hygiene Philosophique*. Paris, France: Crochard; 1828.

105. Jenner E. *An Inquiry Into the Causes and Effects of the Variolae Vaccine: A Disease Discovered in Some of the Western Counties of England, and Known as the Cow Pox*. Birmingham, Ala: Classics of Medicine Library; 1978.

106. Ilza Veith. Huang Ti Nei Ching Su Wen. *The Yellow Emperor's Classic of Internal Medicine*. Baltimore, Md: Williams and Wilkins; 1949:253.

107. Lao-tzu. *Tao Te Ching* (The Way) Circe 500 BC: Chuang-tzu. In: Dubos R, ed. *Mirage of Health: Utopias, Progress and Biological Change*. New York, NY: Harper and Row; 1959:10.

108. Pao Ching-yen. In: Needham J, ed. *Science and Civilisation in China. Vol 2. History of Scientific Thought*. New York, NY: Cambridge University Press; 1956.

109. Coon CS. *The Hunting Peoples*. London, England: Jonathan Cape Ltd; 1972:390.

110. Dobson A. People and disease. In: Jones S, Martin R, Pilbeam D, eds. *The Cambridge Encyclopedia of Human Evolution*. New York, NY: Cambridge University Press; 1992:411-412.

111. Meindel RS. Human populations before agriculture. In: Jones S, Martin R, Pilbeam D, eds. *The Cambridge Encyclopedia of Human Evolution*. New York, NY: Cambridge University Press; 1992:410.

112. Cannon WB. *Bodily Canges in Pain, Hunger, Fear and Rage*. Boston, Mass: CT Branford; 1929, 1953.

113. Sigerist HE. *A History of Medicine. Vol 1. Primitive and Archaic Medicine*. New York, NY: Oxford University Press; 1955:254-255.

114. Allport GW. The open system in personality theory. *Journal of Abnormal and Social Psychology*. 1960;61:301-311.

115. McDougall W. *The Energies of Men*. London, England: Methuen; 1932.

116. McDougall W. *Social Psychology*. 23rd rev ed. London, England; Methuen; 1936.

117. Lewin K. *A Dynamic Theory of Personality*. New York, NY: 1935.

118. Murray HA. *Explorations in Personality*. New York, NY: 1938.

119. Hull C. *Principles of Behavior*. New York, NY: Appleton-Century-Crofts; 1943.

120. Madsen KB. *Theories of Motivation*. 4th ed. Ohio: Kent State University Press; 1968.

121. Alderfer CP. *Existence, Relatedness and Growth: Human Needs in Organizational Settings*. New York, NY: Free Press; 1972.

122. Maslow AH. *Motivation and Personality*. 2nd ed. New York, NY: Harper and Row; 1970.

123. Young PT. Drives. In: Sills DL, ed. *International Encyclopedia of the Social Sciences*. The Macmillan Co and The Free Press; 1968:275-276.

124. Dashiell JF. *Fundamentals of Objective Psychology*. Boston, Mass: Houghton Mifflin; 1928:233-234.

125. Eysenck HS, Arnold W, Meili R. *Encyclopedia of Psychology*. New York, NY: Continuum Books, The Seabury Press; 1979:705-706.

126. Snell GD. *Search for a Rational Ethic*. New York, NY: Springer Verlag; 1988:147.

127. Wolman B, ed. *Dictionary of Behavioral Science*. New York, NY: Van Nostand, Reinold Co; 1973:250.

128. Anscombe GEM. Modern moral philosophy. *Philosophy*. 1958;33(124):1-19.

129. Watts ED. Human needs. In: Kuper A, Kuper J, eds. *The Social Science Encyclopedia*. London, England: Routledge; 1985.

130. von Bertalanffy L. *General Systems Theory*. New York, NY: George Baziller; 1968:27.

131. Wilcock AA. A theory of the human need for occupation. *Journal of Occupational Science: Australia*. 1993;1(1):17-24.

132. Izard CE. *Human Emotions*. New York, NY: Plenum; 1977.

133. Izard CE, Kagan J, Zajonc RB. *Emotions, Cognition, and Behavior*. New York, NY: Cambridge University Press; 1984.

134. Frijda NH. *The Emotions*. New York, NY: Cambridge University Press; 1986.

135. Csikszentmihalyi M, Csikszentmihalyi I, eds. *Optimal Experience: Psychological Studies of Flow in Consciousness*. New York, NY: Cambridge University Press; 1988:20-25.

136. Knight R, Knight M. *A Modern Introduction to Psychology*. London, England: University Tutorial Press Ltd; 1957:56-57,177.

137. Meyer A. The philosophy of occupational therapy. *Archives of Occupational Therapy*. 1922;1:1-10.

138. Carrel A. *Man, the Unknown*. London, England: Burns and Oates; 1935:178-179.

139. Leone RE. Life after laughter: one perspective. *Elementary School Guidance and Counselling*. 1986;21(2):139-142.

140. Ornstein R, Sobel D. *Healthy Pleasures*. Reading, Mass: Addison-Wesley Publishing Co Inc; 1989.

141. Simon JM. Humor and its relationship to percieved health, life satisfaction, and moral in older adults. *Issues in Mental Health Nursing*. 1990;11(1):17-31.

142. Southam M, Cummings M. The use of humour as a technique for modulating pain. *Occupational Therapy Practice*. 1990;1(3):77-84.

143. Buxman K. Make room for laughter. *American Journal of Nursing*. 1991;91(12):46-51.

144. Mallett J. Use of humour and laughter in patient care. *British Journal of Nursing*. 1993;2(93):172-175.

145. Fromm E. *The Sane Society*. New York, NY: Rinehart; 1955.
146. Marcuse H. *One Dimensional Man*. London, England: Routledge; 1964.
147. Wolff RP, Moore B, Marcuse H. *A Critique of Pure Tolerance*. London, England: Cape; 1969.
148. Bay C. Politics and pseudopolitics. *American Political Science Review*. 1965;59.
149. Bay C. Needs, wants and political legitimacy. *Canadian Journal of Political Science*. 1968;1:241-260.
150. Macpherson CB. *The Real World of Democracy*. Oxford, UK: Clarendon Press; 1966.
151. Macpherson CB. *Democratic Theory: Essays in Retreival*. Oxford, UK: Clarendon Press; 1973.
152. Fitzgerald R, ed. *Human Needs and Politics*. Sydney, Australia: Permagon; 1977.
153. Lorenz K. *The Waning of Humaneness*. Munich, Germany: R Piper and Co Verlag; 1983:124.

Suggested Reading

Blaxter M. *Health and Lifestyles*. London, England: Tavistock/Routledge; 1990.

Csikszentmihalyi M. Activity and happiness: towards a science of occupation. *Journal of Occupational Science: Australia*. 1993;1(1):38-42.

Csikszentmihalyi M. *Flow: The Psychology of Optimal Experience*. New York, NY: Harper and Row; 1990.

Csikszentmihalyi M, LeFevre J. Optimal experience in work and leisure. *Journal of Personality and Social Psychology*. 1989;56(58):5-22.

do Rozario L. Ritual, meaning and transcendence: the role of occupation in modern life. *Journal of Occupational Science: Australia*. 1994;1(3):46-53.

Doyal L, Gough I. *A Theory of Human Need*. Houndmills, Hampshire: Macmillan; 1991.

Dubos R, ed. *Mirage of Health: Utopias, Progress and Biological Change*. New York, NY: Harper and Row; 1959.

Hetzel BS, McMichael T. *L S Factor: Lifesyle and Health*. Ringwood, Victoria: Penguin; 1987.

Lukes S. *Individualism*. Oxford, UK: Basil Blackwell; 1973.

Maslow A. *The Farther Reaches of Human Nature*. Viking Press; 1971.

Maslow AH. *Toward a Psychology of Being*. 2nd ed. New York, NY: D Van Nostrand Co; 1968.

McNeill WH. *Plagues and People*. London, England: Penguin Books; 1979.

Ornstein R, Sobel D. *Healthy Pleasures*. Reading, Mass: Addison-Wesley Publishing Co Inc; 1989.

Ornstein R, Sobel D. *The Healing Brain: A Radical New Approach to Health Care*. London, England: Macmillan; 1988.

Wilcock AA, van der Arend H, Darling K, et al. An exploratory study of people's perceptions and experiences of well-being. *British Journal of Occupational Therapy*. 1998;61(2):75-82.

World Health Organization. *Primary Health Care*. Report of the International Conference on Primary Health Care, Alma Ata, USSR, 1978.

World Health Organization, Health and Welfare Canada, Canadian Public Health Association. *Ottawa Charter for Health Promotion*. Ottawa, Canada, 1986.

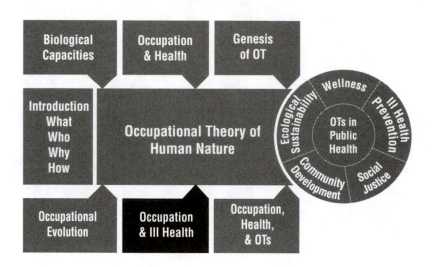

Chapter 6
Ill Health: Occupational Risk Factors

This chapter presents the reader with ideas about:
- Public health, medical science, and occupational health
- The history of patterns of morbidity, social structures, and population size from an occupational perspective
- Occupational determinants of ill health, such as occupational imbalance, deprivation, alienation, and stress

Early humans used occupational behavior to improve survival odds and decrease the experience of ill health. Although this is still the case in many instances, the current complexity of occupational behavior may conceal detrimental effects of human occupation. This chapter focuses on identifying "occupational" risk factors to health and well-being. In doing so, it is in line with public health conventions aimed at the "absence of illness" through preventive approaches based on known risks. As this can be regarded as a first step in the promotion of health, it is appropriate to consider whether occupational risk factors can be prevented even though they are very complex. The chapter focuses particularly on occupational imbalance, deprivation, and alienation as risks to health, so studies not only in health care literature but also from education and sociopolitical fields that address these issues have been analyzed. This was done because there is inadequate understanding and consideration, as well as a lack of research about occupation as it relates to illness or the prevention of occupational risk factors in a holistic sense.

The chapter begins by exploring why public health researchers, given their particular interest in the prevention of illness, have paid scant attention to either the illness prevention or the health promoting benefits of engagement in occupation, despite the fact that a variety of risk factors to health can result from less than optimal balance, use, choice, or opportunity in occupation. There are, perhaps, two major reasons:

1. Throughout most of its recent history, public health has been tied, conceptually, to medical science, as noted in Chapter 1
2. The notion of occupation has been associated with paid employment, rather than with the human need for purposeful activity as a requirement for health

These two issues will be discussed briefly.

Public Health and Medical Science

Public health's close association with medical science is illustrated by the emphasis on the "absence of illness" view of health in public health and health education texts. The topics that are most frequently addressed—cigarette smoking, alcohol and drugs, eating habits, exercise and fitness, stress control, safe sex, and occupational (paid employment) hazards—are clearly identified as risk factors in illness.[1,2]

Such topics, along with issues of social justice and equity, are also prominent in social health texts. The medical view of illness is so pervasive that the pursuit of a disease-free state is the idea that prevails, and the difference between helping people to be healthy and stopping them from being unhealthy, which are different operations, based on different premises, is poorly appreciated. Indeed, from my own experience, even most health care workers concerned with social or community health appear to assume that prevention of illness is the same as the promotion of health. For example, all health promotion centers I have seen in public hospitals provide the same type of information as the texts noted above. Additionally, in conversation with health care workers involved in prevention, I have found they commonly and strongly assert their field of endeavor is health promotion. So dominant is this idea that health is used as the identifying descriptor for services aimed at ill health, such as health care, health science, health professionals, and even public health.

Current research priorities and health resource expenditure also support the claim that health care is dominated by medical science's preoccupation with illness, that healing takes priority over preventing illness, and that preventing illness takes precedence over maintaining and enhancing wellness. For example, there is substantial criticism that curative and technological health programs receive too great a percentage of resources aimed at health despite evidence of highly developed, industrialized societies having a decreasing margin of return on continued investments in conventional, curative medical care against the improvement of health status.[3] That criticism is often levelled from the perspective of preventive medicine. Katz, Hermalin, and Hess suggest that:

> *Health professionals and institutions are often justly criticized for devoting too much attention and money to curative programs, while down-playing or ignoring preventive activities. Government planners and policy makers at all levels emphasize treatment intervention programs to the relative neglect of preventive efforts.*[4]

While clearly differentiating between curative and preventive approaches to health, this suggests that health resources would be equitably shared if those approaches were the only recipients. Such a suggestion ignores other than "absence of illness" approaches and maintains public health's long-time association with reductionist, as opposed to holistic, concepts of health. Because public health tends to consider risks at population levels, it is easy to be seduced into thinking that its approach is holistic.

The pervasiveness of "absence of illness" approaches, exemplified by the modern phenomena of medical science, such as organ transplants, have created a myth that all illness can be overcome. In fact, the Better Health Commission of Australia suggests that we live in a society that continues to foster the belief that, with the aid of modern technology, we can control our bodies and the environment and expect health and wellness as our right.[5] The Better Health Commission itself has been criticized for fostering the same belief in its detailed recommendations. Such beliefs have reinforced "healing" rather than "health" ideologies and confused curative medicine with health. With such beliefs, the most logical way to promote health would be a regimen of following medical rules, such as regular medical check-ups, a balanced nutritional diet, adequate exercise, an appropriate amount of sleep, and obeying as far as possible those mandates that are said to decrease risk of ill health. In many ways, the majority of public health initiatives and how they are reported in the media support the message that this is indeed the case. For example, the emphasis given to "screening" suggests that if whatever is wrong can be found it can be fixed. While these are important adjuncts to health, even if such rules are followed, illness is not necessarily avoided, and "health," nor, indeed, well-being, is not the inevitable reward. Although lifestyle and bad habits (i.e., smoking) are blamed for many of today's chronic diseases,[6-8] with apparent support from numerous public health studies such as the 20-year Framingham Cohort study,[9] they are insufficient to explain who gets sick and who stays healthy. Research concentrating on why people succumb to unhealthy lifestyles and habits is necessary but is rare. Additionally, health is so complex that studies carried out at population level can only establish probable links. There are as yet many unknown determinants of illness, and even fewer of wellness.

Clearly, not all risk factors have been established. Other possibilities, and the underlying determinants of risk factors, need to be studied with the rigor applied to the study of risks already known about. The occupational nature of humans is one example that merits closer scrutiny and can be seen as having many of the same requirements as inquiry into the social nature of ill health. In recent years, public health has recovered the notions of social medicine, which studies the "social behavior of human beings and their external environment" and, occasionally, how people "work and play" in many different cultures. While this type of research embraces some, but not all, notions about occupation and health, at least it is now accepted that there are "associations between much of this human behavior and human health and disease."[10] Douglas Gordon, who was a medically trained pioneer of social medicine in Australia, suggests that the practice of social medicine includes coming to understand the motives, values, social organizations, and structures of different cultures as well as the "philosophies and essential mysteries of human behaviors insofar as these affect health."[10]

Public health maintains a long tradition of epidemiological research. This type of exploration, viewed as normative by the research establishment, empirical in nature and greatly influenced by positivism, is appealing to funding bodies. Epidemiology does not embrace the most suitable research methods to explore complex interactive determinants of health, such as motives, values, social organizations, and structures of different cultures, and that can be applied to the relationship between occupation and health from individual to global perspectives. This necessitates qualitative, phenomenological methodologies being recognized as valid research tools in conjunction with conventional quantitative epidemiology. Qualitative methodologies are well suited to exploring the occupational aspects from this wider view of public health, as well as the more restricted perspective of the relationship between illness and occupational hazards. Using qualitative methodologies, along with critical research approaches, it is possible to extend both the direction and the range of exploration to include underlying determinants based on long-held occupational beliefs and structures.

Public Health and Occupational Health

Recent tendencies in the public health specialty of "occupational health and safety" indicate the limited focus of public health in matters pertaining to health and occupation.[11] Occupational medicine is, perhaps, older than public health, with at least two texts on "mining" diseases being published in the 16th century and classical texts on occupational diseases being published by Ramazzini in 1700 and Thackrah in 1831.[12-15] The focus has historically been on ill health, and the current public health interest reflects this emphasis. For example, in the BBC documentary *Skeletons of Spitalfields*, occupational health experts expressed their surprise at finding that the skeletal remains of hands belonging to 19th century weavers did not display evidence of undue degeneration as a result of overuse. The alternative point of view, that the variety of hand exercise inherent in the activity may be a health benefit, was not even mentioned.[16]

The present emphasis in occupational health also mirrors the current societal, political, and economic value given to paid employment above other occupations. While leisure and recreation are given some attention in relation to healthy lifestyle through programs such as the "Life: Be In It" campaign, the amount of research and resources allocated to this topic relegates it to a much lesser status than paid employment. Other aspects of occupation are effectively ignored or studied in isolation. The major problem in such approaches is that if the phenomenon of occupation is not studied as an entity broader than paid work, the likelihood of understanding the true relationship between occupation and health is lessened, just as reductionist approaches within preventive medicine lessens the likelihood of appreciating interactive and compounding factors in disease processes.

The public health preoccupation with risk factors of ill health suggests that it may be necessary to demonstrate the linkages between engagement in occupation and the prevention of illness if research pertaining to these are to be valued and resourced by public health authorities. A broad, contextual picture of the interaction between occupation and ill health might begin with the changing occupational behaviors of humans, which can be seen as central to changes in morbidity and mortality. To this end, the next few pages review briefly the occupational history of patterns of morbidity.

Occupational History of Patterns of Morbidity

McNeill explains how early hominids, as other animals, fit into a self-balancing, self-regulating ecological system, preying on other forms of life, as they were preyed upon by large-bodied organisms, parasites, and micro-organisms. They were, in fact, "caught in a precarious equilibrium between the microparasitism of disease organisms and the macroparasitism of large-bodied predators." In a natural state, some microparasites provoke acute disease, killing the host; some provoke immunity reactions; others achieve a stable relationship with the host who perhaps experiences continuous, low-level malady; and yet others are carried by the host and are the cause of disease in others. Yet, as was intimated in the last chapter, for early hominids, apart from occasional disturbances such as drought, fire, and floods, which set limits to population imbalance, "a tolerable state of health can be supposed, such as exists among wild primates of the forest today." Within this natural scenario, any change to one living creature is compensated for by genetic or behavioral change in co-organisms. "Undisturbed" biological evolution is a slow process, but when humans began to evolve culturally, and to adapt, as well as adapt to, different habitats by changes in their occupation, they transformed the balance of nature and patterns of disease altered along with this occupational transformation. As human hunter-gatherers began to dominate the food chain, populations increased; as they became able to overcome cold through use of clothing, shelter, and fire, they were able to expand into colder environs, leaving behind many of the parasites and disease organisms. In new environments, populations escalated and occupations proliferated.[17] This was aided by the circumstance that in nomadic life "the small collections of human beings were too scattered to sustain micro-organisms which do not readily achieve a carrier state."[18,19]

It would seem, however, that the world's resources can support only limited numbers of hunter-gatherers and that social strategies to control population numbers, such as abandonment of unwanted infants, probably were used.[18] The modern assumption that life must be preserved at all costs sits uncomfortably with a natural ecological point of view. In contrast, although stability, better access to food, and improved shelters during the agricultural era reduced comparatively morbidity and mortality due to starvation, as well as providing better facilities to nurture and care for infants, the sick, and the aged, low life expectancy remained the common experience because of the increased incidence of infectious diseases.[2] The continual development of agriculture, which prevented the re-establishment of natural ecosystems, along with the rise of villages, towns, and cities, provided ideal conditions for hyperinfestations of various potential disease organisms. Throughout the world, diseases such as diphtheria, scarlet fever, malaria, typhus, smallpox, syphilis, leprosy, and tuberculosis caused ongoing morbidity, along with various plagues that caused a periodic but devastating toll. Indeed, the bubonic plague, at its peaks, killed 10,000 people daily in Constantinople during the 6th and 7th centuries,[20] and in the 14th century, within only a few years, between one third and one half of the population in Europe and Britain.[21]

Such epidemics and infectious diseases occurred because, with increased population density as well as more travel and contact from trade, diseases that had been checked by generations of adaptation gained new leases of life. As occupations such as oceanic exploration, trading, and conquest grew, so did the spread of disease, sometimes with disastrous consequences. For example, in 1520 smallpox arrived in Mexico along with the relief expedition for Cortez and played a major role in the outcome of the Spanish conquest[17]; in Australia, Aboriginals having "no racial experience with diseases such as measles, mumps, smallpox, chickenpox, and influenza" were devastated when exposed to these disorders along with white settlement.[10]

During most of human existence, the population increase has only been about 0.1% annually, compared with a present global increase of approximately 2% annually.[22] Based on what occurs in modern primitive economies, the small growth of human populations can be attributed to factors such as primitive forms of birth control, disease, famine, war, and high mortality rates in infants and children,[10] particularly as infectious diseases did not cease to be the major threat to health until this century. The industrial revolution initially provided few health benefits for the vast majority of people who moved to towns and cities to find paid employment. In 1780, only 15% of the population in the United Kingdom, 0% in Australia, and 5% in the United States lived in towns or cities. This had risen to 50% in the United Kingdom by 1851, in Australia by 1870, and in the United States by about 1910.[23] Perhaps the most obvious result of this urban population explosion was overcrowding in environments not constructed for comfortable and sanitary living, which, aggravated by industrially polluted working conditions, led to a widespread increase in ill health. Eversley suggests:

> *We who live in the 20th century can hardly imagine the significance of pain, disfigurement, and the loss of near relations as a constant factor in every day life. Slight wounds became infected and suppurated for weeks. Fractures healed badly. Minor irritations like toothache and headache became major preoccupations, paralyzing ordinary activity...Even where no acute injury or identifiable major disease was involved, common colds, gastric upsets from the consumption of rotten foodstuffs, and permanent septic foci such as those provided by bad teeth were common, if not universal.[24]*

Many factors have brought about an improvement in this state of affairs including public health initiatives from the mid-19th century, particularly the improvement of sanitary conditions, water supply, and housing. Other social and economic changes, such as improved nutrition, smaller families, less overcrowding, and improved education, along with major advances in medical and pharmaceutical science, have also contributed to a decrease in disease.[25] Indeed, it is possible to appreciate Gordon's suggestion that medicine's role in making life more bearable "is probably its major achievement and for this it receives little credit."[10]

Occupational Structure and Population Size

This overview of the interaction between changing occupational structures and behaviors and morbidity and mortality opens a window onto a variety of recurring themes. One that emerges as important in terms of occupational structure is population size, so it is pertinent to consider the present trend toward urbanization for economic reasons associated with paid employment as an example of a potential underlying risk factor to health.

Although only 3% of the world's population lived in cities as late as 1800, centralization of occupational efforts started with the acquisition and possession of land following the adoption of agriculture. However, only a small proportion of people have lived in towns and cities for the thousands of years since then, and these urban centers were much smaller than modern cities, which usually have in excess of 1 million people living in them. The Greeks "mistrusted aggregations of more than 10,000 people since they considered anything larger hard to govern and keep healthy." Medieval and Renaissance cities were also small, yet are said to have been "architecturally, economically, and intellectually satisfactory and satisfying social entities even though their hygiene was poor and their infant mortality high."[10] This picture changed as paid employment became segregated from family life, and home base and urbanization escalated dramatically during the past 200 years. From roughly 1730 until the turn of this century, urban conditions were appalling.[26] Urbanization has continued to rise and by 1980 reached 80% in the United Kingdom, 86% in Australia, and 76% in the United States.[23]

Overcrowding itself has been described by Lorenz as deleterious to health: people subjected to the overpopulation of city life experience "exhaustion of interhuman relationships," which causes them to lose sight of the innate friendliness and social nature of humans that is apparent "when their capacity for social contact is not continually overstrained." He argues that "superabundance of social contacts forces every one of us to shut himself off in an essentially 'inhuman' way, and which, because of the crowding of many individuals into a small space, elicits aggression."[27]

In some cities, the inhabitants deem it wise to restrict some occupations, such as walking, because of such aggression. However, it may be that, for many people, the constant stimulation and change that accompanies city living compensates for the disadvantages, such as the lack of freedom to pursue such a simple, basic occupation as walking. In such a vein, Dubos, in the Foreword to Hinrichs' *Population, Environment and People*, comments: "I love crowds and cities...All over the world the largest and most polluted cities are also the ones with the greatest appeal even though their inhabitants uniformly complain of congestion and pollution."[28]

There may also be some truth in the claim that city living "provokes to activity those attributes of the brain which are essentially human, namely the capacity to devote major resources of human endeavor to pursuits and goals that are not material."[10] People tend to express strong feelings about their attachment to city living or their desire to "get away from it all," yet whether or how changes in the size of population groupings affect health has not been the topic of intensive inquiry and may be a major, largely unrecognized factor in occupational imbalance, deprivation, and alienation.

Occupational Risk Factors

In the next section of the chapter, occupational imbalance, deprivation, and alienation will be discussed as risk factors that occur as a result of the underlying factors described in Chapter 5. The type of economy, national priorities and policies, and cultural values create occupational institutions and activities that may not only promote health and well-being but can also lead to risk factors such as overcrowding, loneliness, substance abuse, lack of opportunity to develop potential, imbalance between diet and activity, and ecological breakdown. They can also result in ongoing unresolved stress from occupational imbalance, deprivation, or alienation, which are risk factors in themselves, may result from other risk factors, or lead to the development of health risk behaviors. These risk factors can lead to early, preclinical health disorders such as boredom; burnout; depression; decreased fitness, brain, or liver function; increased blood pressure; and changes in sleep patterns, body weight, and emotional state, and ultimately to disease, disability, or death. Figure 6-1, which was prompted by the Better Health Commission's graphic of the Social Determinants of Health, encapsulates this overview.

Occupational Imbalance

The first of the risk factors to be considered is occupational imbalance. Balance, as a result of "heeding" physiological messages such as the urge to use physical, mental, social capacities, or rest is seldom, if ever, the primary concern of sociocultural structures, yet a balance between and within intrinsic and extrinsic factors appears to be a key concept in achieving health and well-being. In fact, Friedman suggests that Cannon's ideas about homeostasis "may well come to dominate medical thinking in the 21st century...as the interdependence of the internal bodily systems is revealed, and as the role of harmony between the person and the environment is documented."[29]

The idea of balance was central to the Greek view of health. They believed that illness resulted from imbalance of the four humors and that a physician's job was to advise on due proportion, to "restore a healthy balance," and to aid "the natural healing powers believed to exist in every human being."[30] This was recognized in Hippocratic writings[31] and by Plato who espoused balance of mind and body by avoiding "exercising either body or mind without the other, and thus preserv[ing] an equal and healthy balance between them." He advocated that those engaged in "strenuous intellectual pursuit" must also exercise the body, and those interested in physical fitness should develop "cultural and intellectual interests."[32] In the same way, engagement in occupations must be "properly proportioned" so that a balance exists in the exercise of individual human capacities. To this end, imbalance, in occupational therapy terms, is often taken to refer specifically to a lack of balance between work, rest, and play.[33-37] Defining this is no easy task because what is considered work or play is a social rather than a biological construct and because what people feel about

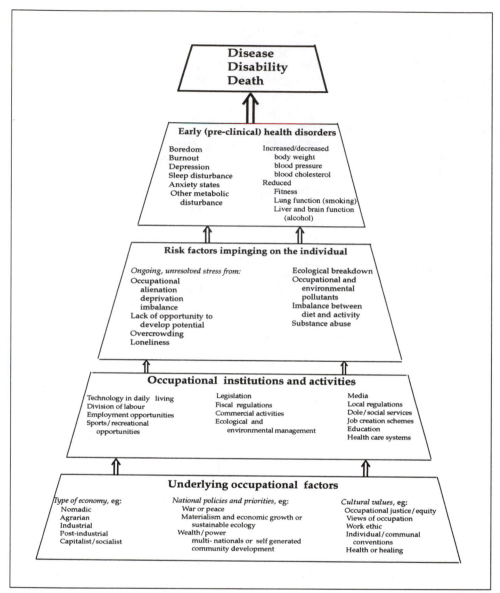

Figure 6-1. Occupational factors leading to ill health. Adapted from Better Health Commission. *Looking Forward to Better Health*. **Vol 1. Canberra: Australian Government Publishing Service; 1986:5.**

or do in their work, rest, or play differs for everyone. The evolutionary perspective and health focus of my theory suggest that imbalance involves a state that occurs because people's engagement in occupation fails to meet their unique physical, social, mental, or rest needs and allows insufficient time for their own occupational interests and growth as well as for the occupations each feels obliged to undertake in order to meet family, social, and community commitments.

It follows, from the standpoint of my theory, that imbalance will therefore differ for each individual, just as their capacities, interests, and responsibilities differ, and that imbalance can be viewed as a factor in disease processes. For example, in terms of infectious diseases, when "our responses to problems in life are excessive or deficient, ...the balance is upset between us and our resident pathogens" because "the central nervous system and hormones act on our immune defenses in such a way that the microbes aid and abet disease"[38,39]; and in terms of the so-called lifestyle disorders of the present day, imbalance can be a cause of the production of "excessive stress hormones—cortisol and catecholamines—which can lead to artery damage, cholesterol buildup, and heart disease."[38,40] From this point of view, physiological imbalance and ill health result from individual responses to, and coping with, the vicissitudes of everyday life, which are closely tied to people's engagement in occupations.

Contemporary occupational structures and the social environment and political agendas that support these structures may not provide people with opportunities for health enhancing, balanced yet stimulating use of capacities, because occupational value in post-industrial cultures (and many other cultures striving to emulate post-industrialism) usually centers around paid employment. Within paid employment, there is little commonality in physical, mental, social, and obligatory requirements or opportunities for choice, so, for the majority of people, engagement in other occupations is necessary, in most instances, to ensure that all capacities are exercised and balanced to a point equating to health and well-being. However, a limited understanding of this concept of balance suggests that it is chance, rather than design, that leads to balanced lifestyles.

In part, this is because massive and rapid changes in society result in ongoing alterations to use of capacities. For example, on the whole, people are no longer required to undertake either sustained or substantial physical exercise. They undertake it at will rather than for necessity. This contrasts markedly with the situation that existed until fairly recent times.[2] Hetzel and McMichael report that:

> *Vigorous physical activity was part of everyday life for most people, at home, at work, and in transit between them. Even as recently as 1850, human muscles provided up to one third of the energy used by workshops, factories, and farms. Today the figure is less than 1%; the human body is becoming redundant as a source of energy in the workplace [with physical activity having become] largely a recreational option rather than a survival necessity.*[2]

Very few modern people would run or walk for several hours every day, as early humans did, despite considerable media exposure to the claims that exercise of sufficient vigor and regularity is protective of cardiovascular disease and conducive to general well-being. Lack of physical activity and coronary heart disease is as strong a risk factor as increased blood pressure, smoking, and high levels of cholesterol, and adults who are inactive are twice as likely to die from cardiovascular disease than those who are very active.[41] Commonly accepted standards about what this protective level of fitness entails is vigorous, repetitive, rhythmical activity such as walking, running, swimming, or cycling, for at least 20 minutes, three to four times a week.[42] In Britain, the United States, and Australia, less than half the adult population meet that standard, with women less likely to engage in physical activity than men (see boxed aside on page 140).[2,43-45]

While the Australian government is implementing programs within schools that actively encourage women to participate in sports,[46] Green, Hebron, and Woodward suggest that women give a different meaning and structure to leisure that represents to them time for relaxation and a physical and mental recharging.[47,48] As meaning and

- According to Hetzel and McMichael, in a 1983 Australian survey of "approximately 6,000 study subjects aged 25 to 64, half of the men and two thirds of the women rarely or never exercised...at the level sufficient to maintain heart-lung endurance fitness."
- According to the 1985 American National Health Interview Survey, discussed by Caspersen et al, only 7% of the women and 8% of the men exercised according to a level recommended by the American College of Sports Medicine.
- In the Blaxter study in the United Kingdom, which defined exercise solely as a leisure time activity, 63% of males and 69% of females reported no vigorous activity.
- A study by Clee on self-reported patterns and attitudes toward leisure of 138 participants over the age of 18 years, and from a variety of settings such as home, schools, sports clubs, and retirement villages, supports the notion that men indulge in more physically active leisure pursuits, such as sports, than females, many of whom prefer more sedentary recreation including reading and craftwork.

structure can be learned, a change of societal emphasis, values, and opportunities may result in women becoming more interested in sport as a leisure or work occupation. In fact, Boutilier and SanGiovanni report a dramatic increase of women's participation in sports in America since the 1970s, which they see as a result of both the feminist movement and "the emergent mid-century emphasis on physical fitness."[49]

The protective effect of vigorous activity is part of the occupational health mechanism of biological evolution. The protective effects include strengthening of heart muscle,[50,51] increased production of protective HDL cholesterol,[52,53] reduction in triglycerides,[54] reduced blood pressure,[55,56] improved glucose metabolism,[57] increased resting metabolic rate, maintenance of weight loss,[58] and reduction of fibrin stickiness (and therefore the formation of blood clots).[59] Apart from cardiovascular disease, several studies have shown the protective effect of physical activity against osteoporosis, some cancers,[60] anxiety, and depression.[61] However, as Kaplan, Sallis, and Patterson suggest "the study of physical activity as it relates to health is in its infancy," and it is difficult to estimate and measure, as most studies use different criteria to define physical activity, or describe and quantify its many variations.[54] Apart from gender, many studies have also found differences between groups according to age, ethnicity, sociocultural status, education, and paid employment.[62-65]

All of these factors relate to differences in occupational behavior: simply recommending an exercise regimen that meets predetermined health criteria is not effective for everybody. Physical activity in the past met many other occupational needs and societal values; what is recommended to replace "superseded" occupations in the present age has also got to meet the ever-changing needs and values of humans' occupational nature in the future. Instead, in a reductionist way and counter to the notion of "balance," the expenditure of physical energy, its components, and the specificity of each to perceived health functions have been put under the microscope, and people are now given reductionist advice on aspects of physical activity that are deemed to be good or bad for selected issues. For example, the American College of Sports

Medicine makes a distinction between physical activity for "fitness" or for "health,"[42] and fitness has been similarly divided by the American Alliance for Health, Physical Education, Recreation, and Dance, into "motor skill related fitness" and "health related fitness." In the latter:

> *Components appear to be related to the development of cardiovascular-respiratory health, maintenance of an optimal body weight, and the development of adequate flexibility and muscular strength and endurance important for the prevention of low back injury and pain.*[66]

While the research that provides the basis for such division is valuable, its presentation in both professional and popular media leads to the assumption that other types of physical activity are of less value. It is hardly surprising that people hearing this type of rhetoric do not equate the physical activities of daily living, nor more general occupational behaviors with their health. In a retrospective study conducted on 100 people older than 60, it was found that the majority of the sample did not associate their life's occupations with their health.[67] This finding appears to be indicative of a "medicalized" understanding of health by the general public, which is, perhaps inadvertently, being reinforced by health education strategies and the media.

This modern reductionism can be contrasted with the holistic nature of hunter-gatherer lifestyles in which physical activity and nutrition were part of an ecological healthy "whole."[68] In the present day, weight gain and obesity are common health concerns in post-industrial societies, and many widely differing circumstances associated with occupation affect the prevalence of weight disorders, yet in the multitude of articles and texts about diets there is scant reference to the need to consider diet and occupation as closely related. For example, although it has been estimated that an individual per 121 pounds of body weight will expend approximately 1.5 calories per minute employed as a typist, in contrast to 3.5 if engaged in domestic work, nutritional intake seldom varies when occupations change, with a resultant imbalance between energy input and output.[69-71] (Grades are according to the obesity index based on the ratio W/H^2 devised by JS Garrow in *Treat Obesity Seriously.*)

It is often the small percentage of people who are committed to physical exercise regimens and "physical health" who are very aware of how their food intake affects their occupation. However, even these are subject to breakdown of health because of imbalance. For example, it has recently been reported that although athletes generally experience a high level of physical fitness and well-being, they frequently suffer some form of breakdown of health at the time of major competition. Evidence about the cause of pathophysiology of such overtraining syndrome is limited, but it has been suggested that the stress of training can cause depression and decreased immune function.[72] This gives rise to the notion that too much exercise, taken to reach peak performance in this case, is detrimental to health as is too little exercise, which can lead to atrophy of body tissue and organs. Kenneth Cooper, who is credited with coining the term "aerobics," now suggests that over-exercising can trigger the overproduction of free radicals, which could be linked with many lifestyle disorders and even death.[73] Indeed, from a study of cases of sudden death during exercise, Siscovick, Weiss, Fletcher, and Lasky found that the risks of death during exercise are increased by 700%, despite men who exercise having half the death rate of those who do not exercise.[74] Moderate, rather than strenuous, exercise is now being seen, by some, as a more sensible physical fitness regimen, and this recommendation fits in well with notions about occupational balance.

Despite this changing view, another aspect of balance, that between activity and rest, is also poorly understood, even though the "sleep" research discussed in Chapter 3 points to them being part of the same continuum. When the natural balance between active and rest occupations is considered (apparent from studies of more primitive cultures), it would seem that artificial constructs, such as the 8-hour day or 5-day work week, have little to recommend them. Within these constructs, people are engaging in activity for socially, economically, or politically based "temporal" reasons. There is a lack of understanding of how biologically based temporal rhythms impact upon occupation and on occupation's relationship to ill health, despite studies that have found that shift work, which disrupts sleep-wake patterns, can lead to irritability, malaise, fatigue, stomach complaints, diminished concentration, diminished functional capabilities, mood changes, and increased susceptibility to accidents.[75-77]

In evolutionary terms, rest between occupations appears to be an early survival mechanism. From personal, close, and ongoing observations of habitual rest/activity patterns of domestic animals, I note that much of their time is spent in rest and watchfulness. This is contrasted with periods of intense activity. (Such observation has included six dogs, one cat, two goats, four lambs, one cow, three calves, about 100 fan tail pigeons, and innumerable bantam hens.) This biological balancing function serves a survival purpose whereby energy is conserved and stored during resting, while the watchfulness informs so that the animal is ready for action should a need arise. The watchfulness remains as a dominant behavior, although its original survival function is obscured under the sociocultural guise of entertainment or minding other people's business. While assuming that humans retain vestiges of the resting mechanism, Hetzel and McMichael suggest that, although contemporary Western society "has largely eliminated" the need for "recreational inactivity (as) a natural means of resting tired limbs or conserving hard won energy, ...the instinct for it remains."[2] This may, in some way, account for the often expressed desire of people "to stop working, to go for a holiday, to have a rest, to retire if they could afford to do so, to be anywhere other than at work" and that society's arbitrary temporal constructs and constraints are counter to biological activity patterns.

Late in the evolutionary chain, as human capacities increased, the need to keep more diverse "intellectual" capacities exercised for when they were required demanded increased and more flexible activity patterns. These activity patterns were superimposed on and integrated with the older activity/rest rhythms. These patterns often compete, and inactivity or passive activity, which seldom provides for the newer "top of the hierarchy" needs for satisfaction, purpose, and meaning, can become the easier option. For example, watching television is one of the most common "resting" occupations of present times, and Kubey and Csikszentmihalyi found that it is universally reported as involving practically no challenges and no skills and does not provide flow experiences.[78-80] Csikszentmihalyi suggests the low level of energy expenditure may be a factor in its popularity, along with the notion that "a mismatch between opportunities and abilities leads to a progressive atrophy of the desire for new challenges."[81] This notion has some merit, but in addition it is modern "watchfulness" during which time people learn about and reflect on their world for similar survival reasons to earlier times. In combination with this, choice of passive, unsatisfying, and what are frequently described as unhealthy pursuits may be a particular, but unconscious, problem for those who, because of early deprivation or lack of learning and opportunity, do not develop their innate capacities and potential, and need to be more watchful. As well, in present occupational structures, the amount of time people have available for restful occupations may not meet their overall needs in terms of biological balance, because among other factors, many people are obliged to use their mental capacities differently than in earlier times. That is, there is probably a decrease of time and opportunity for intellectual or spiritual reflection and much more time required to attend to routine, but demanding paperwork that has to be filled in for work, social security, and taxation purposes. For many, this is stressful, and a common complaint is that people lack energy and are tired by the mental and social demands of their occupations. So in spite of widespread dissemination of information that sedentary lifestyles jeopardize long-term health and survival, many people still choose sedentary occupations for their leisure time, and imbalance between physical, mental, social, and rest occupations is an ongoing occurrence.

In 1992, with a small group of student researchers from the Adelaide School of Occupational Therapy, I undertook a pilot study to explore perceptions of occupational balance and its relationship to health. Using a cluster sampling method and with 146 respondents, the results indicated that, for many, ideal occupational balance is approximately equal involvement in physical, mental, social, and rest occupations. A significant relationship, using one-way analysis of variance (p=0.0001), was found between the closeness of current occupational patterns to those perceived by the respondent to be ideal and their reported health. A comparison of mean scores for three categories of health—poor, fair, or excellent—revealed that the less the difference between current and ideal occupational balance, the healthier the group was. Eighteen of the respondents (12.3%) had identical current and ideal balances, and each of these reported their health to be fair or excellent, while none of the respondents who reported poor health rated their current balance as identical to their ideal balance.[82]

The arbitrary dividing of occupation impedes the conscious awareness of the need to balance mental, physical, social, rest, chosen, and obligatory occupations as integral aspects of health. For many people, lack of such balance results in boredom or burnout. Boredom is the most common emotional response to lack of occupation, and burnout is the widely reported emotional response to overstimulation and too much occupation. Both boredom and burnout are forms of stress that have been linked with ill health. While overload has received more attention than insufficient occupation as a cause of illness, if energy systems are not used they deteriorate. Both "highly conditioned endurance athletes who go through a period of detraining" and people who are bedridden experience huge "decreases in the oxygen energy system in relatively short periods of time."[66] This phenomenon can decrease immune responses and increase susceptibility to ill health.[83-86] In parallel, and probably associated with the opposite of boredom, more than 10 studies have demonstrated that physical activity has a protective effect against certain cancers.[60]

Ornstein and Sobel assert that "the brains mechanism for adaptation can be overwhelmed and blitzed by too much change and challenge"[87] but that "a certain amount of stimulation and information" is needed "to maintain its organization." They observe that:

> As the brain evolved, its ability to handle the world became increasingly comprehensive...The paradox is that as the human brain matures and develops it both enormously increases its ability to find out new things and, at the same time, develops an enormous capacity for getting bored.[87]

Ardell claims that "boredom is the arch-enemy of wellness" and that "it is the leading cause of low level worseness." He argues that it can be held responsible for health risk behaviors, such as smoking, drug and alcohol abuse, and "a failure to take the positive initiatives associated with potent lifestyles."[88]

There are many reasons for the apparent increase in boredom and burnout caused by occupational imbalance. This includes societal pressure to pursue particular occupations that may impose upon individuals the apparent need to do more than they are capable of, or to do less than they achieve personal satisfaction from. Ornstein and Sobel suggest there is an optimal set point for stimulation "in the middle of an organism's response level" maintained "through feedback processes similar to the homeostatic mechanisms of the body" and that when there is either "too much or too little, instability results and disease may follow."[87] Similarly, Csikszentmihalyi has found that an optimal state relating to health and well-being occurs when individuals are challenged by their occupations and have the personal capacities to meet the challenge.[89] If this does not occur, ill health may be a consequence. These views support the "needs construct" described in the last chapter.

Until the industrial revolution, as Jones observed, "labor/time-absorbing employment was the norm in human experience."[23] In earlier times, many people grew or made most of the products they required by virtue of both physical exercise and creative endeavor. By practicing and mastering skills from beginning to end, they were able to use their capacities to the extent that each felt comfortable and as a consequence benefited from a sense of achievement, satisfaction, and well-being, which assisted their resistance to disease and illness. This allowed a more cohesive perspective of occupation that, it is argued, enabled greater awareness of too much or too little exercise of capacities. However, at times of environmental crisis or ecological change when the challenges became too demanding, despite this more holistic awareness, susceptibility to disease would have increased. As Sigerist suggests:

> *Work...may also be harmful to health, may become a chief cause of disease, when there is too much of it, when it is too hard, exceeding the capacity of an individual, when it is not properly balanced by rest and recreation, or when it is performed under adverse circumstances.*[90]

Apart from individual experience of imbalance, there is an imbalance in health opportunities through occupation throughout the community, between the haves and the have nots, between the rich and the poor, between the informed and the illiterate, and between the employed and the unemployed. This imbalance is becoming a cause for concern to the extent that it is a common topic of conversation in many community venues and is being addressed in popular media. For example, *The Weekend Australian Review*, dated April 8-9, 1995, devoted more than a page to an article addressing the age of overwork. This presented evidence from several major post-industrial nations to suggest that many people in paid employment are now expected to take on increased duties, to spend longer hours on work tasks without extra rewards, and that health breakdowns from this cause are increasing.[91,92] Women are particularly at risk as they often undertake a double role of domestic and paid employment occupations.

This is the case not only in post-industrial societies. Barrett and Browne assert that African women have a triple workload as biological, social, and economic producers, which is deleterious to their health,[93] and Ferguson found that women in a marginal area of Kenya experience stress-related ill health because of the demands of their many occupations, as well as poor nutrition, high fertility rates, and limited access to health care.[94] At the other end of the spectrum is the rising numbers of unemployed with decreased opportunity for engagement in satisfying and valued occupation. Inequities of this type cause not only individual illness but community disease. This disease is compounded by the present-day need to adapt and cope with an ever-changing social, occupational, and ecological environment. If individuals need to have some degree of stability for the human system to remain healthy, there could come a time when maintaining the balance between development, particularly occupational development, and physiological processes is a major issue in health.

Despite affluent societies having an abundance of occupational choices that offer opportunity for the exercise and development of physical, mental, and social skills, the structures, material costs, and values placed upon different aspects of occupation may well affect how successfully individuals access these opportunities. People may also be restricted in their choice by factors as various as time, lack of resources, lack of awareness, or, perhaps, because the focus of their occupations appears irrelevant to survival, health, or well-being. Such obstacles can cause occupational imbalance because of occupational deprivation, which is another major risk factor.

Occupational Deprivation

Deprivation implies the influence of an external agency or circumstance that keeps a person from "acquiring, using, or enjoying something."[95] The external agency or circumstance that causes occupational deprivation may be technology, the division of labor, lack of employment opportunities, poverty or affluence, cultural values, local regulations, and limitations imposed by social services and education systems, as well as ill health and disability. Familiar examples spring to mind, such as the person confined to a bed and wheelchair because of physical handicap, the reluctant retiree, numerous individuals engaged in caregiver duties, the school leaver or middle-aged process worker unable to find paid employment, or the lonely, battered child with little access to toys or stimulus.

Infants deprived of the opportunity for learning through doing because of lack of sensory stimulation within their environments fail to develop normally or to thrive.[96-101] Indeed, all types of biological and social deprivation have been associated with failure to make use of occupational opportunities,[102] poor health,[103] and with dysfunction in adolescence.[104] In extreme examples where children have been left alone in almost empty rooms and provided with only food and a place to sleep, they have failed to develop even basic occupational skills of walking and self-care. The classic example of child deprivation is the "wild boy of Aveyron" who appeared from the woods of Caune, in France, in the late 18th century, after, probably, at least 7 of his 12 years living alone. Despite 5 years of experimental education by Jean Itard, he never attained normal language or robust health, although he did develop in many ways.[105] A more recent example is provided by the prolonged deprivation experienced by children in Romanian orphanages, in which "every child who has been in these institutions for 6 months or longer has significant developmental delays."[106] In a pilot study exploring the effects of sensory deprivation and the changes that can occur following enrichment of the environment, infants were initially found to be functioning at a level between the "at risk" and "deficiency" categories of the total Test of Sensory Functions.[107] Following a 6-month program within an enriched environment, children improved in all but "adaptive motor functions."[108]

Another group of people who experience extreme occupational deprivation are prisoners of war. The importance of finding meaning through occupation is one factor in the survival odds of prisoners. For example, Dimsdale, in a study of the coping behavior of Nazi concentration camp survivors, identified purpose as essential to those who survived. One of his subjects focused on "where I could find a blanket, something to chew, to eat, to repair, a torn shoe, an additional glove,"[109] and Frankl, an existential psychiatrist, observed about his own concentration camp experiences that mortality rates were highest among those unable to find purpose.[110] Prisoners in jails often face similar, if not so extreme, states of occupational deprivation, which has been linked with both community and individual disorders, such as prison riots[111] and suicide while in custody.[112] Supporting the link between lack of purposeful occupation and ill health is a longitudinal study of long-term prisoners, which found the opposite to be the case as, over a period of 7 years, the prisoners being studied became increasingly involved in a variety of occupations that led to decreases of dysphoric emotional states, stress-related medical problems, and disciplinary incidents.[113]

Many people experience reduced occupational options because they are deprived of paid employment and may, as a result, have reduced opportunity to use physical, mental, or social capacities and may thereby suffer a decrease in health. However, it would appear that there may be more than this simple explanation to consider. One important characteristic of paid employment at present, noted in the chapter on occupational evolution, is the value placed upon it by society, which is probably as great as skill in obtaining the requirements for sustenance would have been among hunter-gatherers. In other words, significant work will be more conducive to mental and social health and well-being if it involves both meeting a primary urge and complying with societal values. Lack of significant work may cause mental and social ill health, which can result in physical illness as well because of the integrative nature of the nervous system. Research data seem to support that decreased health status is linked with unemployment.

Richard Smith's summary account suggests that unemployment and poor health are strongly associated, that unemployment itself causes some illness, and that health problems are compounded by unemployment; that the poverty, low socioeconomic status, poor education, and housing conditions, associated frequently with both ill health and unemployment, cause difficulties in clarifying the strength of the associations. Unemployment is also associated with high divorce rates, child and spouse abuse, unwanted pregnancies, abortions, reduced birthweight and child growth, perinatal and infant mortality, and increased morbidity in families, though for none of the associations can it be assumed that unemployment itself is the cause.[114]

Smith is supported by many detailed studies. About one fifth of the unemployed report a deterioration in their mental health since being out of work.[115-117] Studies using standardized questionnaires consistently show that the mental health of the unemployed is poorer than those with work[117,118] and that there is a link between unemployment, suicide, and deliberate self-injury.[119] There is less evidence associating unemployment with psychoses.[120] Fryer and Payne found that 5% of the unemployed they studied reported an improvement in their mental health—some because they escaped from jobs they disliked—while others had found positive aspects to unemployment.[121] The studies linking unemployment with physical illness are limited. However, the British Regional Heart Study has shown higher rates of bronchitis, chronic obstructive lung disease, and ischemic heart disease among the unemployed than among the employed.[122] Beale and Nethercott found a statistically significant 20% increase in medical consultation rates for families of 80 men and 49 women who lost their jobs when a local factory closed, compared with controls who did not lose their jobs.[123] A 60% increase in referrals to hospital outpatients was also found. In a 1992 Australian paper, unemployed men were reported as experiencing a 66% higher prevalence of disability, 21% prevalence of recent illnesses, 101% more days of reduced activity because of illness, and of diabetes and respiratory disorders as a cause of death than employed men. Women followed the same trends but not to the same extent.[124] Brenner, a professor at Johns Hopkins University, found a relationship between downward fluctuations in the American economy between 1940 and 1973 and physical and emotional illness.[125,126] He calculated that an unemployment increase of about 1 million people (1% of the population) sustained for 6 years could be linked with increases of 36,887 in total deaths, 4,227 in mental hospital admissions, and 3,340 in prison admissions. His study indicated that health is vulnerable to subtle economic fluctuations and that it improves and declines with the economy. Scott-Samuel and Moser found unemployment may also be associated with premature death[127-130]; however, Gravelle is unconvinced that this is the case.[131]

Other people who are at risk of ill health from occupational deprivation include disadvantaged groups within the community, such as the poor, the disabled, minority ethnic groups, and the aged. There are differences in the risks of ill health between such social groupings and others,[132-134] and it is argued here that occupational deprivation plays a part in this equation. For example, Australian Aboriginal elders, particularly from remote areas, disturbed by "self-destructive activities such as drinking [and] violence," poor health, along with loss of traditional occupations, "asked that 'sit-down' money be replaced by money for work done by those who were unemployed."[135] The Community Development Employment Project Scheme came into being providing "an increase in the health of communities, ...more people involved in physically active tasks, a decrease in alcohol consumption, an increase in cleanliness, and better nutrition."[136] This is a rare example of an "occupational" initiative being implemented for combined health, social, and economic benefits.

Very few initiatives are being implemented for those with ongoing health problems, such as many of the disabled. In fact, programs aimed at promoting their health through opportunities to encourage growth of occupational potential are the first to be axed when health resources become scarce. This is even though such programs are not expensive when compared with technologically brilliant life-saving procedures that may condemn a brain injured victim to an unresourced, unsatisfying, and unhealthy life in the future. Hodges asks, "Are service needs for the promotion of health among the disabled different than for the non-disabled, and are they adequately met?" He identifies the lack of development of strategies for the disabled as a major void and suggests that for this "significant portion of society...the concept of health promotion and disease prevention takes on added dimensions and heightened need."[137]

Women, too, have generally suffered occupational deprivation for hundreds of years but the industrial revolution brought the differences and divisions of labor between men and women to a point seen by Mackie and Pattullo as destroying the vitality of women.[138] Equality of occupational opportunity between men and women had declined from the Paleolithic era on, yet during particular eras some women enjoyed some respite. For example, in the medieval period, it was possible for women entering a nunnery (usually upper class, unmarried women, and later from the merchant classes) to receive a better education and the chance to engage in a greater range of occupations than those who married, and women in towns were able to engage in many trades.[139-142] The number of medieval English words ending in "ster" or "ess," such as "webster" (woman weaver), "baxter" (woman baker), and "seam-stress" (woman sewer), are worth noting. So too is the fact that women worked in 86 of 100 trade and professional guilds in Paris as listed in Etienne Boileau's 13th century *Book of Trades*. Women did not, however, have political equality and were subservient to their fathers or their husbands. Although accepted as of lesser value than the roles men undertook, women's occupations, which were often "gruelling and virtually unending," were also productive, rich in variety, self-expression, responsibility, achievement, satisfaction, and not "compartmentalized, isolated, or solitary."[138] Not all women were engaged in paid employment, but the restricted occupational role of affluent women was hazardous to health in a different way. Their physical activity was slight, the use of their mental capacities restricted, and their "social usefulness was never recognized or recompensed. Instead their dependence on the male bread-winner and their work in the family reduced their capacity to organize."[143] Florence Nightingale at the age of 26 observed that "women don't consider themselves as human beings at all" and said that she knew of some who had gone mad for lack of things to do[144]; similarly Elizabeth Garrett Anderson suggests that "there is no tonic in the pharmacopoeia to be compared with happiness, and happiness worth calling such is not known where the days drag along filled with make-believe occupations and dreary sham amusements."[145]

The strong preference for women to follow domestic and child-raising occupations in the home, in Victorian times, was linked with infant health. Indicative of the period, Jones concluded that:

> *The children of women engaged in industrial occupations suffer from the effects of maternal neglect. They are handicapped from the moment of birth in their struggle for existence, and have to contend not only against the inevitable perils of infancy but also against perils due to their neglect by their mothers and to the ignorance of those to whose care they are entrusted.*[146]

It was even thought that if married women undertook paid employment outside the home this could be at the sacrifice of infant lives.[147]

Dyhouse reports that during formal discussion of Dr. Jones' paper there was some criticism of this conclusion, such as that statistics linking women who took jobs outside the home with infant mortality rates provided conflicting evidence, that overcrowding and insanitary conditions were more crucial variables, and that some children might benefit from better food and conditions provided by mother's wages.[148] The 1893-1894 Royal Commission on Labour, which investigated conditions of women's work, including "the effects of women's industrial employment on their health, mortality, and the home" found Jones's association between women's employment and infantile mortality were imprecise and impressionistic.[149]

The inequality of opportunity that has characterized women's occupations for thousands of years as a result of the type of economy and dominant cultural ideas, such as about social justice and equity, humanism, individualism, and familism, is still evident today, although in post-industrial societies it has improved greatly.[150] Even so, as recently as 1976, Douglas Gordon, in his book *Health, Sickness and Society,* expresses occupational gender bias in observing:

> *It is said that a man's job provides him with a means to satisfy his ego by*

preserving his personal integrity and by maintaining his place in the world. On average a man's occupation is more important to his mental health than is outside occupation to a woman. She gains status as a wife and mother and from her home...Some women need to work outside: a lot do not wish to do so. At least that is what they say.[10]

The remarkable improvements in women's morbidity and mortality since the 19th century appear to be multifactorial, including reduced birth rate, greater understanding of obstetric and gynecological disorders, emancipation, a change of attitudes, and, it is argued, the increased opportunity for women to exercise capacities and develop potentials. Indeed, a few studies point to this being the case.[151,152] However, despite the growing numbers of women participating in other than domestic work, the study of the relationship between women's occupations and health are limited, on the whole, to job stress,[153-156] reproductive hazards,[156-160] and the threat to family function and maternal responsibilities.[161]

Occupational deprivation and imbalance have been variable and, generally, gradual as occupation evolved in the course of human adaptation to challenge. It has been noted that adaptation is being called for at a rapidly increasing rate at present, and Ornstein and Sobel suggest that the technological possibility of more radical changes in occupation could result in serious health consequences. They say that, because parts of the brain are rooted in earlier species' inheritance, people are only able to respond with biological reactions that are either "obsolete" or "inappropriately illicited."[87] Similarly, Dubos warns that although humans may appear to adapt to new environments, their biological inheritance only enables adaptation up to a point and that chronic disease states can develop over time.[162] These warnings are an echo of some of Dunn's anxiety as to whether individuals and families can "attain and maintain wellness while riding the crest of a social millrace"[163] and Maslow's concerns that mankind is "at a point in history unlike anything that has ever been before" with "huge acceleration in the growth of facts, of knowledge, of techniques, of inventions, of advances in technology." Maslow suggested that the rapidity of the changing world calls for "a different kind of human being...who is comfortable with change," because "societies that cannot turn out such people will die."[164] The Ottawa Charter also recognizes that there are health concerns associated with socioecological change and calls for a "systematic assessment of the health impact of a rapidly changing environment, particularly in areas of technology, work, energy production, and urbanization."[165] Such an assessment would need to take into account the concept of alienation or "estrangement," which is the third occupational risk factor to be considered.

Occupational Alienation

Since the time when people lived in harmony with the natural environment early in the species history, with only the simplest of technology to assist them to meet their needs, mankind has sought to challenge and master nature by developing more and more sophisticated technology to meet their occupational wants, to conquer ill health and to delay death by ever-increasingly sophisticated medical science. Such technological change is seen, by some, as alienating. Alienation is defined in *The Standard English Desk Dictionary* as "estrangement; transference of ownership; diversion to a different purpose." It is a term much debated by 20th century Marxists, as it is a theme that surfaced as important in the early humanist period of Marx's work since first being published in English in 1932.[166,167]

As a central concept of Marx's philosophy, alienation is intimately connected with his views about activity and human nature.[168] Individual, group, institutional, or societal activity can result in alienation when it is not in accordance with our species' nature. Marx saw our species' nature as a unity of naturalism and humanism; that is, he viewed humans in evolutionary terms, as part of nature, and, in humanist terms, as praxic beings who both change nature and create themselves. He regarded as potentially alienating any productive, economic, social, or spiritual activity, as well as the products of activity such as philosophies, morals, money, commodities, laws, or social institutions.[166] He argues that because of "cultural" and "capitalist" history such activities and products have become estranged from the natural creativity of human species' nature, resulting in feelings of alienation toward self and others and the activities and products themselves. These alienating activities, along with division of labor, are "forced upon individuals by the society which they themselves create"[169] and as long as "activity is not voluntary...man's own deed becomes an alien power opposed to him, which enslaves him instead of being controlled by him."[170]

To illustrate this concept of alienation, consider the analogy of an animal born in captivity—a lion, for example, who has only ever known a world of a cage, of other animals living solitary lives in their own cages, and of people who feed and care for him, but who demand particular activity and behavior from time to time. It is possible to understand that the lion will experience needs and instincts that relate to the natural environment in which he would have lived in the wild but with no means of really appreciating or satisfying them. He is estranged or alienated from his species' nature, from his activities, and from other animals but because he has never known a natural lifestyle does not understand why he feels unhappy, frustrated, or the need to escape to something different. Humans because of their occupational species' nature have constructed, over time, their own cages. The bars are the products and results of their occupations, such as the social values of any culture or society, its laws and rules, its political direction, and its economic structure including the day-to-day occupational opportunities and demands on each individual. Like the lion, humans are estranged from their species nature, from others, from what they do, and from the results of their activities. Daniel Miller even suggests that the status given to the medical profession and its scientific values can be alienating factors in the way that they exert control over the procedures aimed at rapid repair of body parts decontextualized from the recipient's mental or social needs.[171]

Marx particularly linked feelings of alienation with the restrictions imposed upon the ordinary worker by capitalism and industrial processes. He pondered on the contrast between the craftsmen who worked skillfully with tools that were often handmade and the factory workers who in many instances were subservient to their tools—the machines. He wrote that far from freeing humans from toil "the lightening of the labor, even, becomes a sort of torture, since the machine does not free the laborer from work, but deprives the work of all interest."[172] He envisaged that factory workers "robbed thus of all real life-content, have become abstract individuals, ...the only connection which still links them with the productive forces and with their own existence—labor—has lost all semblance of self-activity and only sustains life by stunting it."[173] Marx perceived this stunting outcome as less than health-giving and suggested a direct illness connection associated with the processes of industrialization because "factory work exhausts the nervous system to the uttermost, it does away with the many sided play of the muscles, and confiscates every atom of freedom, both in bodily and intellectual activity."

Smith suggests in *Unemployment and Health* that, for many, these problems continue to the present, as "most employment for most people has, since the industrial revolution, been hard, exhausting, boring, dirty, degrading, and, as Marx said, alienating."[174] These alienating changes were compounded, during the industrial revolution, by "the terrific destruction of human values," with Dubos suggesting that if ever people "lived under conditions completely removed from the state of nature dreamed of by the philosophers of the enlightenment, it was the English proletariat of the 1830s."[175]

Those conditions are now regarded as so unhealthy that it is difficult to understand why people made the mass exodus from country to town, until it is appreciated that "the move from farm to factory was based on social trends that the individual could not control," and "it is far from clear that it was individual preference...that led to urban migrations," but economic need.[176] It is also worth noting that the conditions of most people in the 18th century were far from idyllic, with laborers working from dawn to dark in "poverty and darkness."[177] Huge numbers of the population changed not only their habitats but the structure of their social networks from small, cohesive groupings, which worked and played together, to large populations where individuals knew or were close to few people. Jones observes that a "new concept of 'going to work'" emerged as "employment based at or near home" was "replaced by work at central locations such as factories and shops."[23] Centralization separated men and women, altering the value of their occupations and experiences of social and mental well-being; it separated adults from children, altering teaching and learning roles; and children, unless engaged in child labor with their parents, no longer observed or participated with them as they engaged in the daily round of socially valued roles and skills. Instead they learned from strangers.

Such changes to basic human relationship patterns may well have gradually impacted on some of the family loneliness and social alienation problems common in the modern world and that lead directly or indirectly to ill health. Mijuskovic puts a case that alienation and individual loneliness are more pronounced and prevalent in "atomistic societies," such as America and other post-industrial societies than in "organic communities." In the latter, natural functions, role perspectives, mutual interdependence, and intrinsic relations are stressed in contrast to individual freedom, external connections, causal and reductionistic explanations, rule orientation, and artificial frameworks of the former.[178] His view has some merit when it is observed how current post-industrial values and changing occupational structures, language, and technologies can restrict freedom of action by ever-increasing rules, regulations, and bureaucracy; replace ongoing human endeavor with labor-saving technology, which often creates work of a mundane variety; reduce the availability of paid employment, which has interest, meaning, or meets individual needs for growth and challenge; and create a materialistic way of life out of step with sustaining the natural world of which humans are a part. All of these changes have the potential to create environments that are alienating enough to spawn discontent and disease (Figure 6-2).

Since Marcuse renewed attention to Marx's theme of alienation in 1932, others, such as Fromm, have continued widespread and intense discussion, which links the notions of alienation with sickness or ill health for individuals and for societies.[179] In numerous recent studies, alienation associated with unsatisfactory occupational factors has been found to be implicated in ill health and risk behaviors, particularly for

Figure 6-2. Work of a mundane variety with little interest or meaning is alienating. An example at the Carolina Cotton Mills in 1908. Courtesy George Eastman House, Rochester, NY.

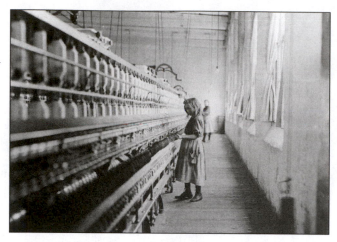

people already disadvantaged.[180-188] While technological change in itself (unless toxic) is unlikely to cause illness, the effects on people's engagement in occupations and their reaction to the changes can lead to illness if the change is alienating, even in high demand jobs.[189] Justice argues that when work is perceived as stressful, boring, or meaningless, the likelihood of "mass illness" is increased,[38] and this is backed up by a review of material from 16 epidemics of illness at various workplaces and schools undertaken by staff from the American National Institute for Occupational Safety and Health.[190] There is convincing evidence that the health benefits of paid employment depend on its quality,[117,191-194] and those who are dissatisfied with work experience numerous symptoms and stress and tend to drink or smoke more than those who are satisfied.[195]

Alienation for workers, unions, and labor managers will continue to increase as production and service jobs become "deskilled" and lose their capacity to interest those doing them, because "many jobs that have been transformed by new technology are characterized by high levels of boredom."[196,197] Along with this, Naisbitt suggests that people are experiencing turbulence that may well have health implications hard to anticipate as they are caught in the rapid, "mega" change from an industrial to an information society. For those employed in intellectual occupations, such as educators, administrators, scientists, and health professionals, stresses caused by what he calls the "chaos of information pollution" are frequently described as overwhelming.[198]

"Technological change is often hailed as a signpost of human progress and a vehicle for human liberation."[199] Pollard observes that the belief in progress is an assurance that science and technology will continue to provide more and more material benefits, as well as mastery over the environment.[200] So much respect is progress accorded in today's world that the natural health needs of people pale in significance beside the drive to create more and more sophisticated technology. How technological progress in entertainment equipment has altered the character of many shared social occupations is a case in point. Other leisure occupations also have been influenced by technological advancements, supposedly so that excellence is more attainable. Examples include the sporting activities for which chemical potions as well as mechanical, biophysical, and electronic apparatus have been developed and marketed so that individuals may achieve previously unrealized feats. Such technology subtly alters the elements of human toil, the pure skill, and the mental and social exercise components drawn from within any participant. This is also true in the arena of paid employment, and it is suggested that the way in which technology and division of labor have been used remain as in the industrial revolution "antagonistic to individual growth."[201] This reduction in the use of human energies and potentials via technology, which drastically changes use of human creativity and natural environments, is primarily to meet market purposes rather than human needs and thus is alienating.

Other major and potentially alienating change that goes along with rapid technological advances has been a marked increase in the urge to accumulate material goods and property, without a thought for the potential of materialism to destroy our ecosystem. Many erroneously equate material wealth with happiness and health, mistaking the means for the ends. Mumford suggests that "over-charges of empty stimuli, ...materialistic repletion, ...costly ritual of conspicuous waste, ...and highly organized purposelessness" are part of the "clinical picture of the cultural disease from which the world suffers."[21] He goes so far as to assert that "the supernatural theology of the Middle Ages was closer to reality than the crass materialism of an age which fancies that the achievement of an 'economy of abundance' will automatically ensure a maximum of human felicity."[21]

The acquisition of assets is now seen as a primary need and is regarded, by Lorenz, as having reached a "pathological" state with the potential to cause mental and social disruption deemed to be symptoms of cultural ill health. He asserts that the apparent rush to acquire material wealth undermines health, although "man rushes, not only because he is propelled by greed, for this alone would not induce him to ruin his own health, but because he is driven" by fear.[27]

Throughout this chapter, it has been indicated that occupational alienation, along with deprivation and imbalance, have the potential to lead to stress-related illness, which will now be considered, albeit briefly despite its considerable importance.

Stress

Stress is a basic phylogenic mechanism, which under normal circumstances works to maintain physiological equilibrium in times of physical and emotional pressure. If prolonged at an unacceptable level, susceptibility to illness is increased. Adolph Meyer is credited with recognizing, early in this century, that disease appeared to occur when this regulatory system became subjected to overload,[202] and Hans Selye, in 1936, described the "general adaptation syndrome"[203] in which he hypothesized that the adaptive response can break down due to "innate defects, understress, overstress, or psychological mismanagement. The most common stress diseases...are peptic ulcers...high blood pressure, heart accidents, and nervous diseases."[204]

Work based on Selye's hypothesis has largely sustained it. A well-publicized study by French and Caplan links stress with coronary heart disease,[205] and others have suggested that stress is associated with disorders of the musculoskeletal, digestive, and immune systems[206] and depressive illness. Roskies and Lazarus propose that the ability to cope with everyday stress has more effect on physical, mental, and social health than stress episodes themselves,[207] and similarly, Moore argues that:

> *Long-term chronic stress and especially chronic unpredictable stress can result in an earlier demise or long-term disability (mental and/or physical), unless therapeutic intervention can reverse the individual's way of coping and/or reverse the situations which are causing the stress.*[208]

She lists some effects of chronic unpredictable stress as increased blood pressure, heart rate, respiration, muscle tension, and blood-glucose levels; decreased peristalsis, lymphocytes, T and B cells, immune response, destabilization of lyosomes, and hyper-alert states.

The type of illness experienced as a result of stress is thought, by Selye, to express any individual's weakest points,[209] so any genetic or familial predisposition, such as mental breakdown, arthritis, or cardiac failure, can be activated by prolonged stress.[210] There is some disputing of the links between stress and illness. Temoshok, for example, argues that there is little empirical evidence either "to support or refute potential biological pathways linking stress factors and disease initiation or progression for any disorder." He suggests that this reflects the complexity of the connections, which probably include person and situation variables, interaction effects including physiological and psychological predispositions, as well as social, cultural, economic, and political contexts.[211]

Moderating factors, such as diet,[212] medication,[213] physical activity, and rewarding occupational roles,[214] as well as relaxation techniques,[215] can provide resistance to stress-related disorders. For example, it has been suggested that playing sports is relaxing because "one is using the mind and body the way they were intended to be used in fighting or running away" in response to the fight or flight reaction.[216] Such argument leads to the view held by Eisler: that health is more likely to be maintained if individuals have the skills and resources to cope effectively with the diversity of life's challenges[217] and, following Selye's lead, to the questions asked by Antonovsky about not whether stress is bad for health, but for whom and under what conditions is it good or bad. He speculates that the mechanisms for the relationship between a sense of coherence and health includes experience of successful coping with stressors. Indeed, moderate stress that augments the functional capacities of all systems is necessary for maintaining positive health and vitality as well as providing a reserve against extreme stress. "Heart attacks are not the result of shoveling snow or running for a train, ...they are the product of a lifetime of not doing things like shoveling snow or running for a train."[218]

Stress-related illnesses as a result of occupational alienation, deprivation, and imbalance have undoubtedly increased during occupational evolution, despite the obvious benefits in living in today's post-industrial world rather than that of hunter-gatherers'. Now, for those living in post-industrial societies, there is longer life expectancy, lower infant mortality, and miraculous advances in technological and pharmaceutical medicine to reverse the effects of much disease, disability, and trauma.

Since the 1940s, ...the impact of scientific medicine and public health administration upon conditions of human life has become literally worldwide. In most places epidemic diseases have become unimportant, and many kinds of infection have become rare where they were formally common and serious. The net increment to human health and cheerfulness is hard to exaggerate.[17]

These advances ensure that more people are provided with a stable base from which to experience positive health and well-being. On the whole, though, health and well-being seem to sit uneasily amid the rush and stresses of present-day occupational structures that humans have constructed over the years, with much morbidity and mortality resulting from lack of individual or community awareness about the relationship between occupation and ill health. This is, in large measure, because of a lack of research based upon a sufficiently broad or holistic perspective of occupation and a resultant dearth of intervention strategies from public health, social, political, or national policies.

In another time of rapidly changing occupational conditions, early this century, a small group of idealists, such as mental hygienists like Adolph Meyer, trade union activist Helen Marot, and founders of the Arts and Crafts movement (based on Morris's ideology) in America recognized and acted on the apparent link between health, well-being, and occupations. This was sufficient to lead to the concept of "health through occupation" being adopted by social activists and pioneer occupational therapists early in the 20th century to counteract the maladaptive effects of industrialization and occupational deprivation, imbalance, and alienation for those who were ill. The next two chapters discuss the genesis of this concept and how the message became dimmed by general acceptance of the changed shape of occupational structures and by a change of emphasis within health services.

References

1. Last J, ed. *Public Health and Preventive Medicine*. Conn: Appleton and Lange; 1987.
2. Hetzel BS, McMichael T. *L S Factor: Lifestyle and Health*. Ringwood, Victoria: Penguin; 1987:186-187.
3. Maddox GL. Modifying the social environment. In: *Oxford Textbook of Public Health*. Vol 2. New York, NY: Oxford University Press; 1985.
4. Katz AH, Hermalin JA, Hess RE, eds. *Prevention and Health: Direction for Policy and Practice*. New York, NY: The Haworth Press; 1987.
5. Better Health Commission. *Looking Forward to Better Health*. Vols 1-3. Canberra: Australian Government Publishing Service; 1986.
6. Department of Health and Human Services. *The Health Consequences of Smoking: Cancer*. Rockville, Md: 1982.
7. Department of Health and Human Services. *The Health Consequences of Smoking: Cardiovascular Disease*. Rockville, Md: 1983.
8. Department of Health and Human Services. *The Health Consequences of Smoking: Chronic Obstructive Lung Disease*. Rockville, Md: 1984.
9. Gordon T, Sorlie P, Kannel WB. *Section 27, Coronary Heart Disease Atherothrombotic Brain Infarction. Intermittent Claudication. A Multivariate Analysis of Some Factors Related to Their Incidence: Framingham Study, 16 Year Follow Up*. US Department of Health, Education and Welfare, Public Health Service. NIH Pub. No. 1740-0320, 1971.
10. Gordon D. *Health, Sickness and Society: Theoretical Concepts in Social and Preventive Medicine*. St. Lucia, Queensland: University of Queensland Press; 1976:5,157,164,311,337,378.
11. Parmeggiani L, ed. *ILO Encyclopedia of Occupational Health and Safety*. 2 Vols. 3rd rev ed. Geneva, Switzerland: International Labour Organisation; 1983.
12. Agricola (George Bauer). *De re Metallica 1556*. Hoover HC, Hoover HL, trans. New York, NY: Dover Publications; 1950.
13. Paracelsus. *Four Treatises of Theophrastus von Hohenheim Called Paracelsus. 1567*. Sigerist HE, ed. Temkin CL, Rosen G, Zilboorg G, Sigerist HE, trans. Baltimore, Md: Johns Hopkins Press; 1941.
14. Ramazzini B. *Disease of Occupations*. New York, NY: Collier-MacMillan; 1980.
15. Thackrah CT. *The Effects of the Principle Arts, Trades, and Professions, and of Civic States and Habits of Living, On Health and Longevity*. London, England: Longman, Rees, Orme, Browne and Green; 1831.
16. Skeletons of Spitalfields. UK: BBC Television Documentary, circa 1990.
17. McNeill WH. *Plagues and People*. London, England: Penguin Books; 1979:13,25,192.
18. Douglas M. Population control in primitive peoples. *British Journal of Sociology*. 1966;17:263-273.
19. Birdsell JB. On population structure in generalized hunting and collecting populations. *Evolution*. 1958;12:189-205.
20. Procopius. Persian wars 23:1. *History of the Wars*. 5 Vols. Dewing HB, trans. Cambridge, Mass: Harvard University Press; 1914.
21. Mumford L. *The Condition of Man*. London, England: Heinemann; 1963:148,380.
22. Cipolla CM. *The Economic History of World Populations*. 5th ed. Harmondsworth: Penguin; 1970.
23. Jones B. *Sleepers, Wake! Technology and the Future of Work*. Melbourne, Australia: Oxford University Press; 1982:16,83.
24. Eversley DEC. Epidemiology as social history. In: Creighton CA, ed. *History of Epidemics in Britain*.

2nd ed. London, England: Cassell; 1965:1-35.

25. Doll R. *Preventive Medicine: The Objectives in "The Value of Preventive Medicine."* Ciba Foundation Symposium 10. London, England: Pitman; 1985.

26. Mumford L. *The Culture of Cities*. New York, NY: Harcourt, Brace; 1938.

27. Lorenz K. *Civilized Man's Eight Deadly Sins*. Latzke M, trans. London, England: Methuen and Co Ltd; 1974:8-9,76.

28. Hinrichs N, ed. *Population, Environment and People*. New York, NY: McGraw-Hill; 1971:xi.

29. Friedman HS, ed. *Personality and Disease*. New York, NY: John Wiley and Sons; 1990:7,11.

30. Risse GB. History of Western medicine from Hippocrates to germ theory. In: Kiple KF, ed. *The Cambridge World History of Human Disease*. New York, NY: Cambridge University Press; 1993:11.

31. Hippocrates. *Regimen*. In: *Hippocratic Writings: On Ancient Medicine*. William Benton; 1952.

32. Plato. *Timaeus*. Lee HDP, trans. Penguin Classics; 1965:116-117.

33. Meyer A. The philosophy of occupational therapy. *Archives of Occupational Therapy*. 1922;1:1-10. In: *American Journal of Occupational Therapy*. 1977;31(10):639-642.

34. Levin HL. Occupational and recreational therapy among the ancients. *Occupational Therapy and Rehabilitation*. 1938;17:311-316.

35. Llorens L. Changing balance: environment and individual. *American Journal of Occupational Therapy*. 1984;38:29-34.

36. Marino-Schorn JA. Morale, work and leisure in retirement. *Physical and Occupational Therapy in Geriatrics*. 1986;4:49-59.

37. Spencer EA. Toward a balance of work and play: promotion of health and wellness. *Occupational Therapy in Health Care*. 1989;5:87-99.

38. Justice B. *Who Gets Sick: Thinking and Health*. Texas: Peak Press; 1987:28-29,31-32,179.

39. Wolf S, Goodell H. *Behavioural Science in Clinical Medicine*. Springfield, Ill: Charles C Thomas; 1976.

40. Price VA. *Type A Behaviour Pattern: A Model for Research and Practice*. New York, NY: Academic Press; 1982.

41. Powell KE, Thompson PD, Caspersen CJ, Kendrick JS. Physical activity and the incidence of coronary heart disease. *Annual Review of Public Health*. 1987;8:253-287.

42. American College of Sports Medicine. *Guidelines for Exercise Testing and Prescription*. 4th ed. Philadelphia, Pa: Lea and Febiger; 1991.

43. Caspersen CJ, Christensen GM, Pollard RA. Status of the 1990 physical fitness and exercise objectives—evidence from NHIS 1985. *Public Health Reports*. 1986;101:587-592.

44. Blaxter M. *Health and Lifestyles*. London, England: Tavistock/Routledge; 1990.

45. Clee J. Unpublished study. University of South Australia; 1991.

46. Department of Sport, Recreation and Tourism. *Annual Report. 1985/86*. Canberra: Australian Government Publishing Service; 1986.

47. Green E, Hebron S, Woodward D. *Women's Leisure in Sheffield: A Research Report*. Sheffield Department of Applied Social Studies; 1987.

48. Green E, Hebron S, Woodward D. *Women's Leisure. What Leisure?* London, England: Macmillan Educations Ltd; 1990.

49. Boutilier M, SanGiovanni L. Women and sports: reflections on health and policy. In: Lewin E, Olesen V, eds. *Women, Health and Healing: Toward a New Perspective*. New York, NY: Tavistock Publications; 1985:209.

50. Blair SN, Kohl HW, Paffenbarger RS, Clark DG, Cooper KH, Gibbons LW. Physical fitness and all-cause mortality: a prospective study of healthy men and women. *JAMA*. 1989;262:2395-2401.

51. Ekelund LG, Haskell WL, Johnson JL, Whaley FS, Criqui MH, Sheps DS. Physical fitness as a predictor of cardiovascular mortality in asymptomatic North American men. *N Engl J Med*. 1988;319:1379-1384.

52. Haskell WL. Exercise induced changes in plasma lipids and lipoproteins. *Preventive Medicine*. 1984;13:23-36.

53. Wood PD, Haskell WL, Blair SN, et al. Increased exercise level and plasma lipoprotein concentrations: a one-year randomised study in sedentary middle-aged men. *Metabolism*. 1983;32:31-39.

54. Kaplan RM, Sallis JF, Patterson TL. *Health and Human Behavior*. New York, NY: McGraw-Hill Inc; 1993:350.

55. Hicky N, Mulcahy R, Bourke GJ, Graham I, Wilson-Davis K. Study of coronary risk factors relating to physical activity in 15,171 men. *British Medical Journal*. 1975;5982:507-509.

56. Siegel WC, Blumenthal JA. The role of exercise in the prevention and treatment of hypertension. *Annals of Behavioural Medicine*. 1991;13:23-30.

57. Vranic M, Wasserman D. Exercise, fitness and diabetes. In: Bouchard C, Shephard RJ, Stephens T, Sutton JR, McPherson GD, eds. *Exercise, Fitness and Health: A Concensus of Current Knowledge*.

Champaign, Ill: Human Kinetics; 1990:467-490.

58. Epstein LH, Wing RR, Thompson JK, Griffin W. Attendance and fitness in aerobic exercise: the effects of contract and lottery procedures. *Behavior Modification*. 1980;4:465-479.

59. Haskell WL, Leon AS, Caspersen CJ, et al. Cardiovascular benefits and assessment of physical activity and fitness in adults. *Medicine and Science in Sports and Exercise*. 1992;24:S201-S220.

60. Calabrese LH. Exercise, immunity, cancer and infection. In: Bouchard C, Shephard RJ, Stephens T, Sutton JR, McPherson GD, eds. *Exercise, Fitness and Health: A Concensus of Current Knowledge*. Champaign, Ill: Human Kinetics; 1990:567-579.

61. Stephens T. Physical activity and mental health in the United States and Canada: evidence from 4 population surveys. *Preventive Medicine*. 1988;17:35-47.

62. Gilliam TB, Freedson PS, Geenen DL, Shahraray B. *Medicine and Science in Sports and Exercise*. 1981;13:65-67.

63. Stephens T, Jacob DR, White CC. A descriptive epidemiology of leisure time physical activity. *Public Health Reports*. 1985;100:147-158.

64. Shea S, Basche CE, Lantigua R, Weschler H. The Washington Heights-Inwood healthy heart program: a third generation community-based cardiovascular disease prevention program in a disadvantaged urban setting. *Preventive Medicine*. 1991;21:201-217.

65. King AC, Blair SN, Bild DE, et al. Determinants of physical activity and interventions in adults. *Medicine and Science in Sports and Exercise*. 1992;24:S221-S237.

66. Williams MH. *Lifetime Fitness and Wellness: A Personal Choice*. 2nd ed. Dubuque: Wm. C. Brown Publishers; 1990:9,27.

67. Wilcock AA, et al. *Retrospective Study of Elderly Peoples' Perceptions of the Relationship Between Their Lifes' Occupations and Health*. Unpublished material, University of South Australia, 1990.

68. King-Boyes MJE. *Patterns of Aboriginal Culture: Then and Now*. Sydney, Australia: McGraw-Hill Book Co; 1977:17,155.

69. Passmore R, Eastwood MA. *Davidson and Passmore, Human Nutrition and Dietetics*. Edinburgh: Churchill Livingstone; 1986.

70. Garrow JS. *Treat Obesity Seriously*. Edinburgh: Churchill Livingstone; 1981.

71. Hafen BQ, ed. *Overweight and Obesity: Causes, Fallacies, Treatment*. Provo, Utah: Brigham Young University Press; 1975.

72. Budgett R. Overtraining syndrome. *British Journal of Sports Medicine*. 1990;24(4):231-236.

73. Cooper K. *Dr Kenneth Cooper's Antioxidant Revolution*. Melbourne, Australia: Bookman; 1994.

74. Siscovick DS, Weiss NS, Fletcher RH, Lasky T. The incidence of primary cardiac arrest during vigorous exercise. *N Engl J Med*. 1984;311:874-877.

75. Monk T. Coping with the stress of shift work. *Work and Stress*. 1988;2:169-172.

76. Dinges D, Whitehouse W, Carota-Orne E, Orne M. The benefits of a nap during prolonged work and wakefulness. *Work and Stress*. 1988;2:139-153.

77. Rosa R, Colligan M. Long workdays versus restdays: assessing fatigue and alertness with a portable performance battery. *Human Factors*. 1988;5:87-98.

78. Kubey R, Csikszentmihalyi M. *Television and the Quality of Life*. Hillsdale, NJ: Erlbaum; 1990.

79. Csikszentmihalyi M, Larson R, Prescott S. The ecology of adolescent activity and experience. *Journal of Youth and Adolescence*. 1977;6:281-294.

80. Larson R, Kubey R. Television and music: contrasting media in adolescent life. *Youth and Society*. 1983;15:13-31.

81. Csikszentmihalyi M. Activity and happiness: towards a science of occupation. *Journal of Occupational Science: Australia*. 1993;1(1):38-42.

82. Wilcock AA, Hall M, Hambley N, et al. The relationship between occupational balance and health: a pilot study. *Occupational Therapy International*. 1997;4(1):17-30.

83. Geschwind N, Galaburda A, eds. *Biological Foundations of Cerebral Dominance*. Cambridge, Mass: Harvard University Press; 1984.

84. Andervont HB. Influence of environment on mammary cancer in mice. *Journal of National Cancer Institute*. 1944;4:579-581.

85. Achterberg J, Collerrain I, Craig P. A possible relationship between cancer, mental retardation and mental disorder. *Social Science and Medicine*. 1978;12:135-139.

86. de la Pena A. *The Psychobiology of Cancer*. New York, NY: Praeger Publishers; 1983.

87. Ornstein R, Sobel D. *The Healing Brain, A Radical New Approach to Health Care*. London, England: Macmillan; 1988:206-207,213-217.

88. Ardell DB. *High Level Wellness*. 2nd ed. Berkeley, Calif: Ten Speed Press; 1986.

89. Csikszentmihalyi M. *Flow: The Psychology of Optimal Experience*. New York, NY: Harper and Row; 1990.

90. Sigerist HE. *A History of Medicine*. Vol 1. *Primitive and Archaic Medicine*. New York, NY: Oxford University Press; 1955:254-255.
91. Gare S. The age of overwork. *The Weekend Australian Review*. 1995;April 8-9:2-3.
92. Schor J. *The Overworked American: The Unexpected Decline of Leisure*. New York, NY: Basic Books; 1991.
93. Barrett HR, Browne A. Workloads of rural African women: the impact of economic adjustment in Sub-Saharan Africa. *Journal of Occupational Science: Australia*. 1993;November(2):3-11.
94. Ferguson A. Women's health in a marginal area of Kenya. *Social Science and Medicine*. 1986;23:17-29.
95. *Funk & Wagnall's Standard Desk Dictionary*. Vol 1 A-M. New York, NY: Harper and Row; 1984:172.
96. Gilfoyle EM, Grady AP, Moore JC. *Children Adapt*. Thorofare, NJ: Charles B Slack; 1981.
97. Short MA. Vestibular stimulation as early experience: historical perspective and research implications. *Physical and Occupational Therapy in Pediatrics*. 1985;5:135-152.
98. Drotar D. Failure to thrive and preventive mental health: knowledge gaps and research needs. In: Drotar D, ed. *New Directions in Failure to Thrive*. New York, NY: Plenum Press; 1985:27-44.
99. Provence S, Lipton RC. *Infants in Institutions*. New York, NY: International Universities Press; 1962.
100. Day S. Mother-infant activities as providers of sensory stimulation. *American Journal of Occupational Therapy*. 1982;36:579-589.
101. Archer PW. Perceptual problem of cerebral palsy children and the occupational therapist. *Canadian Journal of Occupational Therapy*. 1959;26:123-127.
102. Mackie A. Social deprivation and the role of psychological services. *Educational and Child Psychology*. 1992;9(3):84-89.
103. Townsend P, Simpson D, Tibbs N. Inequalities in health in the city of Bristol: a preliminary review of statistical evidence. *International Journal of Health Services*. 1985;15(4):637-663.
104. Mechanic D. Adolescents at risk: new directions. *Journal of Adolescent Health*. 1991;12(8):638-643.
105. Itard J. The wild boy of Aveyron. In: Malson L, ed. *Wolf Children and the Problem of Human Nature*. New York, NY: Monthly Review Press; 1972.
106. Bascom B. Program summary, projects and descriptions. In: *Brooke Foundation Annual Report*. Washington, DC: Brooke Foundation; 1993:12.
107. DeGangi GA, Greenspan SI. *Test of Sensory Functions in Infants (TSFI) Manual*. Los Angeles, Calif: Western Psychological Services; 1989.
108. Haradon G, Bascom B, Dragomir C, Scipcaru V. Sensory functions of institutionalized Romanian infants: a pilot study. *Occupational Therapy International*. 1994;1:250-260.
109. Dimsdale, JE. The coping behavior of Nazi concentration camp survivors. *American Journal of Psychiatry*. 1974;131(7):795.
110. Frankl VE. *Man's Search for Meaning*. Boston, Mass: Beacon Press; 1962.
111. Useem B. Disorganization and the New Mexico prison riot of 1980. *American Sociological Review*. 1985;50(5):677-688.
112. Liebling A. Suicides in young prisoners: a summary. *Death Studies*. 1993;17(5):381-409.
113. Zamble E. Behavior and adaptation in long term prison inmates: descriptive longitudinal results. *Criminal Justice and Behavior*. 1992;19(4):409-425.
114. Smith R. *Unemployment and Health: A Disaster and a Challenge*. Oxford, UK: Oxford University Press; 1987.
115. Colledge M, Bartholomew R. *A Study of the Long Term Unemployed*. London, England: Manpower Services Commission; 1980.
116. Jackson PR, Warr PB. Unemployment and psychological ill health: the moderating role of duration and age. *Psychological Medicine*. 1984;14:605-614.
117. Warr P. Twelve questions about unemployment and health. In: Roberts R, Finnegan R, Gallie D, eds. *New Approaches to Economic Life*. Manchester: Manchester University Press; 1985.
118. Dowling PJ, De Cieri H, Griffin G, Brown M. Psychological aspects of redundancy: an Australian case study. *Journal of Industrial Relations*. 1987;29(4):519-531.
119. Platt S. Unemployment and suicidal behaviour: a review of the literature. *Social Science Medicine*. 1984;19:93-115.
120. Jaco EG. *The Social Epidemiology of Mental Disorders*. New York, NY: Russell Sage Foundation; 1960.
121. Fryer D, Payne R. Proactive behaviour in unemployment: findings and implications. *Leisure Studies*. 1984;3:273-295.
122. Cook DG, Cummins RO, Bartley MJ, Shaper AG. Health of unemployed middle aged men in Great Britain. *Lancet*. 1982;i:1290-1294.
123. Beale N, Nethercott S. Job loss and family morbidity: a study of factory closure. *Journal of Royal College General Practitioners*. 1985;280:510-514.
124. *Enough to Make You Sick: How Income and Environment Affect Health*. Australian National Health

Strategy Research paper, No 1, Sept 1992.

125. Brenner MH. Health costs and benefits of economic policy. *International Journal of Health Services*. 1977;7:581-593.

126. Brenner MH. Mortality and the national economy: a review, and the experience of England and Wales. *Lancet*. 1979;ii:568-573.

127. Scott-Samuel A. Unemployment and health. *Lancet*. 1984;ii:1464-1465.

128. Moser KA, Fox AJ, Jones DR. Unemployment and mortality in the OPCS longitudinal study. *Lancet*. 1984;ii:1324-1329.

129. Moser KA, Goldblatt PO, Fox AJ, Jones DR. Unemployment and mortality: comparison of the 1971 and 1981 longitudinal census sample. *British Medical Journal*. 1987;294:86-90.

130. Kerr C, Taylor R. Grim prospects for the unemployed. *New Doctor*. 1993;Summer:23-24.

131. Gravelle H. *Does Unemployment Kill?* Oxford, UK: Nuffield Provincial Hospitals Trust; 1985.

132. Hart JT. The inverse care law. *Lancet*. 1971;February 27:405-412.

133. Martin GS. *Social/Medical Aspects of Poverty in Australia*. Australian government inquiry into poverty. Canberra: Australian Government Publishing Service; 1976.

134. Opit LJ. Economic policy and health care: the inverse care law. *New Doctor*. 1983.

135. Jensen H. What it means to get off sit-down money: Community Development Employment Projects (CDEP). *Journal of Occupational Science: Australia*. 1993;1(2):12-19.

136. Aboriginal and Torres Strait Islander Commission. *No Reverse Gear: A National Review of the Community Development Projects Scheme*. 1993.

137. Hodges A. Health promotion and disease prevention for the disabled. *Journal of Allied Health*. 1986;November.

138. Mackie L, Pattullo P. *Women at Work*. London, England: Tavistock Publications; 1977:10.

139. Stavrianos LS. *The World to 1500: A Global History*. 4th ed. Englewood Cliffs, NJ: Prentice Hall; 1988:273-275.

140. Boileau E. *Livre de Metiers (Book of Trades)*. 13th century.

141. Power E. The position of women. In: Crump CG, Jacob EF, eds. *The Legacy of the Middle Ages*. Oxford, UK: Clarendon Press; 1926:401-434.

142. Gross SH, Bingham MW. *Women in Medieval-Renaissance Europe*. St. Louis Park, Minn: Glenhurst; 1983.

143. Rowbotham S. *Hidden from History*, London, England: Pluto Press; 1973:58.

144. Woodham-Smith C. *Florence Nightingale*. London, England: The Reprint Society; 1952:71.

145. Anderson EG. *Fortnightly Review*. London, England; 1874:590.

146. Jones H. The perils and protection of infant life. *Journal of the Royal Statistical Society*. 1894;1(vii):1-98.

147. Hewitt M. *Wives and Mothers in Victorian Industry*. London, England: Rockcliff; 1958.

148. Dyhouse C. Working class mothers and infant mortality in England, 1895-1914. *Journal of Social History*. 1978;xii:248-267.

149. Collett CE. The collection and utilization of official statistics bearing on the extent and effects of the industrial employment of women. *Journal of the Royal Statistical Society*. 1898;219-261.

150. Frumkin RM. Occupation and major mental disorders. In: Rose AM, ed. *Mental Health and Mental Disorder*. London, England: Routledge; 1956.

151. Wheeler AP, Lee ES, Loe HD. Employment, sense of well-being, and use of professional services among women. *American Journal of Public Health*. 1983;73(8):908-911.

152. Pepitone-Arreola-Rockwell F, Somner B, Sassenrath EZN, Rozee-Koker P, Stringer-Moore D. Stress and health in working women. *Journal of Human Stress*. 1981;7(4):19-26.

153. Waldron I. The coronary-prone behavior pattern, blood pressure, employment and socio-economic status in women. *Journal of Psychosomatic Research*. 1978;22:79-87.

154. Lemkau JP. Women and employment: some emotional hazards. In: Beckerman CL, ed. *The Evolving Female*. New York, NY: Human Sciences Press; 1980.

155. Haw MA. Women, work and stress: a review and agenda for the future. *Journal of Health and Social Behavior*. 1982;23:132-144.

156. Lewin E, Olesen V. Occupational health and women: the case of clerical work. In: Lewin E, Olesen V, eds. *Women, Health and Healing: Toward a New Perspective*. New York, NY: Tavistock Publications; 1985.

157. Bell C. Implementing safety and health regulations for women in the workplace. *Feminist Studies*. 1979;5(2):286-301.

158. Hunt VR. A brief history of women workers and hazards in the workplace. *Feminist Studies*. 1979;5(2):274-285.

159. Petcheky R. Workers, reproductive hazards, and the politics of protection: an introduction. *Feminist*

Studies. 1979;5:233-245.

160. Wright MJ. Reproductive hazards and "protective" discrimination. *Feminist Studies.* 1979;5(2):302-309.

161. Fogarty MP, Rapoport R, Rapoport RN. *Sex, Career, and Family.* Beverly Hills, Calif: Sage Publications; 1971.

162. Dubos R. Changing patterns of disease. In: Brown RG, Whyte HM, eds. *Medical Practice and the Community: Proceedings of a Conference Convened by the Australian National University, Canberra.* Canberra: Australian National University Press; 1968:59.

163. Dunn HL. *High Level Wellness.* Arlington, Va: RW Beatty; 1961.

164. Maslow A. *The Farther Reaches of Human Nature.* Viking Press; 1971.

165. World Health Organization, Health and Welfare Canada, Canadian Public Health Association. *Ottawa Charter for Health Promotion.* Canada: Ottawa; 1986.

166. Marx K. *Economic and Philosophical Manuscripts, 1844 (1932).* In: Livingstone R, Benton G, trans. *Karl Marx: Early Writings.* Penguin Classics; 1992.

167. Marx K. *Grundisse* (1857). Penguin Classics; 1970.

168. Petrovic G. Alienation. In: Bottomore T, ed. *A Dictionary of Marxist Thought.* 2nd ed. Oxford, UK: Blackwell; 1991:11-16.

169. Mohun S. Division of labour. In: Bottomore T, ed. *A Dictionary of Marxist Thought.* 2nd ed. Oxford, UK: Blackwell; 1991:155.

170. Marx K, Engels F. *The German Ideology. 1845-46.* London, England: Lawrence and Wishart; 1964.

171. Miller D. Dissociation in medical practice: social distress and the health care system. *Journal of Social Distress and the Homeless.* 1993;2(4):243-267.

172. Marx K. *Capital* (1867). Vol I. Hamburg: Otto Meisner; 1867:422-424.

173. Fischer E. *Marx in His Own Words.* London, England: Allen Lane, The Penguin Press; 1970:43-44.

174. Smith R. *Unemployment and Health: A Disaster and a Challenge.* Oxford, UK: Oxford University Press; 1987:2.

175. Dubos R. *Mirage of Health: Utopias, Progress and Biological Change.* New York, NY: Harper and Row Publishers; 1959:147.

176. Triplett T. Hebrides women: a philosopher's view of technology and cultural change. In: Wright BD, Ferree MM, Mellow GO, et al, eds. *Women, Work and Technology.* Ann Arbor, Mich: The University of Michigan Press; 1987:147.

177. Bronowski J. *The Ascent of Man.* London, England: British Broadcasting Corporation; 1973:260.

178. Mijuskovic B. Organic communities, atomistic societies, and loneliness. *Journal of Sociology and Social Welfare.* 1992;19(2):147-164.

179. Fromm E. *The Sane Society.* New York, NY: Rinehart; 1955.

180. Yates A. Current status and future directions of research on the American Indian child. *American Journal of Psychiatry.* 1987;144(9):1135-1142.

181. Burke RJ. Career stages, satisfaction, and well-being among police officers. *Psychological Reports.* 1989;65(1):3-12.

182. Winefield HR, Winefield AH, Tiggemann M, Goldney RD. Psychological concomitants of tobacco and alcohol use in young Australian adults. *British Journal of Addiction.* 1989;84(9):1067-1073.

183. Nutbeam D, Aaro LE. Smoking and pupil attitudes towards school: the implications for health education with young people: results from the WHO study of health behaviour among schoolchildren. *Health Education Research.* 1991;6(4):415-421.

184. Mosher A, Pearl M, Allard MJ. Problems facing chronically mentally ill elders receiving community based psychiatric services: need for residential services. *Adult Residential Care Journal.* 1993;7(1):23-30.

185. Nah KH. Percieved problems and service delivery for Korean immigrants. *Social Work.* 1993;38(3):289-296.

186. Semyonova ND. Psychotherapy during social upheaval in the USSR. Special section: in times of national crisis. *Group Analysis.* 1993;26(91):91-95.

187. Hammarstrom A. Health consequences of youth unemployment: review from a gender perspective. *Social Science and Medicine.* 1994;38(5):699-709.

188. Rodenhauser P. Cultural barriers to mental health care delivery in Alaska. *Journal of Mental Health Administration.* 1994;21(1):60-70.

189. Haynes SG. Type A behavior, employment status, and coronary heart disease in women. *Behavioural Medicine Update.* 1984;6(4):11-15.

190. Colligan MJ, Murphy LR. Mass psychogenic illness in organizations: an overview. *Journal of Occupational Psychology.* 1979;52:77-90.

191. Warr P. *Work, Unemployment and Mental Health.* Oxford, UK: Oxford Science Publications; 1987.

192. Winefield A, Tiggerman M. A longitudinal study of the psychological effects of unemployment and

unsatisfactory employment on young adults. *Journal of Applied Psychology.* 1991;76(3):424-431.

193. Winefield A, Tiggerman M, Winefield H. Unemployment distress, reasons for job loss and causal attributions for unemployment in young people. *Journal of Occupational and Organizational Psychology.* 1992;65:213-218.

194. Winefield A, Tiggerman M, Winefield H, Goldney R. *Growing Up with Unemployment.* London, England: Routledge; 1993.

195. Verbrugge LM. Work satisfaction and physical health. *Journal of Community Health.* 1982;7(4):162-283.

196. Farnworth L. An exploration of skill as an issue in unemployment and employment. *Journal of Occupational Science: Australia.* 1995;2(1):22-29.

197. Adler P. Technology and us. *Socialist Review.* 1986;85:67-96.

198. Naisbitt J. *Megatrends; Ten New Directions Transforming Our Lives.* New York, NY: Warner Books; 1982:24.

199. Haddad CJ. Technology, industrialisation, and the economic status of women. In: Wright BD, Ferree MM, Mellow GO, et al, eds. *Women, Work and Technology.* Ann Arbor, Mich: The University of Michigan Press; 1987:33.

200. Pollard S. *The Idea of Progress: History and Society.* Oxford, UK: Alden and Mowbray; 1968.

201. Marot H. *The Creative Impulse in Industry: A Proposition for Educators.* New York, NY: EP Dutton and Co; 1918:135.

202. Adams JD, ed. *Understanding and Managing Stress: A Book of Readings.* Calif: University Associates Inc; 1980.

203. Selye H. A syndrome produced by diverse nocuous agents. *Nature.* 1936;138:32.

204. Selye H. In: Monat A, Lazarus RS, eds. *Stress and Coping: An Anthology.* 2nd ed. New York, NY: Columbia University Press; 1985:25.

205. French JRP, Caplan RD. Organizational stress and individual strain. In: Marrow AJ, ed. *The Failure of Success.* New York, NY: Amacon; 1972:30-66.

206. McQuade W, Aikman A. *Stress.* New York, NY: EP Dutton and Co; 1974.

207. Roskies E, Lazarus RS. Coping theory and the teaching of coping skills. In: Davidson PO, Davidson SM, eds. *Behavioural Medicine: Changing Health Lifestyles.* New York, NY: Brunner/Mazel; 1980.

208. Moore JC. *Neurosciences and Their Application to Occupational Therapy.* Unpublished lecture notes. Neuroscience Conference, Adelaide, 1989:185.

209. Selye H. *The Stress of Life.* New York, NY: McGraw-Hill; 1976.

210. Kobasa SC, Maddi SR, Courington S. Personality and constitution as mediators in the stress-illness relationship. *Journal of Health and Social Behavior.* 1981;22:368-378.

211. Temoshok L. On attempting to articulate the biopsychosocial model: psychology-psychophysiological homeostasis. In: Friedman HS, ed. *Personality and Disease.* New York, NY: John Wiley and Sons; 1990:211.

212. Olson RE. *Nutritional Reviews: Present Knowledge in Nutrition.* 5th ed. Washington, DC: Nutrition Foundation; 1984.

213. Weiner H. *Psychobiology and Human Disease.* New York, NY: Elsevier; 1977.

214. Hazuda H. Women's employment status and their risks for chronic disease. Colloquium presentation, University of Texas School of Public Health, Houston. Reported in: Justice B. *Who Gets Sick: Thinking and Health.* Texas: Peak Press; 1987.

215. Pelletier KR. *Mind as Healer, Mind as Slayer.* New York, NY: Delta; 1977.

216. Maddi SR. Issues and interventions in stress mastery. In: Friedman HS, ed. *Personality and Disease.* New York, NY: John Wiley and Sons; 1990:132.

217. Eisler RM. Promoting health through interpersonal skills development. In: Mattarazzo JD, Weiss SM, Herd JA, Miller NE, Weiss SM, eds. *Behavioural Health: A Handbook of Health Enhancement and Disease Prevention.* New York, NY: John Wiley and Sons; 1984.

218. Klump TG. How much exercise to avoid heart attacks? *Medical Times.* 1976;4(104):64-74.

Suggested Reading

Barrett HR, Browne A. Workloads of rural African women: the impact of economic adjustment in Sub-Saharan Africa. *Journal of Occupational Science: Australia.* 1993;November(2):3-11.

Blaxter M. *Health and Lifestyles.* London, England: Tavistock/Routledge; 1990.

Dubos R. *Mirage of Health: Utopias, Progress and Biological Change.* New York, NY: Harper and Row Publishers; 1959.

Haradon G, Bascom B, Dragomir C, Scipcaru V. Sensory functions of institutionalized Romanian infants: a pilot study. *Occupational Therapy International.* 1994;1:250-260.

Hetzel BS, McMichael T. *L S Factor: Lifestyle and Health.* Ringwood, Victoria: Penguin; 1987.

Lorenz K. *Civilized Man's Eight Deadly Sins.* Latzke M, trans. London, England: Methuen and Co Ltd; 1974.

McNeill WH. *Plagues and People*. London, England: Penguin Books; 1979.

Mumford L. *The Condition of Man*. London, England: Heinemann; 1963.

Ornstein R, Sobel D. *The Healing Brain, A Radical New Approach to Health Care*. London, England: Macmillan; 1988.

Risse GB. History of Western medicine from Hippocrates to germ theory. In: Kiple KF, ed. *The Cambridge World History of Human Disease*. New York, NY: Cambridge University Press; 1993.

Smith R. *Unemployment and Health: A Disaster and a Challenge*. Oxford, UK: Oxford University Press; 1987.

Wilcock AA, Hall M, Hambley N, et al. The relationship between occupational balance and health: a pilot study. *Occupational Therapy International*. 1997;4(1):17-30.

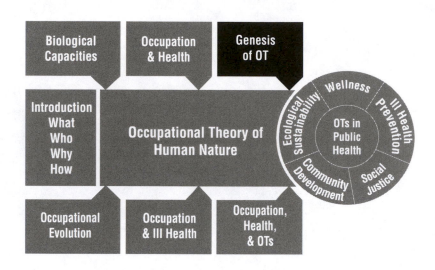

Chapter 7
The Genesis of Occupational Therapy

This chapter presents the reader with ideas about:
- The distinctive role of occupational therapy, and its difference from other health professions, in order to establish its place in the pursuit of health
- Ideologies generated by the work of 19th century social reformers and philosophers which are behind the genesis of occupational therapy
- Moral treatment, the Arts and Crafts movement, feminism, and pragmatism
- Stories of some people who were influential in developing the profession's ideological base including Adolph Meyer, Jane Addams, and Eleanor Clarke Slagle
- The social context of the profession's birth and its influences on ideological development

As occupational therapy claims to be fundamentally concerned with people attaining health through occupation, it is useful, from a public health perspective, to consider the distinct philosophical and practice base of occupational therapists, with a view to using their expertise in the drive to enable "health for all." To this end, this chapter explores the genesis of occupational therapy at the beginning of the 20th century in America, its predecessor, "moral treatment," and some of the ideas that influenced its emergence, such as industrialization, the Arts and Crafts movement, pragmatism, and feminism.

Occupational therapy is a profession of the 20th century although the philosophies and rationales on which it is based have a very long history. Hopkins' and Smith's and McDonald's historic perspective on occupational therapy states that the importance of occupation in health was recognized and used thousands of years ago by the Chinese, the Greeks, the Persians, and the Egyptians.[1,2] McDonald[1] provides as one of several examples Homer's tale of Hephaistos, the noble craftsman god who was lame, being given equipment by Thetis and Euronyme that enabled him to become skilled in much "cunning handiwork."[3]

Occupational therapy reflects natural, biological, and common sense truths about health and well-being. Its simplest claim is that occupation, or any form of human activity, has effects upon the health of the individual engaged in the activity. Human occupation may be chosen wisely to enhance or maintain health, to reduce ill health, or to help the adaptation process should handicap appear irreversible. Occupational therapy was originally more concerned with promoting or maintaining health for those without access to normal human activity because of chronic illness than being remedial for people with acute illness. Nor was it applied to well individuals or the community at large, although it appears to have grown from community programs addressing social problems, as well as moral treatment for the insane.

It is a complex profession that is poorly understood by the public, other health workers, educational institutions, and governments. From its beginnings, it has been peripheral to conventional medicine and health care, probably because, although it has always been associated with medicine, and much of the impetus for its establishment came from psychiatrists and physicians, it does not share the same reductionist base of practice. Views of illness and perspectives of treatment possibilities between occupational therapy and medicine began to differ shortly after the genesis of occupational therapy from the 1920s on. From about that time, changes in medical services occurred in which reductionist practice, pharmaceutical intervention, and technology-based skills gained importance, and personal skill development of a simpler kind, in which occupational therapy specialized, became devalued. Despite this, occupational therapy is recognized as a health profession compatible with conventional medicine. It is perhaps remarkable that the profession is still attached to health care systems centered on the short-stay acute hospital, as many interventions thought essential by occupational therapists address problems that demand time and long-term programs to achieve results.

The complexities of the relationship between occupation, ill health, health, and well-being have already been discussed, so how it is viewed and defined by the profession is of interest. The World Federation of Occupational Therapists defines it:

> *As assessment and treatment through the specific use of selected activity. This is designed by the occupational therapist and undertaken by those who are temporarily or permanently disabled by physical or mental illness, by social or by developmental problems. The purpose is to prevent disability and to fulfill the person's needs by achieving optimum function and independence in work, social, and domestic environments.*[4]

This fairly traditional definition can be applied to occupational therapy practitioners throughout the world. In some ways, particularly by its reference to "assessment and treatment" to be "designed by the occupational therapist," it reflects the association that occupational therapy has had with the medical model. Each country tends to further define its practice according to local needs and conditions. One of the definitions adopted by the Australian Association of Occupational Therapists in 1987 stated that:

> *Occupational therapy is concerned with human occupation and its importance in health for persons of all ages. Occupational therapists evaluate the physical, psychosocial, and environmental factors that reduce a person's ability to participate in everyday activities or occupation. Therapeutic objectives are achieved through techniques or activities designed to:*
> 1. *Diminish or control pathology*
> 2. *Restore and/or reinforce functional capacity*
> 3. *Facilitate learning of skills and function essential for adaptation or productivity*
> 4. *Promote and maintain health*[5]

Early definitions and descriptions were simpler. For example, in 1917 the American National Society for the Promotion of Occupational Therapy was formed when architects George Edward Barton and Thomas Bessell Kidner, social worker Eleanor Clarke Slagle, physician William Rush Dunton, and teacher Susan Cox

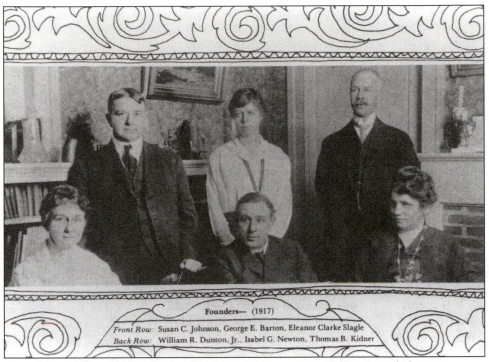

Founders— (1917)

Front Row: Susan C. Johnson, George E. Barton, Eleanor Clarke Slagle
Back Row: William R. Dunton, Jr., Isabel G. Newton, Thomas B. Kidner

Figure 7-1. Founders of the National Society for the Promotion of Occupational Therapy (NSPOT), 1917, Clifton Springs, NY. Box 123, File No. 1016. Bethesda, Md. Reproduced courtesy of the Archives of The American Occupational Therapy Association Inc, Bethesda, Md.

Johnson, who were all working in the field, met at Clifton Springs, New York, to write the Certificate of Incorporation (Figure 7-1).[6] The objectives of the Society were "the advancement of occupation as a therapeutic measure; the study of the effect of occupation upon the human being; and the scientific dispensation of this knowledge."[7] Those particular objectives could well be seen as having current value to public health, so it is useful to explore the historical context in which the notions developed.

Moral Treatment

It is moral treatment that many people describe as the forerunner of occupational therapy today. As one product of the Age of Enlightenment, this humane approach to the insane revolutionized psychiatric institutions during the 18th and 19th centuries. The genesis, success, and demise of moral treatment is a fascinating but cautionary tale.

The fascination starts with the nomenclature moral, which implies that what it replaced was immoral. In today's terms, it certainly appears so, as the traditional treatment meted out to "lunatics in madhouses," in Europe, prior to the 19th century, included whipping and chaining, along with many other approaches for "coercing patients into straight thinking and accepting reason" such as "vomits, purges, ...surprise baths, copious bleedings, and meager diets."[8] Eminent doctors of the mad, such as William Cullen, argued that "restraining the anger and violence of madmen is always necessary for preventing their hurting themselves or others; but this restraint is also to be considered as a remedy."[9] This treatment, far from being condemned by people of the time, provided entertainment for the curious, when, for a penny, the inmates were exhibited through the open doors of Bethlem Hospital. In fact, even George III, during bouts of mania, was subjected to similar treatment by his physician Francis Willis. "He was sometimes chained to a stake. He was frequently beaten and starved, and at best he was kept in subjection by menacing and violent language."[10]

Whether or not behavior is perceived as humane or inhumane, moral or immoral depends on the context, the world view, and the values of those perceiving. Scull argues that "the subjugation of the madman [and] the breaking of his will by means of external discipline and constraint" were consistent with the view that "in losing his reason, the essence of his humanity, the madman had lost his claim to be treated as a human being."[11] In turn, this view was congruent with the theological and supernatural beliefs and values of an agrarian economy in which God and nature dominated, and humans, on the whole, did not seek, or think possible, self-transformation. Moral treatment, he suggests, arose as a result of a change in "the cultural meaning of madness," which emerged along with the change from agriculture to industry, from reliance on nature to reliance on human activity, and invention in the transformation of natural resources into marketable products. In fact, as industrialists sought to "make such machines of man that cannot err," they cultivated in workers a new belief in "'rational' self-interest [that was] essential if the market system were to work."[12] So too, in moral treatment, were "lunatics...made over in the image of bourgeois rationality."[11]

At about the same time as Pinel liberated and removed the prison chains of the insane constrained in the dungeons of Bicêtre in France, William Tuke established moral treatment in Britain, specifically for Quakers at the York Retreat.[13-16] Others such as John Ferriar of the Manchester Lunatic Asylum and Edward Long Fox from Bristol were among practitioners who followed essentially similar approaches. Tuke based his revolutionary approach on beliefs that self-discipline and hard work, rather than external control, were the keys to rehabilitation of the insane, just as they were the keys to education of children for success in a world that had begun to recognize the capacity for human improvement. (Prior to setting up the York Retreat, William Tuke established Ackworth, a school for girls.) Reflecting the Quaker work ethic, as well as religious discipline, treatment at the Retreat encouraged individuals to regain self-control through occupation, as "of all the modes by which the patients may be induced to restrain themselves, regular employment is perhaps the most generally efficacious."[14] Tuke recognized that "in itself, work possesses a constraining power superior to all forms of physical coercion" because of "the regularity of the hours, the requirements of attention, [and] the obligation to produce a result."[13] It is also a requisite of self-esteem, which Tuke valued highly.

Pinel's "moral" approach differed in several ways from Tuke's, particularly in that his asylum was "a religious domain without religion, a domain of pure morality, of ethical uniformity"[13] but it, too, recognized the value of occupation:

It is the most constant and unanimous result of experience that in all public asylums, as in prisons and hospitals, the surest and perhaps the sole guarantee of the maintenance of health and good habits and order is the law of rigorously executed mechanical work.[17]

The occupation theme continued after Pinel's time; we read, for example, of Leuret, a 19th century French psychiatrist, who included exercise, drama, music, reading, and manual labor and stressed improvements of habits and the development of a consciousness of society within his treatment programs.[18] It was from Tuke's and Pinel's programs that "madness" became associated with medicine and from these 18th century ideas that modern notions of rehabilitation have grown.

Despite the fact that America still retained a predominantly agricultural economy, it was "rapidly developing a new liberal philosophy of the individual," and it, too, embraced the concept of moral treatment,[19] in part, through the efforts of William Tuke's son Samuel,[20] and also through the reforms of Benjamin Rush, who, like Pinel, was inspired by the writings of physician-philosopher John Locke (1632-1704). (John Locke's main philosophical works are *An Essay Concerning Human Understanding* and *Two Treatises of Civil Government*, both published in 1690.) Hopkins suggests it may well be significant that the development of this person-centered treatment began at a time when the rights and equalities of men were being fought over on both sides of the Atlantic.[2]

The Worcester State Hospital in Massachusetts, which opened in 1833, served as a proving ground for moral treatment in America, demonstrating "beyond doubt that recovery was the rule."[21] Thomas Story Kirkebride, who, in 1844, was one of 13 founders of the Association of Medical Superintendents of American Asylums for the Insane, also played an important role in establishing moral treatment, not least by his writings about the construction of asylums.[22,23] He implemented moral treatment in the Pennsylvania Hospital for the Insane, a prestigious private institution that he headed for 40 years. He wrote annual reports aimed at prospective customers and their families, among others, in which he detailed more than 50 occupations available to inmates. They included light gymnastics, fancy work, magic lantern displays, and lecture series, and, in order to meet the intellectual and artistic needs of more cultivated clients, "intelligent and educated individuals with courteous manners, and refined feelings" were employed to encourage reading, handiwork, and music on the wards.[24] He assured prospective patrons that cure could be expected in many cases, especially if treatment was prompt, but that even in cases requiring long-term care, moral and humane conditions would apply. In fact, moral treatment was reported as curative by the superintendents of the asylums who ran the programs, with some hospitals, such as the Hartford Retreat, recording success rates of up to 90%.[25] An example of the recovery statistics of patients admitted to the Worcester State Hospital between 1833 and 1852 and used to attract prospective customers is provided in Table 7-1.

The cautionary part of the tale lies in the decline of moral treatment despite its reputed success. As most of the American asylums in which it was used were small private hospitals, access was limited to the affluent, but with the touting of the curative effects of moral treatment, social reformers pushed for it to be available to all, not just the well-to-do. They were so successful in their endeavors that the asylums became overcrowded, often with immigrant "insane paupers."[19] Activity rooms became wards, and as resources were limited, due to a Civil War-taxed economy, the treatment deteriorated into custodial care.[25] Indeed, in the aftermath of the Civil War, and the change from agriculture to industry, both social values and the economy were in a state of flux. Humanistic social values were being gradually replaced by "reductionist, mechanical" values associated with industrialization and in some

5-Year Period	Patients Admitted	Patients Discharged, Recovered	Patients Discharged, Improved
1833-1837	300	211 (70.0%)	39 (8.3%)
1838-1842	434	324 (74.6%)	14 (3.2%)
1843-1847	742	474 (63.9%)	34 (4.6%)
1848-1852	791	485 (61.3%)	37 (4.7%)

Table 7-1. Outcome in Patients Admitted to Worcester State Hospital Who Were Ill Less Than 1 Year. Data from Annual Reports of the Hospital. Used by permission from Bockoven JS. *Moral Treatment in Community Mental Health.* 1972;14. Springer Publishing Co Inc, New York, NY 10012.

quarters by social Darwinism.[26] Peloquin also suggests that as occupational programs deteriorated because of these factors, medicine was reconsidering the causes of insanity in the light of new physiological knowledge in which ideas about occupation did not seem important. Indeed, it seems almost inevitable that as positivist, medical science developed, doctors would try to make their role in the treatment of the insane fit with their view of their own skills, beliefs, and purpose. The doctor's role in moral treatment in the early days was as a wise authority figure, Pinel and Tuke both asserting that "his moral action was not necessarily linked to any scientific competence."[13] Foucault, who describes psychiatric practice as a "certain moral tactic contemporary with the end of the 18th century, preserved in the rites of asylum life, and overlaid by the myths of positivism, points to a gradual "magical" belief in psychiatrists and ultimately to the transfer of the potential to cure from asylum to doctor.[13] It was unavoidable that the natural would be overtaken by the scientific. The reported success of moral treatment was challenged as exaggeration and disappeared from psychiatric practice. Peloquin concludes that:

Moral treatment's decline relates closely to a lack of inspired and committed leadership willing to articulate and redefine the efficacy of occupation in the face of medical and societal challenges. The desire to embrace the most current trend of scientific thought led to the abandonment of moral treatment in spite of its established efficacy. The failure to identify and address the social and institutional changes that had gradually made the practice and success of moral treatment virtually impossible led to the erroneous conclusion that occupation was not an effective intervention.[25]

Industrialization

As the effects of the industrial revolution accumulated, ideas about humans being regarded as "cogs in a machine" gained respectability. Such ideas were promoted during the late 19th century by the work of people such as Frederick Taylor, who developed the scientific management movement.[27] This movement sought ways to use people effectively in industrial organizations and viewed behavior from the vantage point of job analysis focused on work efficiency, particularly from a physiological perspective.[28] Before Taylor, though, "the drive for maximum productivity and control led managers to divide labor into repetitive, minute tasks. Individual workers could neither envision the larger purpose of their labor nor exert much control over their working lives." Even for professionals and white-collar workers, "the new bureaucratic view of work often fragmented their labor and reduced their sense of autonomy."[29]

The rhetoric of Helen Marot's *Creative Impulse in Industry* provides an indication of the mood of the industrial era: "Industry is the great field for adventure and growth. If America wants industrial efficiency, it must have efficient workers if it holds its place among nations."[30] The machine age appeared to herald a new way of thinking, working, living, and researching. Ackoff suggests that, as the three dominant intellectual styles of this time were reductionism, analysis, and mechanism (in terms of cause and effect), consideration of environmental factors was deemed irrelevant.[31] In medicine, as in other sciences, "machine age thinking" led to a reductionist view that everything could best be studied by considering component parts. In psychiatry and psychology, for example, "the observation by pathologists of microscopic lesions in the central nervous system of patients who had been mentally ill" led to their conclusion that the study of behavior and environmental factors would not yield understanding of disease processes because it was "looked upon as a result of mechanical defect."[19]

Therapeutic Occupations: A New Start

As the therapeutic use of occupation diminished, it seems that, at least in some instances, it was again replaced by restraint in hospitals for the insane. In *Occupation as a Substitute for Restraint in the Treatment of the Mentally Ill: A History of the Passage of Two Bills Through the Massachusetts Legislature*,[32] Vernon Briggs explains that in 1911 three bills proposing the introduction of occupation into mental institutions, along with training in occupation for attendants, were "strenuously opposed by certain men in high positions, most of them connected with private hospitals as proprietors, or with the State service for the care and treatment of the mentally ill as officials or trustees." In the opening address to the Committee on Public Charitable Institutions, he described how patients' engagement in occupation has a positive effect on their health and improves the work environment of attendants. This information was based on several "occupational" initiatives occurring in various parts of the country: a training school for nurses and attendants in Illinois; New York supervisors and Maine nurses sent to receive training at the Chicago School of Philanthropics; and in turn New York hospitals providing training for nurses from Boston. With the passing of the first of the bills, Dr. Mary Lawson Neff, a psychiatrist, was appointed as director or instructor of occupational therapy. Apart from establishing programs for patients, she reported in her *Résumé of Work of 1912 in Developing Therapeutic Occupations in the State Hospitals of Massachusetts* on the staging of an education exhibition that visited eight hospitals and was attended by more than 2,000; invitations to lecture at a variety of hospitals, universities, and public departments; a course of lectures for nurses delivered at Danvers, Worcester, Taunton, Westborough, Medfield, Boston, and Waverley; and a conference on occupational therapy that was attended by nearly 100 people.[33]

Another occupation training scheme that was occurring about that time was provided by Susan Tracey, who some credit as being the first occupational therapist of the 20th century.[6] A trained nurse and teacher, she established a course in invalid occupations for nurses in 1906 at the Adams Nervine Asylum in Jamaica Plains,

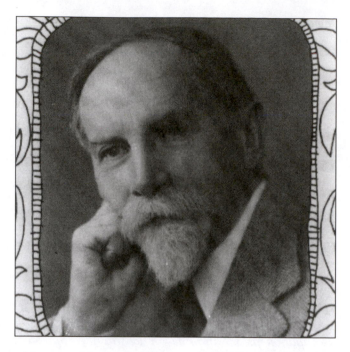

Figure 7-2. Adolph Meyer. Reprinted with permission from the Archives of the American Psychiatric Association.

Massachusetts, and presented her teaching materials in a book first published in 1910. In the introduction to this text, Daniel Fuller explains how Tracey stimulated the interest of the nurses she trained, how graduates in private practice came back to consult, and how exhibitions and lectures were provided to superintendents of other training schools. One interesting observation made by Fuller, is that "the elimination from the patient's mind of the idea of 'prescription' or 'remedy' in connection with the occupation is doubtless often much to be desired." He recognized that interest developed for its own sake enabled patients to make it an ongoing part of their lives and to maintain and enhance their health.[34] This valuable concept became lost as reductionism and professionalism grew, so that "prescribed occupation" became the accepted norm.

When presenting the proposed legislative change, Vernon Briggs called upon several experts to support his claims, including Adolph Meyer (Figure 7-2). This "mental hygienist" is so important to the history of occupational therapy that a brief biography is in order.

Adolph Meyer

Adolph Meyer was born in Zurich, Switzerland in 1866 and migrated to America in 1892 after completing his medical studies in Zurich and studying in England, Scotland, and Paris with eminent neurologist Hughlings Jackson and others. He worked first at the Illinois Eastern Hospital for the Insane at Kankakee and then at Worcester Lunatic Hospital in Massachusetts. In both institutions, he instigated far-reaching institutional reforms and "began to impose himself as the leader of the advanced guard in American Psychiatry" with a then-radical viewpoint which held that life experiences play an important role in the etiology of mental diseases.[35] In repudiating the reductionist, analytical, and mechanistic view, Meyer was one of "the new breed of humanists" who took a holistic view that was strongly influenced by the ideas of pragmatism propounded by William James and the related theories of the newly emerging Chicago School of Functionalism led by John Dewey.[35] Meyer was committed to the development of a science of psychology that was both academic and practical. He embraced James' revolutionary view that the chief purpose of the mind "is to enable individuals...to pursue specific interests and achieve specific goals" and that psychologists should study the mind in use "in the ordinary, practical situations of everyday life."[35] Along with Mead and Dewey, Meyer professed that "doing, action, and experience are being" and that the activities expressed in living demonstrate mind-body synthesis.[36,37] This view rejected commonly held Descartian notions of the time.

Muncie describes the fundamental concept of Meyer's psychobiological approach as being "integration," with the view that living individuals can only be studied as whole people in action, which of necessity includes society as part of the whole.[38] Meyer also made use of the "concept of habit" as formulated by Pierce, James, and Dewey, arguing that the "cumulative effect of early faulty habit patterns was to produce abnormal or inefficient behavior in later life."[35]

Meyer was appointed professor of psychiatry at Johns Hopkins University in 1908, a position he held until 1941. His psychobiological model of human nature was fundamental to the mental hygiene movement in which he played an important role. This movement expanded the scope of psychiatry into community settings, such as the family, schools, workplace, and prisons, and ascribed education as an important component of mental health. Estelle Breines explains that it was Meyer's participation in the mental hygiene movement that linked him with social activists Jane Addams and Julia Lathrop, who worked at Hull House in Chicago and were teachers of Eleanor Clarke Slagle, a pioneer occupational therapist who later worked with Meyer at Phipps Clinic in Baltimore.[36]

The work of Adolph Meyer is not well known today despite the assertion made by some medical historians that he dominated American psychiatry for the first 20 years of this century and remained influential until his death in 1950.[35] His interest in occupation was demonstrated early in his career. He remarked in his 1921 paper "Philosophy of Occupational Therapy," given at the 5th annual meeting of the National Society for the Promotion of Occupational Therapy, that the first medical paper he presented in the early 1890s sought ideas from his colleagues about appropriate occupations for use with American patients. He described a long association with occupational programs that his wife, Mary, among others, organized during the first decade of the 20th century as well as an interest in the types of education programs being offered at Hull House to train nurses in play and occupation. Meyer's paper on occupational therapy philosophy was later published in the first edition of the *Archives of Occupational Therapy*.[39,40] Occupational therapists claim him as their philosopher but, despite his obvious interest, there is little evidence in his mainstream writings that he considered occupational therapy to be the focal point of his life's work. Ironically, occupational therapists are still espousing his philosophies today, while mainstream psychiatry has bypassed his ideas in favor of psychoanalysis, behaviorism, and neurochemistry. His approaches were, however, remarkably congruent with many new values pertaining to health and well-being.

Several factors alluded to in the outline of Meyer's work require further discussion. These include elaboration of the roles of Hull House in Chicago, the people who worked there such as Jane Addams and Eleanor Clarke Slagle, and the philosophy of pragmatism.

Hull House

Hull House was a "settlement" house developed to meet the social, economic, and health problems of new immigrants and assist them to adjust into the American industrial society of the turn of the century. The settlement movement, which aimed at developing and improving community or neighborhood life as a whole, rather than providing particular social services, began when Samuel Barnett, his wife, and invited university students settled at Toynbee Hall in a poor area of London in 1884. The movement quickly spread to America—Neighbourhood Guild, New York (now University Settlement) being established in 1886 and Hull House in Chicago in 1889.[41] The movement continued to grow throughout Europe and Asia, and it can be seen as a forerunner to today's community development movement. Hull House was central to many of Chicago's ethnic communities and served as a second home to Greek, Italian, Jewish, German, Polish, Russian, and Bohemian immigrants. It provided the venue for many mutual aid, professional, trade, educational, athletic, theatrical, and musical organizations and groups[42] and was a center in which, from its inception, civic betterment, investigative research, and joint ventures with activist scholars from the University of Chicago toward social reform took place.[43]

Feminism

Hull House was founded and developed by women. As such, it was an important stepping stone in the history of feminism and women in the helping professions. Feminism grew from the same Enlightenment ideas that sparked humane and moral treatment, so it is not surprising to discover that Mary Wollstonecraft's document *A Vindication of Rights of Women* was published as early as 1792.[44] Early feminist activists concerned themselves with securing legal rights for women in education, marriage, and employment; with anti-slavery; with evangelical movements; and later with the struggle for votes.[45] By the end of the 19th century, educational opportunities were beginning to open up for women, although courses on the status of women were in their infancy.[46] (One of the earliest known courses on the status of women was offered by the Department of Sociology at the University of Kansas in 1892.) Jane Addams (Figure 7-3) was educated at one of numerous women's colleges in the American northeast, which, it has been suggested, provided women with the confidence needed to forge a new type of lifestyle for themselves. It is interesting, from the perspective of this book, to note her description of her own experience of occupational deprivation and imbalance, which colored her later beliefs and approaches at Hull House. In a paper given to the Ethical Culture Societies in Plymouth, Massachusetts, in 1892, she applied her own experience to that of other educated young people who "have been shut off from the common labor by which they live which is a great source of moral and physical health. They feel a fatal want of harmony in their lives, a lack of coordination between thought and action," which can be provided by "a proper outlet for active faculties." She recognized that lack of occupational opportunity is not restricted to the poor and that "this young life, so sincere in its emotion and good phrases and yet so undi-

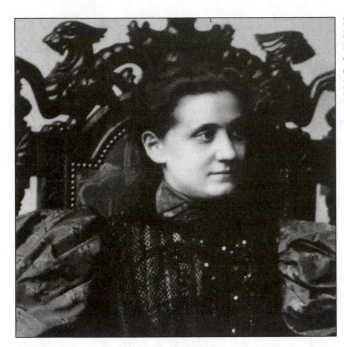

Figure 7-3. Jane Addams. Reprinted with permission from Jane Addams Memorial Collection, Special Collections, The University Library, The University of Illinois at Chicago.

rected, seems to me as pitiful as the other great mass of destitute lives." She described the Hull House Settlement as:

> *An experimental effort to aid in the solution of the social and industrial problems which are engendered by the conditions of life in a great city...It is an attempt to relieve at the same time, the over accumulation at one end of society and the destitute at the other.*[47]

Arts and Crafts Movement

Addams' beliefs about meaningful occupation, formed by her experience, also led to her involvement in the establishment of the Chicago Arts and Crafts Society in 1897, along with prominent business and professional people, faculty members from the University of Chicago, and the co-founder of Hull House, Ellen Gates Starr.[29] Charles Norton, the first professor of fine arts at Harvard and a close friend of John Ruskin, is credited with bringing the ideology of Ruskin's and Morris' Arts and Crafts movement to America. Morris' views about work and a simple life on a "human scale," away from materialistic, alienating cities, found "particularly fertile ground in late 19th century America," which had long been influenced along similar lines by functionalist religious groups such as Puritans and Shakers.[48] Different groups accepted the ideology in different ways.

> *While Simple-Lifers stressed familiar virtues of discipline and work, aesthetes embodied a new style of high consumption appropriate to the developing consumer economy, and educational reformers offered manual training as a therapeutic mode of adjustment to the corporate world of work.*[29]

However, because the Puritan work ethic was so central to American culture, Ruskin's and Morris' conceptualization of a pre-industrial craftsperson, unhurried and absorbed in his own creativity, became reinterpreted in America so that eventually no distinction was made between modern and pre-industrial work habits.

"Labor! All Labor is noble and holy," Edward Pearson Pressey, Unitarian minister and the founder of the New Clairvaux handicraft community, proclaimed.[49] (This community was named after St. Bernard of Clairvaux, a 12th century hero of simplicity.) He was not alone in this view, a view that enabled Arts and Crafts leaders, along with their progressive contemporaries,[50,51] to draw back from fundamental social change for social justice in favor of "a new kind of reform" that fitted individuals into emerging hierarchies and aimed instead at "manipulating psychic well-being."[29]

This notion of "mental and moral growth" was compatible with 19th century American ideas about individualism, which was central to capitalism, its liberal democracy ideology, and values focusing on human rights.[52,53] Indeed, individualism, in Arieli's view, "supplied the nation with a rationalization of its characteristic attitudes, behavior patterns, and aspirations. It endowed the past, the present, and the future with the perspective of unity and progress,"[54] and it provided an exciting and challenging dream for each of its citizens. Historian John William Draper describes the "wonderful, unceasing" activity and social development of the North, following the Civil War, as "the result of individualism; operating in an unbounded theatre of action. Everyone was seeking to do all that he could for himself."[55] For Ralph Waldo Emerson, America's favorite poet of the late 19th century, individualism was "the route to perfection—a spontaneous social order of self-determined, self-reliant, and fully developed humans."[56] Not for Draper and Emerson the belief of Marx, Ruskin, and Morris, that socialism was the path to fully developed humans in tune with their creative natures.

Similarly, even in Hull House, where Ruskin's and Morris' photographs had pride of place, as evidence of its founder's respect for their work, the Arts and Crafts ideology was reinterpreted from a socialist to an individualistic focus.[48] For example, Starr, who demonstrated her understanding of Morris' ideals in her essay "Art and Labor," devoted herself in her work with immigrants to "the solace of art" rather than "the freeing of the art power of the whole nation and race by enabling them to work in gladness and not in woe."[57] Likewise, Addams dismissed anti-modernism and accepted the inevitability of the industrial system, so that instead of fighting for social justice against the division of labor and occupational inequities produced by mass production, she sought to revitalize working class lives by education toward best using the industrial economy and personal fulfillment.[29] Like other Arts and Crafts leaders, she accepted that manual training was the solution for industrial problems, focusing on the "factory hand's need for fulfillment" in contrast to others who "began with the factory owner's need for efficiency. They presented manual training as a practical business proposition—a way to replace shiftless or incompetent employees with conscientious graduates of trades schools."[29] This focus helped the transformation to the 20th century work culture, which separates work from living and from joyful occupation, reinforcing the belief that the work people do for a living will is, and indeed should be, tedious and demanding.[29]

In terms of the role of women in American society at the time, the direction taken by the women leaders at Hull House was inevitable. To establish positions in which they could exercise their previously untapped capacities and potential, women needed to demonstrate their ability to work within dominant social values, rather than lead massive social change, even if they had perceived this to be necessary, which is

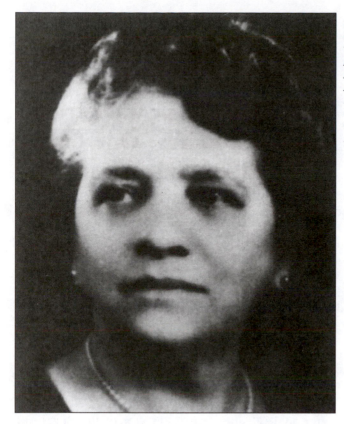

Figure 7-4. Eleanor Clarke Slagle. American Occupational Therapy Association. *A Professional Legacy: The Eleanor Clarke Slagle Lectures.* **Rockville, Md: Author; 1985:vii. Reproduced courtesy of the American Occupational Therapy Association Inc, Bethesda, Md.**

doubtful. Establishing a female workforce in the professions and bringing to these a feminine, caring, moral viewpoint that flowed over from their earlier, often unacknowledged, family or charitable duties was in itself sufficiently challenging to the social order. Indeed, these strong women demonstrated their abilities and right to be where they were, through developing their "professionalism" in a way that was adaptive and politically expedient.

However, neither the capitalist, individualist growth focus nor the anti-modern socialist revolution focus was successful in creating global awareness of the need to consider people's occupational nature in future social planning, although both went some way in that direction. The choice of individual education rather than social revolt can be viewed as one factor that led to the diminution of the development of a broadly based, lasting "occupational perspective," and delayed the consideration of this view until the present post-industrial difficulties once more raised some collective consciousness as to its importance. Despite the enormous energy and commitment of strong leaders, the exploration of humans as occupational beings was lost in their zeal to establish practical programs that were based on their own concepts of how humans' occupational natures could be best fitted to emerging social environments. As part of this process, the burgeoning occupational therapy that grew from humanist and socialist ideas became bound to individualist, medical, or other models for years to come.

Eleanor Clarke Slagle

It is not surprising that workers in such an environment, in which the therapeutic benefits of occupation were so well recognized and used, instigated classes for attendants and nurses of the insane to learn about invalid occupations. In 1908, Julia Lathrop, Rabbi Hirsch, and Dr. Graham Taylor held the first Special Course in Curative Occupations and Recreation at Hull House.[36] Eleanor Clarke Slagle (Figure 7-4) completed the fourth class, in 1911, following her enrollment in the Chicago School of Civics and Philanthropy as a social work student.[6] "Her vigorous and unrelenting teaching, organizing, and championing of 'occupational training'...came from exposure to this course and a subsequent commitment to these principles."[58] She immediately assumed a teacher role herself, before being "borrowed" to work with Adolph Meyer in establishing "the Phipps Clinic for Action."[59] In 1915, she returned to Hull House to become director of the Henry B. Favill School of Occupations, which is said to be the first formal school of occupational therapy. (Favill was a Chicago physician with an interest in social issues.) This started as a Community Workshop for cases of "doubtful insanity," whom the courts considered might return to usefulness if given a "proper environment and trade,"[60] and incorporated a program of study in curative occupations and recreation. Slagle built upon the foundation established by Julia Lathrop, incorporating the ideas of Addams, James, and Meyer into a program that focused on "'habit training' through meaningful use of time and purposeful activity,"[58] including the concept that "for the most part, our lives are made up of habit reactions" and that "occupation usually remedially serves to overcome some habits, to modify others, and to construct new ones to the end that habit reactions will be favorable to the restoration and maintenance of health."[61]

Following the school's closure in 1920, she became director of the Bureau of Occupational Therapy of the New York State Department of Mental Hygiene. (It is of interest that this Bureau by 1941 boasted a staff of 255.) She concentrated much of her effort on "re-education in decent habits of living," following "the same growth and development as normal education," for patients who had deteriorated for many years in the "back wards" of mental institutions.[62] Her training programs, which spanned 24 hours each day, had the stated purpose of re-education of "the patient, (a) mentally, (b) physically, and (c) socially according to the individual need and to the highest capability of the patient," with the ultimate aim of the patient's return to the community.[62] During her illustrious career, she developed and demonstrated her professionalism and furthered the feminist cause by serving in all the offices of the American Occupational Therapy Association (AOTA). She is commemorated by the prestigious Eleanor Clarke Slagle Lectureship awarded annually by the AOTA to an occupational therapist who is regarded as having made an outstanding contribution to the profession.

Pragmatism

The philosophy of pragmatism propounded by William James was central to Slagle's work.[63] She even quoted his words in her syllabus: "The moment one tries to define what habit is, one is led to the fundamental properties of matter...Habit diminishes the conscious attention with which our acts are performed."[62] (Habit training is adopted from pragmatism through the Meyer influence,[64] but is also central in the Arts and Crafts movement.) This use of James' philosophy is not surprising because of the close association between the University of Chicago, in which, at this time, the study of pragmatism flourished, and Hull House, which was a center where the themes of pragmatism were tried on the community.[65]

Although a philosophy of pragmatism was first articulated by Charles Sanders Pierce (1839-1914), who believed that an idea or the significance of meaning could be understood best by examining its consequences on human activity,[66] William James is the better known pragmatist philosopher.[67] This philosophy, with functionalist and utilitarian overtones, was the antithesis of European metaphysical philosophies and was closely associated with the American way of life at the turn of the century. James, like Marx, was much influenced by Hegel and Darwin, and occupational therapy was influenced by these same ideas through two routes: one from Hegel and Darwin to Marx to Morris to Hull House; the other from Hegel and Darwin to James to Meyer and Dewey to Hull House.

The pragmatists John Dewey and George Herbert Mead worked at the University of Chicago, and Dewey, along with Meyer and James, had significant influence on occupational therapy. This trio's influence was perhaps because of their particular interpretations of pragmatism. While Pierce focused on a scholarly and general concept of the philosophy and Mead emphasized the "subjective and relational role of the individual in society," James focused on a psychological approach as it affected individuals. Meyer focused on psychiatric practice, which saw "personality is fundamentally determined by performance" and stressed the integration of mind and body, activity and habit, time and environment in real life, and Dewey focused on education and social reconstruction, seeing knowledge as the result of "experience in life tasks."[36]

Dewey was a trustee of Hull House and worked there as counselor and lecturer. Although he left Chicago in 1904, his influence remained strong and undoubtedly was absorbed into occupational therapy theory.[68] Indeed, Tracey cites Dewey in her text of 1910,[69] and it is also easy to appreciate that his beliefs in active occupation as a modifier of learning and health, his view that a child's mind is "possessed of a number of faculties, such as 'perception, memory, reasoning,' and that these powers develop by training like that required for the fixing of a muscular habit," and that "to learn through work, one experienced happiness, to win that point of view as a daily habit is perhaps the greatest gift bestowed"[64] were accepted as central tenets of the profession. So, too, is the practical understanding that people as creatures of this world spend their lives with a "succession of here-and-now problems to be solved." The solving of these problems result in adaptation and growth.[70] In his early texts, he used words such as "purposive activity" and "active occupations,"[71] and with Meyer anticipated a "holistic systems approach," all of which remain part of occupational therapy theory and rhetoric today. For a graphic representation of the many influences on the genesis of occupational therapy, see Figure 7-5.

Education and Philosophical Base

Despite the threefold objectives formulated at the foundation of the National Society in 1917, it appears from papers and books written around the time that interest was much more centered on the therapeutic application of occupation than upon research and dissemination of knowledge so generated. The founders of occupational therapy and their associates who influenced this focus were them-

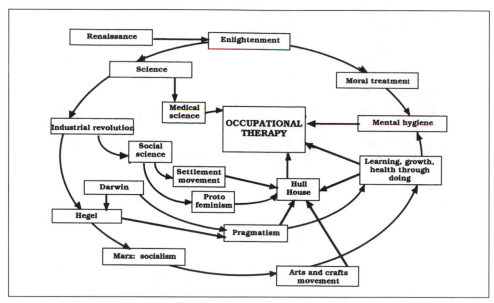

Figure 7-5. Influences on the genesis of occupational therapy.

selves educated, on the whole, in disciplines with a reflective, philosophical orientation. The value of such a base seems to have been taken for granted, so that training programs became based on practice. Slagle, who had a firm concept of the profession's founding philosophies, was responsible for approving all curricula until the 1930s when *The Essentials of an Acceptable School of Occupational Therapy* were adopted by the Council on Medical Education and Hospitals of the American Medical Association in 1935. "The original 'Essentials' stipulated content, but did not stipulate why that content was to be included," and the "principles upon which the 'Essentials' were based became increasingly obscure."[36] This is true not only of the American scene, but of occupational therapy education worldwide. The complexity of ideas that culminated in occupational therapy were perhaps difficult to piece together into a cohesive whole by a small group of people, coming from different backgrounds and working in different centers, miles apart. Indeed, the importance of documenting the foundation of the ideas that contributed to occupational therapy may well have been largely unappreciated as they formed part of the mass consciousness of the era, and because of the seeming truth of the value of occupation to health, it may not have been recognized that there was a need to conceptualize this value in philosophical terms. Unfortunately, "the diversity of organization and perspective, ...in the absence of a well-analyzed and encompassing philosophical conceptualization, contributes to the confusion and insecurity experienced by occupational therapists."[36]

The lack of a formalized philosophical base did not inhibit the zeal of early workers who, through their actions, demonstrated their assumption that opportunity for expression and self-actualization through activity is necessary for health. In those formative years, occupational therapy was focused toward activity programs in institutions where inhabitants stayed long-term for one cause or another. What the occupants of the institutions were able to do was limited by the physical environment of the institutions and by the reason for the inmates' confinement, such as psychotic disorders, tuberculosis, or violent crime. Programs varied from "real" work, such as in the garden or laundry, to physical training or dance. Leisure activities such as music or handcraft were also used regularly. The effects of the Arts and Crafts movement remained powerful, and it is of interest to note that of the 13 American states known to have at least one Arts and Crafts Society in 1904, nine developed occupational therapy programs before 1920.[72,73] The seeds were laid early of the widely held belief that occupational therapy is limited to certain types of activity, despite the fact that the assumption relating health with human occupation is of much wider application. This limitation to what was perceived as pleasurable activity not linked to the realities of life led to the myth that occupational therapy is solely involved in diverting patients' minds from their problems. Because of the impetus to meet the needs of those deprived of occupation, the profession became associated, also at an early date, with people with long-term problems, such as the chronically handicapped. The emphasis, whether reality or myth, on diversion and chronicity eroded the idea of using occupational programs for health and social problems in a wider community context. Many of the ideas about the value of human occupation in community adaptation, in giving a purpose to life, in maintaining a balance in life, and as a modifier of learning and health were hidden in hospital-bound remedial programs, and its potential value to public health on a broad scale appeared to diminish with the passage of time and events. Exploring how these issues, and others, affected the development of the profession's fundamental ideas about occupation and about health will be a focus of the next chapter.

References

1. McDonald EM, ed. *Occupational Therapy in Rehabilitation*. London, England: Bailliere, Tindall and Cassell; 1964.
2. Hopkins HL, Smith HD, eds. *Willard and Spackman's Occupational Therapy*. 7th ed. Philadelphia, Pa: JB Lippincott Co; 1988.
3. Homer. *The Iliad*. Book XVIII.
4. World Federation of Occupational Therapists. Paris, France; 1976.
5. Australian Association of Occupational Therapists. 1987.
6. Reed KL, Sanderson SR. *Concepts of Occupational Therapy*. 2nd ed. Baltimore, Md: Williams and Wilkins; 1983.
7. Certificate of Incorporation of the National Society for the Promotion of Occupational Therapy, Inc. (1917). *Then and Now: 1917-1976*. Rockville, Md: American Occupational Therapy Association; 1967:4-5.
8. Hunter RA, MacAlpine I, eds. *Three Hundred Years of Psychiatry*. London, England: Oxford University Press; 1963:475.
9. Cullen W. First lines in the practice of physics. In: Hunter RA, MacAlpine I, eds. *Three Hundred Years of Psychiatry*. London, England: Oxford University Press; 1963:478.
10. Bynum W. Rationales for therapy in British psychiatry, 1780-1835. In: Scull A, ed. *Madhouses, Mad-Doctors and Madmen: The Social History of Psychiatry in the Victorian Era*. Philadelphia, Pa: University of Pennsylvania Press; 1981.
11. Scull A. Moral treatment reconsidered: some sociological comments on the episode in the history of British psychiatry. In: Scull A, ed. *Madhouses, Mad-Doctors and Madmen: The Social History of Psychiatry in the Victorian Era*. Philadelphia, Pa: University of Pennsylvania Press; 1981:108,115.
12. Wedgwood J. Cited in McKendrick N. Josiah Wedgwood and factory discipline. *Historical Journal*. 1964;1:46.
13. Foucault M. *Madness and Civilization: A History of Insanity in the Age of Reason*. New York, NY: Random House; 1973:247,275-276.
14. Tuke S. *Description of the Retreat*. York: Alexander; 1813:141,156.
15. Ferriar J. *Medical Histories and Reflections*. London, England: Cadell and Davies; 1795:2,111-112.

16. Fox EL. Brislington House, an asylum for lunatics, situated near Bristol. In: Scull A, ed. *Madhouses, Mad-Doctors and Madmen: The Social History of Psychiatry in the Victorian Era*. Philadelphia, Pa: University of Pennsylvania Press; 1981.

17. Pinel P. Traite medico-philosophique sur l'alienation mentale. In: Foucault M. *Madness and Civilization: A History of Insanity in the Age of Reason*. New York, NY: Random House; 1973:258.

18. Leuret F. 1840. On the moral treatment of insanity. In: Licht S. *Occupational Therapy Source Book*. Baltimore, Md: Williams and Wilkins; 1948.

19. Bockoven JS. *Moral Treatment in American Society*. New York, NY: Springer; 1963:14,172,189.

20. Corsini RJ, ed. *Encylopedia of Psychology*. Vol 2. New York, NY: John Wiley and Sons; 1984:162.

21. Bockoven JS. *Moral Treatment in Community Mental Health*. New York, NY: Springer Publishing Co, Inc; 1972:14.

22. Tomes NJ. A generous confidence: Thomas Story Kirkebride's philosophy of asylum construction and management. In: Scull A, ed. *Madhouses, Mad-Doctors and Madmen: The Social History of Psychiatry in the Victorian Era*. Philadelphia, Pa: University of Pennsylvania Press; 1981.

23. Kirkebride TS. *On the Construction, Organization and General Arrangements of Hospitals for the Insane*. Philadelphia, Pa: Lindsay and Blakiston; 1854.

24. Kirkebride TS. *Annual Report of the Pennsylvania Hospital for the Insane*. Cited in: Tomes NJ. A generous confidence: Thomas Story Kirkebride's philosophy of asylum construction and management. In: Scull A, ed. *Madhouses, Mad-Doctors and Madmen: The Social History of Psychiatry in the Victorian Era*. Philadelphia, Pa: University of Pennsylvania Press; 1981.

25. Peloquin SM. Moral treatment: contexts considered. *American Journal of Occupational Therapy*. 1989;43(8):537-544.

26. Serrett KD, ed. *Philosophical and Historical Roots of Occupational Therapy*. New York, NY: The Haworth Press Inc; 1985.

27. Taylor FW. The principles of scientific management. In: Taylor FW. *Scientific Management*. New York, NY: Harper; 1947.

28. Hoy WK, Miskel CG. *Educational Administration, Theory, Research and Practice*. 2nd ed. New York, NY: Random House; 1978.

29. Jackson Lears TJ. *No Place of Grace: Antimodernism and the Transformation of American Culture 1880-1920*. New York, NY: Pantheon Books; 1981:60,67,73,79-81,83.

30. Marot H. *Creative Impulse in Industry*. New York, NY: Arno Press; 1977:xix-xx.

31. Ackoff R. *Redesigning the Future*. New York, NY: Wiley; 1974.

32. Vernon Briggs L. *Occupation as a Substitute for Restraint in the Treatment of the Mentally Ill: A History of the Passage of Two Bills Through the Massachusetts Legislature* (1911). New York, NY: Arno Press; 1973.

33. Neff ML. Résumé of work of 1912 in developing therapeutic occupations in the state hospitals of Massachusetts. Presented to the State Board of Insanity, December 27, 1912. Cited in: Vernon Briggs L. *Occupation as a Substitute for Restraint in the Treatment of the Mentally Ill: A History of the Passage of Two Bills Through the Massachusetts Legislature* (1911). New York, NY: Arno Press; 1973:201-204.

34. Fuller DH. Introduction: the need of instruction for nurses in occupations for the sick. In: Tracey SE. *Studies in Invalid Occupations: A Manual for Nurses and Attendants*. Boston, Mass: Whitcomb and Barrows; 1910:2.

35. Leys R, Evans R, Evans B, eds. *Defining American Psychology: The Correspondence Between Adolph Meyer and Edward Bradford Titchener*. Baltimore, Md: The Johns Hopkins University Press; 1990:43-46,59,162.

36. Breines E. *Origins and Adaptations: A Philosophy of Practice*. NJ: Geri-Rehab, Inc; 1986:14,17,46,67.

37. Golley FB. *A History of the Ecosystem Concept in Ecology*. New Haven, Conn: Yale University Press; 1993.

38. Muncie W. The psychobiological approach. In: Arieti S, ed. *American Handbook of Psychiatry*. Vol 2. New York, NY: Basic Books, Inc; 1959.

39. Meyer A. The philosophy of occupational therapy. *Archives of Occupational Therapy*. 1922;1:1-10.

40. Meyer A. The problems of mental reaction types, mental causes and diseases. In: Winters EE, ed. *The Collected Papers of Adolph Meyer*. Baltimore, Md: The Johns Hopkins Press; 1950-1952:2,598.

41. Reinders RC. Toynbee Hall and the American settlement movement. *Social Service Review*. 1982;56(1):39-54.

42. Holli MG, Jones P, eds. *Ethnic Chicago*. Grand Rapids, Mich: William B Eerman's Publishing Co; 1984.

43. Fish VK. Hull House: pioneer in urban research during its creative years. *History of Sociology*. 1985;6(1):33-54.

44. Wollstonecraft M. *A Vindication of Rights of Women*. London, England: J Johnson; 1792. Reprint with introduction by Kramnick MB, ed. Harmondsworth, England: Penguin Books; 1975.

45. Grimshaw A. Feminism. In: Bullock A, Stalleybrass O, Trombley S, eds. *The Fontana Dictionary of Modern Thought*. 2nd ed. London, England: Fontana Press; 1988:312.

46. Chamberlain M. Women's studies. In: Kuper A, Kuper J, eds. *The Social Science Encyclopedia*. London, England: Routledge; 1989:902.

47. Addams J. *The Subjective Necessity for Social Settlement*s. Paper to the Ethical Culture Societies, Plymouth, Mass, 1892.

48. MacCarthy F. *William Morris: A Life for Our Time*. London, England: Faber and Faber; 1994:603-604.

49. Pressey EP. New Clairvaux Plantation, Training School, Industries and Settlement. *Country Time and Tide*. 1903;February:121-122.

50. Link AS, McCormick RL. *Progressivism*. Arlington Heights, Ill: Harlan Davidson, Inc; 1983.

51. Resek C, ed. *The Progressives*. Indianapolis, Ind: The Bobbs-Merrill Co, Inc; 1967.

52. The course of civilization. *United States Magazine and Democratic Review* 1839;VI:208ff,211. Cited in: Lukes S. *Individualism*. Oxford, UK: Basil Blackwell; 1973.

53. Lukes S. *Individualism*. Oxford, UK: Basil Blackwell; 1973.

54. Arieli Y. *Individualism and Nationalism in American Ideology*. Cambridge, Mass: Harvard University Press; 1964:345-346.

55. Draper JW. *History of the American Civil War*. Vol 1. New York, NY: Harper, 1867-1870:207-208.

56. Emerson RW. New England reformers (1844). Summarized in: Lukes S. *Individualism*. Oxford, UK: Basil Blackwell; 1973:29.

57. Starr EG. Art and labor. In: Addams J. *Hull House Maps and Papers*. New York, NY: Thomas Y Crowell; 1895.

58. Cromwell FS. Eleanor Clarke Slagle, the leader, the woman: in retrospect on the 60th anniversary of the founding of the AOTA. *American Journal of Occupational Therapy*. 1977;31(10):645-648.

59. Meyer A. Address in honor of Eleanor Clarke Slagle. In: Serrett KD, ed. *Philosophical and Historical Roots of Occupational Therapy*. New York, NY: The Haworth Press; 1985:109-113.

60. Favill J. *Henry Baird Favill: 1860-1916*. Chicago, Ill: Rand McNally; 1917:87.

61. Slagle EC. *Training Aides for Mental Hospitals*. Paper read at the Fifth Annual Meeting of the National Society for the Promotion of Occupational Therapy, Baltimore, Md, October 20-22, 1921.

62. Slagle EC, Robeson HA. *Syllabus for Training of Nurses in Occupational Therapy*. Utica, NJ: State Hospital Press; 1931:19,30-35.

63. James W. *Pragmatism, and Four Essays from the Meaning of Truth*. Cleveland, Ohio: Meridian Books, The World Publishing Co; 1970.

64. Mayhew KC, Edwards AC. *The Dewey School: The Lab School of the University of Chicago, 1896-1903*. New York, NY: Appleton-Century; 1936:459.

65. Breines E. Pragmatism as a foundation for occupational therapy curricula. *American Journal of Occupational Therapy*. 1987;41(8):522-525.

66. Pierce CSS. *Collected Papers*. Vols 1-6 edited by Hartshornes C, Weiss P. Vols 7-8 edited by Burkes W. Cambridge, Mass: Harvard University Press; 1958.

67. James W. *Pragmatism: A New Name for Some Old Ways of Thinking*. New York, NY: Longmans, Green and Co; 1907.

68. Mills CW. *Sociology and Pragmatism: The Higher Learning in America*. New York, NY: Oxford University Press; 1964:30.

69. Tracey SE. *Studies in Invalid Occupations: A Manual for Nurses and Attendants*. Boston, Mass: Whitcomb and Barrows; 1910:2.

70. Moore TW. *Educational Theory: An Introduction*. London, England: Routledge: 43.

71. Dewey J. *Democracy and Education: An Introduction to the Philosophy of Education*. Toronto, Canada: Collier-MacMillan; 1916.

72. West M. The revival of handicrafts in America. *Bureau of Labor Bulletin*. 1904;55:1573-1622.

73. Reed KL. Tools of practice: heritage or baggage? 1986 Eleanor Clarke Slagle Lecture. *American Journal of Occupational Therapy*. 1986;40(9):597-605.

Suggested Reading

Bockoven JS. *Moral Treatment in Community Mental Health*. New York, NY: Springer Publishing Co, Inc; 1972.

Breines E. *Origins and Adaptations: A Philosophy of Practice*. NJ: Geri-Rehab, Inc; 1986.

Hunter RA, MacAlpine I, eds. *Three Hundred Years of Psychiatry*. London, England: Oxford University Press; 1963.

Jackson Lears TJ. *No Place of Grace: Antimodernism and the Transformation of American Culture 1880-1920*. New York, NY: Pantheon Books; 1981.

Peloquin SM. Moral treatment: contexts considered. *American Journal of Occupational Therapy.* 1989;43(8):537-544.

Reed KL, Sanderson SR. *Concepts of Occupational Therapy.* 2nd ed. Baltimore, Md: Williams and Wilkins; 1983.

Scull A, ed. *Madhouses, Mad-Doctors and Madmen: The Social History of Psychiatry in the Victorian Era.* Philadelphia, Pa: University of Pennsylvania Press; 1981.

Serrett KD, ed. *Philosophical and Historical Roots of Occupational Therapy.* New York, NY: The Haworth Press Inc; 1985.

Tuke S. *Description of the Retreat.* York: Alexander; 1813.

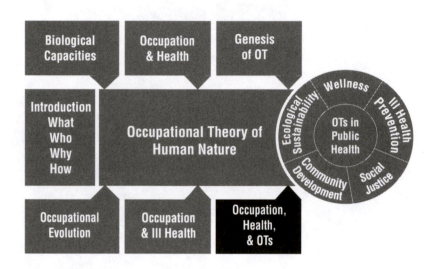

Chapter 8
Occupational Therapy's Relationship with Occupation and Health

This chapter presents the reader with ideas about:
- How occupational therapy's focus on occupation and on health has changed historically as a result of both external and internal pressures
- How attachment to the medical model has influenced the profession's view of occupation and health through prescription, gender bias, patronage, professionalism, and reductionist practices
- Occupational therapy's interest in rehabilitation, the contextual nature of changes to rehabilitation which have resulted in altered practice, and the adaptable nature of the profession
- The profession's rediscovery of "occupation" as a central focus for its view of health
- The profession's developing interest in promoting health and wellness through occupation

Occupational therapy's view of "occupation" and of "health" has fluctuated according to changing values and needs in the community, through its relationship with medicine, and structural demands of health service delivery. In this chapter, those fluctuations and developments will be explored as a response to the World Health Organization (WHO) and Australian and other health authorities' stress on the importance of health professionals reorienting their emphasis of practice toward the positive pursuit of health. (One of the five major imperatives proposed in the Ottawa Charter for Health Promotion is the reorientation of health professionals toward the pursuit of health. The Better Health Commission of Australia accepted this proposal in 1988.) Health professionals who accept that emphasis take on an obligation to review basic ideologies, current practice, and potential for development or change. That kind of review implies an attempt to discover, analyze, and understand the present perceptions and attitudes of the profession toward health promotion. Apart from exploring these by analyzing ideas that are prevalent in debate within the profession, an inquiry to that end has been carried out in a study of Australian occupational therapists reported briefly in this chapter.

The basic ideologies of occupational therapy are congruent with much current health promotion ideology, and the pursuit of healthy and quality lifestyles for clients has always been a major focus of occupational therapy's practice. However, the profession has also been subject to pressures toward reductionist, curative expectations, which have affected the use of and value given to occupation. The following account of those pressures on the development of the profession suggests the profession's reaffirmation of basic ideologies that reflect a health promotion orientation through occupation. It also leads to an appreciation of the ways in which occupational therapists may contribute to community and public health.

Medical Model

"Occupational therapy suffers from a limitation imposed upon it by its origin in the setting of medical care" because it has "regarded itself as part of a larger endeavor masterminded by the medical discipline."[1] Throughout its 20th century life, occupational therapy has been subservient to medicine, which dominates other health professions by "subordination," "limitation," and "exclusion" because it has "control over the work situation, professional autonomy within the medical division of labor, and occupational sovereignty over related and neighboring occupations."[2,3] This unequal relationship has influenced decisively the growth, development, and changing focus of occupational therapy and has contributed to the medical science orientation of its knowledge base. More recently, the reaction of occupational therapists to that inequality has shaped the drive for professional status and the struggle for recognition. The chapter considers four principal dynamics emanating from this association that have shaped occupational therapy:

1. Prescription
2. The feminine gender bias
3. The pursuit of professionalism
4. Scientific reductionism

These will be discussed in some detail in order to clarify the core values of occupational therapy and its potential for development or change.

Prescription

Dunton, one of the founders and second president of the American National Society of Occupational Therapists, played an important role in establishing the tradition of occupational therapists working within a medical model, under the direction of physicians.[4,5] A doctor himself, he gained support from his medical colleagues of the necessity for a prescription or referral for patients to receive occupational therapy, which placed occupational therapists in the role of technicians who would carry out treatment, in much the same way as nurses administer medications on a physician's instructions.[6] Indeed, in his book *Prescribing Occupational Therapy,* which was aimed at educating physicians about occupational therapy's philosophies and principles, Dunton described occupational therapists as technical assistants whom the physicians would direct.[7] In Dunton's prescription, "the division of labor between physicians and occupational therapists followed traditional patterns regarding men and women," with conceptualization and the control being in the hands of men and the "doing" being firmly in the hands of the women. Because the "conceptualizations and the intellectual foundations" were represented as coming from "outside the boundaries of the profession," it was not hard, in addition, to represent outside instruction of the occupational therapist as a necessity.[8]

A long-term effect of this early division of labor has been that, until recently, intellectual foundations and detailed conceptualizations were not addressed as major components of occupational therapy education. Interest in conceptual matters became more important, in part, because the growth of post-graduate programs provided an environment for serious reflection and debate and the beginnings of a research ethic. Evidence of this comes from initiatives such as the American Foundation sponsoring a 1976 seminar on research in occupational therapy in an effort to give impetus and substance to a National research commitment.[9] In Australia, a standing committee on research was established in 1979, and the

Australian Association of Occupational Therapists (AAOT) Research awards were established in 1988.

This interest in conceptual matters led to a renaissance of the original ideas behind the genesis of occupational therapy and a renewed focus on the need to develop a science of occupation. (The first call for a science of occupation was in 1917, as one of the objectives of the American Society for the Promotion of Occupational Therapy.)

The history of occupational therapy as a prescribed therapy has inhibited adequate research or development of its unique view of health. Because prescribed therapy is mechanical, whereas unprescribed therapy is necessarily inquisitive and imaginative, it has restricted the potential evolution of occupational therapists as service providers[10] so that, in many instances, the "potential to help clients...stagnated at the level of applying technical skills."[11] (Within the restrictions imposed by prescription, occupational therapists have been very imaginative.) Additionally, because the service was prescribed by another discipline, much of the specialization that has occurred has "not arisen from, and do[es] not appear to support the development of a core concept or paradigm," which is unique to occupational therapy.[12]

Although Dunton recognized the need for prescribers to understand the nature and scope of the services requested when he addressed his text to referring physicians, it is unlikely that it became compulsory reading in many medical schools. Perhaps, for some years, there was a degree of commitment to "occupational" treatment programs from those intrigued by this "new" therapy. Indeed, the professional literature of the early years is sprinkled with papers by physicians who describe their occupational therapy programs. However, as the "newness" of occupational therapy wore off, it is probable that most doctors, simultaneously fascinated by an increasing knowledge base within their own sphere, spent little time considering the benefits of peripheral therapies and "enablers," such as occupational therapists, particularly when they operate from a premise and philosophical base other than medical science. In fact, at present, occupational therapy receives only passing mention in undergraduate medical training. As a result, prescriptions, if even considered, are limited to superficial requests either very general or specific to doctors' own treatment interests.

The early literature suggests that occupational therapists welcomed the association with medicine and showed some pride in the "prescriptive" application of occupation, which became part of early definitions. Indeed, the first known formal definition of occupational therapy was by a physician, HA Pattison: "Any activity, mental or physical, definitely prescribed and guided for the distinct purpose of contributing to, and hastening recovery from, disease or injury."[13] This alignment with medicine and acceptance of the need for a medical prescription is considered by Griffin, an Australian occupational therapy educator, to be "a custom in occupational therapy practice" that is now undergoing significant change. Increasingly, therapists recognize that "there are clients who benefit from occupational therapist intervention but who do not need to be referred via medical prescription." For example, medical prescription is inappropriate for people in schools, community centers, local government, or industrial settings, or those presenting "to the medical system with problems (such as occupational performance difficulties) which cannot be identified as a disease process."[14] In such cases, clients likely to benefit from occupational therapy will not be referred because of lack of understanding of possible interventions or outcomes.

Gender Bias

In common with other subordinate health professions, occupational therapy was identified early in the piece as women's work. Indeed, by 1938, only one training school in America accepted male students; and for at least another decade, only about 2.5% of occupational therapists were men.[15] At the University of South Australia, which is typical of Australian schools, even in the 1990s, male students made up, at the most, approximately 10% of the first year intake. Anderson and Bell, among others, suggest that the female nature of the profession may in fact reflect its growth during two world wars when most "able-bodied men" were committed "to the front line," and "their rehabilitation had to be undertaken by women,"[16] but Frank argues with this idea which does not account for the very low representation of men in the profession in subsequent decades.[17] In common with other subordinate health professions, the founding physicians and therapists claimed that women have special aptitude for such work and that assumption remains widely accepted.[18,19]

The female founders, who blazed a trail for "less educated or advantaged women," were, on the whole, from the upper middle class, well educated, and immersed in the advancement of careers for women. (In 1918, candidates for the Boston School of Occupational Therapy were sought through the society pages of Boston and Los Angeles newspapers.[17,20]) Despite their proto-feminist impetus and convictions about occupation, they accepted subordination to medicine in a way similar to the gender segregation that was a part of upper middle class domestic arrangements of the day. From about 1750 to 1950, in America, increasing industrialization, accompanied by a growing demarcation between the world of paid employment and home, generated a "cult of domesticity," a recognition of difference in gender traits and of the feminine ideal.[21] The attributes of this feminine ideal, such as "a kindly voice, gentleness, patience, ability and seeming vision, adaptability...and...an ability to be honest and firm" were deemed important for occupational therapists[22] and fostered a "service to medicine" orientation. The bias cast by the feminine ideal was conducive to therapists tending the sick and infirm, giving particular attention to children and the elderly, and choosing self-care and caregiving, homemaking, and creative occupations in preference to social activism, which challenged occupational practices of the day. In some countries, until recently, this was reinforced, in part, by legislation that separated medical and vocational rehabilitation.[23]

The gender-biased focus remains true of today's practice, although the current emphasis on and legislative changes in occupational health and safety have opened the doors to increasing numbers of occupational therapists working within the employment arena. Another attribute of the domestic cult, which was frequently incorporated into occupational therapy practice until recently, was the skill of "making-do" to save money, for example, making splints out of discarded materials, or begging for equipment or materials for patients' projects.[16] (Irene Hollis, a very skilled occupational therapist specializing in hand rehabilitation at Chapel Hill, took pride in her splint making from metal strips salvaged from packing materials.[23a]) In times of economic hardship, such thrift should be admired, yet the most lauded health services reflect the dominance of materialistic values and are those that are technologically advanced and, hence, very expensive. This privileging of the new and expensive has also contributed to reductions in occupational therapy services whenever economic retrenchment was applied. Similarly, life saving (a medical work) has been protected during retrenchment relative to quality of life (the sphere of subordinate therapies). Such protection is also held to reflect the value given to saving lives (whatever the outcome) over quality of life. (Shannon suggests that the medical model was committed to a science and technology successful in prolonging life but ignoring conditions that make life worth living.[24]) Saving the lives of brain damaged motor vehicle accident victims, at great financial and emotional expense, to live the life of a vegetable is a case in point. The life-saving procedure is given preference over economic commitment to long-term rehabilitation for them or even for others who are chronically disabled. For many following stroke, programs usually stop after the first couple of months, but potential for recovery continues for at least 2 years and probably longer. Occupational therapists who "are driven by a moral concern for the individual"[1] have been largely unheard advocates for the long-term rehabilitation of the chronically disabled. Bockoven describes occupational therapists as veterans "of many battles fought to win respect for the individual." He suggests they have acquired unique and valuable assets as a result of "many decades of adversity," of "first hand acquaintance of every conceivable kind of deprivation endured by imprisoned, insecure people," and of being forced by circumstances to engage in a token performance because they had available to them "only a tiny fraction of what was needed to meet their needs."[1]

In Australia, in a way similar to North America, but a quarter of a century later, "pioneering occupational therapists and members of other female-dominated professions at the time...accepted their role within the health service structure which placed men in the position of power," believing that "only through the medical profession could occupational therapy" receive the status and independence it deserved.[16] This remained true until the more recent challenges of feminism brought about a questioning of health practices based almost wholly on a male view of the world.

Gender segregation has provided some advantages to women occupational therapists in terms of their own "economic empowerment," their success in seeking advancement because they were sheltered from male competition, and their contribution to "a professional environment shaped by women's culture, with its emphasis on care rather than competition."[17] This caring culture was sympathetic to the needs of mothers to work part-time as more and more occupational therapists, in common with other female professionals, remained in or returned to the workforce.[25,26] However, some see that these feminine advantages also weakened efforts to upgrade the profession.[27] Eventually, the predominantly female workforce, the small numbers (there has been a long-term, ongoing shortage of occupational therapists[28-30]), the difference in the discipline's emphasis, aggravated by the division between concept and implementation, led many occupational therapists to perceive that professional colleagues and society undervalued what they had to offer. This in turn led to them undervaluing their own contribution, tending not to broadcast their distinctive and different views and being willing to adapt these to socially valued and dominant practices.

Patronage

The most obvious symbol of medical authority was the long-standing practice of having physicians at the head of occupational therapy professional associations. With the exception of Slagle, the presidents of the American National Society for its first three decades were men, mostly from the medical profession. When the AAOT was formed, the Articles of Association required that the president and one vice president had to be a member of or eligible for membership in the British Medical Association. The South Australian branch of AAOT had a physician as president until 1976. A collegiate association with medicine might have been one manifestation of occupational therapists seeking professional status, although the classic conflict sociology of professionalism equates professional status with autonomy and self-control. Friedson argues that a profession is "defined ultimately by its autonomy from external control and this autonomy is determined by power conflicts and not by the elaboration of knowledge,"[31] and Griffin suggests that "the fact that professionalism is about the exercise of power is often neglected by allied health groups, who strive for professional status by developing its outward trappings."[14]

Medical patronage appeared to provide the security of recognition and acceptance of the "specialty," growth through referral of clients, and allies in the exclusion of potential competitors.[32] It also provided one boundary of professional interdependence from which to negotiate other boundaries with health workers from other disciplines, with whom there was a potential for conflict over division of labor, such as physiotherapists, social workers, nurses, and orthotists.[33] Indeed, tension around issues relating to preservation and expansion of roles among health care workers has continued throughout this century.[34] Medical acceptance, and preference for particular offerings of such professionals, acted in a way that restricted "autonomy and independent decision-making."[14]

Professionalism

Professionalism is a much discussed phenomenon of the health domain in the 20th century.[31,35-38] This paragraph deals briefly with the limited question of whether professionalism has affected occupational therapy's commitment to the association between occupation and health. It is clear that, in order to carry out their work as part of the medical team, it was essential for occupational therapists to aim for parity with other members and therefore to aspire to being a profession. Such parity would give credibility to the proclaimed importance of a relationship between occupation and health and justify "prolonged specialized training in a body of abstract knowledge and a collectivity or service orientation" based on aspects of this relationship.[39] On the debit side, "the striving of occupational therapy toward professionalization, based on a male medical model, has led to mental struggle for its practitioners who feel unclear about their role and where they fit into the health care delivery system."[14,40] Indeed, when responsiveness to professionalism, medicine, and marketplace survival assumed more importance than the original premise of occupational therapy, as it did for the large number of occupational therapists who rejected occupation during the 1960s and 1970s in favor of interventions such as counseling, handling techniques, or biofeedback, occupational therapy reduced its unique contribution to health services. Although a number of key figures in the profession, such as Reilly, Yerxa, and Roberts, argued strongly against the "anti-activity" trends,[11,41,42] the rejection of occupation illustrates how the need for professional recognition acted, in some way, as a deterrent for practice based on the central concept of the profession during these decades. Ironically it was also responsible for prompting the need for an exclusive body of knowledge that culminated eventually in a return to older values associated with occupation.

Reductionism

During the 1960s and 1970s, an interest was also generated in clinical research by pressure for scientific proof of effectiveness from the medical profession as a requirement of their recognition of the profession's worth. Occupational therapists seem to have welcomed the pressure from medicine to be scientific, to develop a reductionist base for practice, and to bring their practice in line with more conventional remedial approaches. Although, in recent times, many are questioning the appropriateness of quantitative, reductionist, research methods in the study of complex and contextual behavior, research within these boundaries began to occur, and methodological appropriateness was seldom debated.

In the light of current thinking, the basic philosophy that actual "doing" provides people with a vehicle for growth, development, achievement, and health appears to be a holistic concept. To earlier occupational therapists, this same philosophy appeared compatible with the reductionist, mechanistic, and prescriptive notions of much of the 20th century. For example, as early as 1914, Barton sought to discover and provide an occupation as specific treatment for diseases of every separate organ, joint, and muscle,[43] and many early texts describe step-by-step procedures for particular occupations for particular problems. Swain and Taylor, a case in point, found that "a joint will increase its range of motion with the correct amount and kind of work, but will stiffen if the treatment is the least bit overdone" and so devised a system of measuring joint movement and muscle strength, which they recorded on charts. The "work [was] governed entirely by these charts and the condition of the joint."[44] This type of measurement was also used with neurological patients and is still deemed important today in neurological, cardiac, and hand rehabilitation. Even in the treatment of patients with tuberculosis or with psychological problems, a reductionist, analytical emphasis was evident. Canton explains that just as a "psychologist analyzes action into steps, emotions into simpler component feelings, a thought process into its various aspects" so should an occupational therapist clearly define and analyze the work into "its various phases."[45]

The practice of "activity analysis," in the "time and motion" tradition of Frederick Taylor and in which occupations were systematically analyzed for component parts that may be useful for particular "treatment" effects, was first implemented in the 1920s.[46-51] Continued growth and diversification of occupational therapy using this methodology was encouraged within the medical model. To ensure the most certain and rapid recovery from disease or injury, occupational therapists became experts in occupational "reductionism," analyzing the rates of respiration and blood circulation resulting from activities; measuring the character, strength, and extent of movements used by activities; and judging the quality of mental processes such as motivation, reasoning, judgment, attention, and emotion, which may be demanded by or result from activities.[7] One of the greatest proponents of activity analysis has been Gail Fidler, who initially focused on the psychodynamic properties of occupations such as creativity, hostile and aggressive components, narcissism, reality testing, and group relatedness. She later expanded her analysis to include other properties such as motor, sensory integrative, cognitive, and sociocultural components.[47-51] Kielhofner and Burke suggest that occupational therapy was limited for many years to psychoanalytical, kinesiological, and neurological treatment models, which provided precise and extensive methodology, despite loss of the profession's underlying philosophy.[52]

This adherence to medical science reductionist models and priorities, Shannon argues, resulted in "the derailment of occupational therapy."[24] However, the reduction

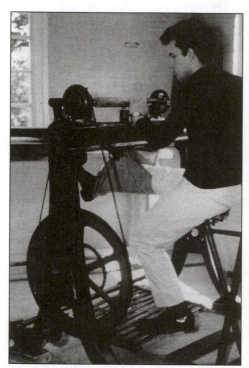

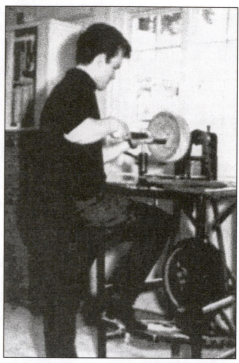

Figure 8-1. Strengthening quadriceps. Courtesy of Windsor Hospital Group.

Figure 8-2. Increasing range of movement. Courtesy of Windsor Hospital Group.

of the profession's basic philosophical premise was probably gradual and never complete; although, following prevalent "medical" model values, most therapists did evaluate and treat symptoms, it was usual practice to view aims of treatment from the perspective of a client's social as well as psychological and physical needs. In 1938, Russell, for example, described activity as nature's best physician because activity also provided a medium for patients to gain self-esteem and happiness, to learn to relate effectively to others, and to re-establish a path toward the realities of community life.[53] This view prevailed in the early 1960s, in an occupational therapy program established by Mary Jones, a founding British occupational therapist who had originally trained as a physiotherapist.[54] Despite a very reductionist orientation that, for the 100 patients who attended 5 days a week for a large part of each working day, included specific attention to a dysfunctional body part, the intervention used occupation for treatment that would lead to "occupational health and wellness" in their everyday lifestyles. For example:

- A 21-year-old fitter and turner who sustained a fracture of the fibula and tibia in a motorcycle accident progressed through an occupational program working on wood and metal turning lathes, seated on a bicycle stool with his leg slung to strengthen his quadriceps during the non-weight bearing period, standing and progressively increasing the range of movement of his leg, maintaining work tolerance and skills, and ensuring that he could return not only to his paid employment but to his major interest in football (Figures 8-1 through 8-6).

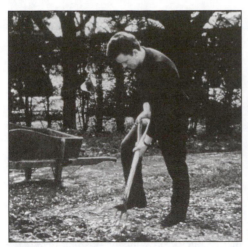

Figure 8-3. Managing uneven surfaces. Courtesy of Windsor Hospital Group.

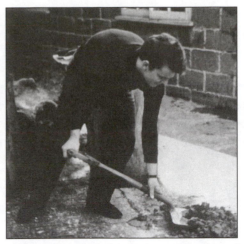

Figure 8-4. Work hardening. Courtesy of Windsor Hospital Group.

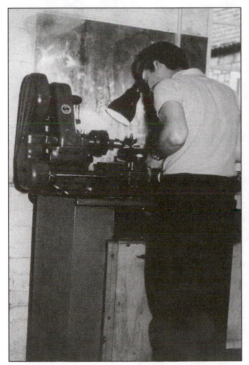

Figure 8-5. Work skills. Courtesy of Windsor Hospital Group.

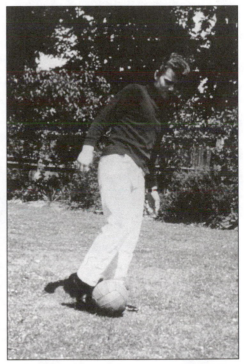

Figure 8-6. Leisure skills. Courtesy of Windsor Hospital Group.

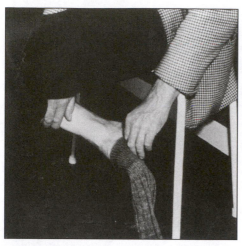

Figure 8-7. Alternative self-care skills. Courtesy of Windsor Hospital Group.

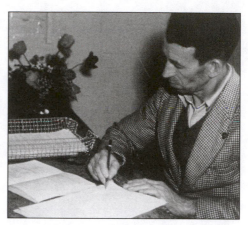

Figure 8-8. Revision of skills for new employment. Courtesy of Windsor Hospital Group.

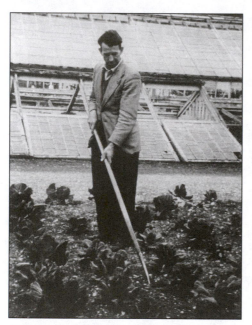

Figure 8-9. Mobility/balance practice. Courtesy of Windsor Hospital Group.

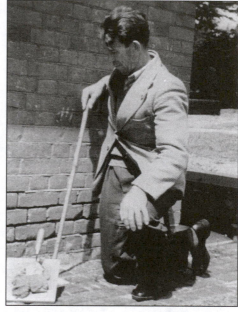

Figure 8-10. Assessing potential to return to previous employment. Courtesy of Windsor Hospital Group.

- A 56-year-old man had an arthrodesis of the hip to reduce pain and dysfunction due to osteoarthritis. His occupational program included alternative methods of self-care to maintain his independence, re-education of mobility patterns using uneven ground in gardening tasks, checking out his potential to return to his former employment as a builder, and developing new skills to enable re-entry into employment in a different capacity as a building site foreman (Figures 8-7 through 8-12).

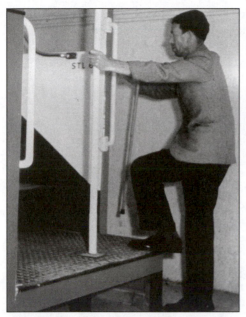

Figure 8-11. Practicing public transport. Courtesy of Windsor Hospital Group.

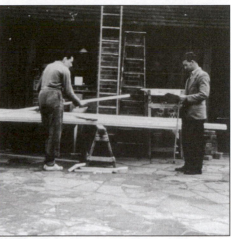

Figure 8-12. New employment. Courtesy of Windsor Hospital Group.

In the foreword to Jones' *An Approach to Occupational Therapy,* CW Guillebaud notes that "the reader is brought to realize how great is the part which occupational therapy...can play in restoring [patients] to an active and productive existence," in providing a "highly useful and valuable economic as well as human service" that is "of the greatest importance for the psychological well-being of the individual."[55] In her final summary, Jones identifies the necessity for occupational therapists to experience "wider opportunities for studying productive activities" and to "spread from the corrective to the preventive fields of study."[54]

Rehabilitation

As part of the "rapid" expansion of knowledge that developed as a result of the work of specialist therapies during the early part of the century, "rehabilitation" developed as a new medical specialty with which occupational therapy aligned itself closely and that remained a clearly identified component of health care for about 20 years.[56] It grew from the earlier notions of "reconstruction," which combined education theories with physical medicine and, especially, from the programs that had been developed to rehabilitate the wounded of World War II. The aftermath of this war led to a rapid growth of allied medical services, including occupational therapy, in many countries including Australia. Although occupational therapy did not get off the ground in Australia until the 1940s, the Arts and Crafts movement was established and influential in Australia as it was in the United States. "The Arts and Crafts Society of Brisbane became involved with remedial teaching for returned servicemen in the early years of the 1914-1918 war and, in fact, went into recess to fully devote itself to these aims."[57]

In part, the growth of allied medical services was aimed at meeting patients' complex, multiple physical, psychological, social, vocational, and economic needs.

Occupational therapy benefited from being obviously in tune with the stated rationale of rehabilitation, but it was the "physical" aspects of rehabilitation that became
the dominant factor, rehabilitation's medical specialty being known as "physical medicine." An indication of this dominance is available in a study by Canadian occupational therapists who reviewed articles published in their national journal between
1950 and 1969 and found 73% focused on some aspect of physical medicine and only
27% on psychosocial concerns.[58]

The biased emphasis on the physical aspects of rehabilitation was part of the reason why the "vogue enjoyed by physical medicine and rehabilitation in the late 1940s
and early 1950s passed quickly. The specialty has since been rejected by much of
mainstream medicine," and by the 1980s only a few "pockets of institutional strong-
holds" remain.[33] In Australia, the huge rehabilitation centers built for the
Commonwealth Rehabilitation Service have been closed down in favor of a "case
management" system, which buys in specialist services according to individual need.
The newer model meets the needs of those with recent problems, rather than those
of the chronically disabled who were seen as a major target group for rehabilitation.
There are now few services for this latter group, but Shannon suggests that the rehabilitation movement was not able to achieve its holistic goal of total care of the chronically disabled because it too was pressed into a reductionist mold and also because
it was poorly resourced. The poor resourcing, even at a time of apparent public affluence, reflects medicine's lack of "professional enthusiasm" in the specialty that, to
some extent, became the "dumping" ground for medicine's castoffs.[24,59,60]

Adaptive Nature

There can be no doubt that ongoing responsiveness to a philosophical base, other
than that which occupational therapy originally espoused and prescriptive interventions applied second hand, encapsulated occupational therapy for many years as a
profession working to remediate sick people within institutional settings operating on
a medical model. During the long association with medicine, occupational therapy
adapted its practice as new ideas and developments occurred. It particularly
embraced the concepts of psychobiology, reconstruction, rehabilitation, neurophysiology, normal development, and, more recently, community health care. Specialist
treatment programs waxed and waned according to medical progress, priorities, interest, and fashion. For example, Meyer's psychobiological theories, which meshed so
well with occupational therapy, were gradually discarded as "naive and oversimpli-
fied" in favor of Freudian psychoanalysis, which fit better with reductionist fervor.[8,61]
Although less comfortable with this approach, occupational therapists worked at
opening "avenues for need fulfillment and ego maturation" and included regression
in treatment activities so that patients could achieve "actual or symbolic gratification"
to meet unsatisfied needs.[62,63] Graduated activity, according to physical and respiratory demands that were developed for the treatment of people with tuberculosis,
declined as chemotherapy reduced the incidence and prevalence of the disease.[16]
With the increase of modern epidemics, such as cardiovascular disease, graduated
programs have been reinvented to assist people affected by such diseases to return
to normal living. Specific techniques that were developed to overcome the physical
problems of children following the polio epidemics of the 1940s and the 1950s
became obsolete for that purpose with the decline of the disease following the Sabin
or Salk vaccine prevention programs. However, these techniques provided the basis

for other work aimed at neurologically impaired children and adults with physical disability. As patients with permanent or temporary physical or psychological disability began to be discharged to their homes and jobs more frequently and earlier,[64] occupational therapists expanded their practice to include activities of daily living (ADL) and work. In the *Bulletin* (July 1955), which was the first official communication of the Sydney Occupational Therapists' Club, Dargan, a Sydney-trained occupational therapist, discusses "startling reversals of old theories" such as patients being encouraged to get out of bed soon after surgery, and being enabled to return to home and work.[64]

From the late 1950s to the present, occupational therapists have increasingly followed compensatory rather than remedial objectives for all types and age groups of clients, as retraining in ADL, aimed at independent self-care, assumed priority in a health care environment committed to fast turnover of patients. It is arguable that ADL is currently the term used by the majority of occupational therapists to describe the central focus of their domain of concern, although it is a term used in a variety of ways according to the focus of the intervention ranging from self-care activities, such as showering and dressing, to the whole range of domestic or vocational pursuits.[65]

Occupational therapy has also been adaptive to the influences of other professions with which it has been closely associated throughout its history, in particular to educators, psychologists, physiotherapists, and social workers. Integrated within the profession's programs are interventions and strategies based around work as diverse as that of Piaget, Erikson, Frostig, Voss, Kabot, Brunnstrom, Bobath, Kübler-Ross, Maslow, Rogers, Skinner, Luria, Benedict Mead, Maxwell Jones, and Travis. Its interest in both remedial and compensatory equipment and devices and splints to aid in overcoming disability has also made it receptive to technological development of new materials and computers. Its commitment to an integrated view of mind, body, and environment has led to a professional belief that it offers holistic therapy, despite its more obvious concern with sick rather than well populations, and individuals rather than communities.

Within the context of the dynamics that have been discussed in the previous paragraphs, I now turn to consider the renaissance of occupation as central to the profession's theory and practice.

Occupation Rediscovered

Against a background of Western society's widespread dissatisfaction with a materialistic, technologically driven society, a new critical social science with an activist conception of human beings began to emerge,[66-68] based on notions propounded by Marx in his earlier works,[69] to a lesser extent on Rousseau's view (c. 1755) that humans in a "state of nature" express "free will" and a capacity for self-improvement,[70] and, more recently, by critical sociologists of the Frankfurt School.[71-73] Fay argues that critical social science assumes that "humans are active creatures," who as a consequence of their "intelligent, curious, reflective, and willful" behavior can "transform themselves and their societies within certain wide limits..."[74]

Similar social and intellectual discontents were expressed by occupational therapists, who had their own perceptions of the inadequacy of reductionism, who began to question the medical establishment and their own direction, and, in some cases, returned to the earlier conception of humans as "occupational [active] beings." Mary Reilly (Figure 8-13), an occupational therapy educator at the University of Southern

Figure 8-13. Mary Reilly. American Occupational Therapy Association. *A Professional Legacy: The Eleanor Clarke Slagle Lectures.* **Rockville, Md: Author; 1985. Reproduced courtesy of the American Occupational Therapy Association Inc, Bethesda, Md.**

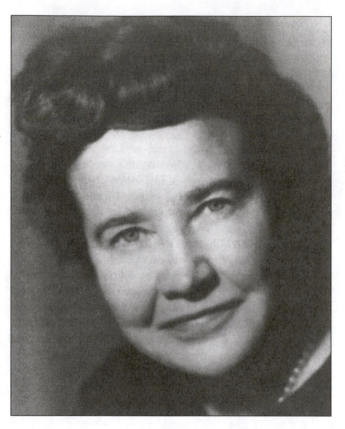

California, led the way by looking backwards at the profession's basic premises. In the 1961 Eleanor Clarke Slagle lecture, she proposed that the original hypothesis of occupational therapy can be stated as "that man through the use of his hands, as they are energized by mind and will, can influence the state of his own health."[41] She postulated that although the First Principle, from which medical science draws its premise, explains that the nature of humans is to be alive, the Second Principle is for humans to grow and be productive, and she maintained that occupational therapy should derive its premise from this principle. The two principles "merge into a concept of function which asserts that both the existence and the unfolding of the specific powers of an organism are one and the same thing." In language in line with my own theories about occupational needs as part of the health-survival package set out in Chapters 2, 5, and 6, she argues that "the power to act creates a need to use the power, and the failure to use the power results in dysfunction and unhappiness." Reilly's concept was based on the sensitivity, adaptability, durability, and creativity of humans in tune with their environments, based on ideas from theorists such as Lerner[75] and Fromm[76] and laboratory testing such as that on sensory deprivation.[77] (Fromm is associated with "critical social science" and the Frankfurt School.)

Following this inspiring lecture, in a series of articles over the span of some 15 years, Reilly initiated the development of an occupational behavior paradigm of practice,[78-80] which other therapists recognized might help overcome occupational therapy's tendency to compromise "its unique philosophical traditions in order to accommodate to the predominant philosophy" of other medical specialties.[81] Reilly defined occupational behavior as "the entire developmental continuum of play and work."[82] The definition acknowledged the importance of economic skills, attitudes, and interests that motivated and enabled clients to survive in an increasingly complex technological world. Her model, which accepted that occupation is wired into humans through the process of evolution,[83] stressed the importance of examining life roles relative to community adaptation; of identifying the various skills that support these roles; of creating an environment where the relevant behavior can be evoked and practiced; and of using occupation as the integrative focus of behavior change. By placing emphasis on interpersonal relationships and on individuals' ability to cope with the community and with changes in life situations, and because "both the well and the sick population" could be accommodated "without altering the model," her paradigm offered appropriate structures for developing community health practice of the time.[81]

Reilly's work re-emphasizing the importance of occupation and the need for occupational therapists to value their unique base of practice introduced new directions for theory development, which recovered some of the profession's philosophical foundation. As director of graduate programs, Reilly also had a huge influence on the work of her graduate students.[84] Gary Kielhofner's papers and books articulating "A Model of Human Occupation," for example, grew out of his work as a master's degree student with Reilly. One of the best known figures of occupational therapy today, Kielhofner, now at the University of Chicago, developed his model from one of Reilly's basic assumptions that "occupation is a central aspect of the human experience" and that "all human occupation arises out of an innate, spontaneous tendency of the human system—the urge to explore and master the environment."[85] According to his Model of Human Occupation, occupational therapy should provide opportunities for directed experiences, that is, participation in life tasks for people described as having occupational dysfunction. The therapeutic aims of such programs include improvement in organization, function, and adaptation within occupational performance, achievable through changes attained in self-image, skill development, new habits, acquired roles, and environmental changes. Some of the most important concepts within this frame of reference are that humans are viewed as open systems,[86] that there is a continuum of occupational function and dysfunction,[87] that engagement in occupation is central to adaptation, so that dysfunction is a threat to health and well-being, and that occupation is governed by three subsystems:

1. Volition
2. Habituation
3. Performance

Progressive levels of occupational function include exploration, competence, and achievement. Progressive levels of occupational dysfunction include inefficacy, incompetence, and helplessness. The concepts are principally applied to occupational therapy practice within traditional health care settings but have potential for wider application. The model entails occupational therapists rethinking their approaches and practices fairly radically and learning a new set of terminology. The recognition Kielhofner's model received following publication established an international trend of the profession back to its philosophical foundation.

In addition to her students, Reilly influenced her colleagues, one of whom, Elizabeth Yerxa (Figure 8-14), in her Slagle lecture, proposed that authentic occupa-

Figure 8-14. Elizabeth Yerxa. American Occupational Therapy Association. *A Professional Legacy: The Eleanor Clarke Slagle Lectures.* **Rockville, Md: Author; 1985. Reproduced courtesy of the American Occupational Therapy Association Inc, Bethesda, Md.**

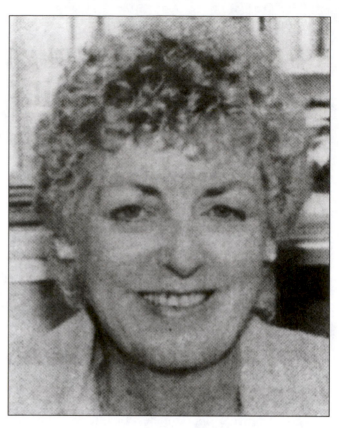

tional therapy should be aimed at client self-actualization through choice, self-initiated purposeful activities, reality orientation, and perception of self and environment.[11] She became a powerful advocate for the development of a basic science of occupation complementary to the applied science of occupational therapy, and developed a doctoral program in occupational science at the University of Southern California. Occupational science is defined by her and her associates at the University of Southern California as "the study of the human as an occupational being, including the need for and capacity to engage in and orchestrate daily occupations in the environment over the lifespan."[88]

She suggested that one of the advantages of such a science to occupational therapy is that:

> *By identifying and articulating a scientific foundation for practice, occupational science could provide practitioners with support for what they do, justify the significance of occupational therapy to health, and differentiate occupational therapy from other disciplines.*[88]

In setting up specifications and criteria for the emerging science, academics instrumental in the establishment of a doctoral program in occupational science at the University of Southern California proposed that it study individuals in interaction with their environment, center on people, "not on a cell or reflex," be developmental in nature, and address the complexities of occupation.[89,90] Those criteria mesh with the central ideas considered in this book, with the proviso that, in order for the discipline to be holistic, it is just as relevant for some occupational scientists to study "occupational humans" at cell or reflex level as it is to study them at the ecological level. What is important is for occupational scientists to make a subtle change from considering humans who use occupation from a biological or cultural perspective to considering biological or cultural issues from the broad perspective of the human need for occupation.

The notion of viewing humans from this different perspective holds a particular promise within the arena of public health, not least in challenging many sociocultural and political structures that deprive or alienate humans from exercising their occupational natures to enhance their health. The following consideration of occupational therapists' response to the development of a science of occupation illustrates this challenge and promise.

Despite a degree of acceptance and excitement around the world—in Australia, Canada, Japan, New Zealand, Sweden, and the United Kingdom, as well as the United States—there is also some diffidence, even conflict, within the profession with regards to the development of a basic discipline of occupational science.[91,92] There are a variety of reasons for this. For example, some occupational therapists view occupational science as just another model or theory that is in competition with their own theory of occupation. They do not support the notion of a many-faceted generic science, into which their own model could fit. Others hold to the clinical tradition and close association with either medicine or other already developed social sciences and see no need for a particular occupational perspective. Still others aspire to a simple, all-embracing theory that can effectively describe their purpose, but individual therapists hold a great variety of views. In addition, they avoid using the word "occupation" because it is so often misunderstood. On both counts, they view with disfavor a generic science of occupation, which may increase the complexity of explanation because of contradictory ideas.

If occupational science grows, there is no doubt that it will increase complexity of understanding because it will include many models, frames of reference, and theories, changing direction according to sociocultural change and advances in biological knowledge. Complexity will lead to heated debate between scientists, just as behavioral, clinical, experimental, humanist, social, occupational, transcendental, or neuropsychologists all argue with each other but collectively contribute to the science of psychology. Heated debate about the profession's foundation beliefs is not part of occupational therapists' tradition, and discussion with therapists reveals a degree of apprehension in moving toward this as a possible scenario. Despite this apprehension, debate and challenge are being voiced in occupational therapy journals about whether there is a need for a science of occupation, whether, indeed, occupation was central in the discipline's early history,[93] or whether occupational science should be developed and resourced by occupational therapists.

Anne Cronin Mosey, who in her Slagle lecture advocates for occupational therapists taking pluralistic rather than monistic approaches, and regards occupational models in the latter light, argues for the complete partition of occupational science and occupational therapy,[94,95] a partition with which Florence Clark and her associates at the University of Southern California disagree strongly.[96] The debate between Mosey and Clark is representative of division within the profession about this issue.

Despite such debate, different theories pertaining to humans' occupational natures have proliferated in recent years,[97-99] and there is a large declaratory literature about occupation. Much of this is linked with notions of health and well-being as discussed

George Mocellin, an Australian occupational therapy educator, in a two-part overview of the beliefs and values of early American occupational therapists, concludes that the concept of "competence" rather than "occupation" provides the philosophical underpinning of occupational therapy.
Mocellin G. An overview of occupational therapy in the context of the American influence on the profession. *British Journal of Occupational Therapy.* 1992;55(1):7-12 and 55(2):5-60.

in earlier chapters. Some examples to illuminate the range of the discipline's conceptions include:

- Fidler's ideas about enabling "doing" to satisfy intrinsic and extrinsic needs and the needs of others; that "doing" skills are dependent upon and change with age, developmental level, biology, and culture[100]; that competency, mastery, adaptation, self-esteem, self-value, and self-worth result from successful "doing" and are interrelated.[47,101]
- Mosey's philosophical assumptions about the maturation, social nature, and structure of the species; each individual's need for occupational balance, to reach potential through purposeful interaction with the environment, each individual's need to be understood within the context of family, community, and culture.[102]
- Moore's linking of humans' occupational behavior with limbic system function so that "the normal system maintains a homeostatic balance in favor of pleasurable rewards and away from painful or non-rewarding stimuli"; that occupational behavioral needs vary because of "individual genetic and biochemical differences as well as...multiple and highly variable relationships with...[the] environment."[103]
- Lloren's emphasis on occupational therapy as a growth model of health.[104]
- do Rozario's conception that occupational therapists focus on "occupational role and performance," the integration of "being and doing," health, and well-being, and that sustainability provides an "'empowering and transformational model of practice' as a process in enhancing people's sense of meaning, value, and satisfaction in daily life."[105]
- Townsend's view of "occupational therapy's social vision," which promotes social justice by enabling development of occupational potential and using practical approaches so that people can "participate as valued members of society despite diverse or limited occupational potential."[106]

Such contributions have led to academic programs based on the study of human engagement in occupation becoming more common in most Western economies.[107,108] Indeed, about 75% of the Australian undergraduate occupational therapy programs have moved in this direction during the past 10 years, and the change toward occupation-based models of practice is the current trend in Australia. Evidence of a change in research interest is also emerging, from purely clinically based studies to consideration of occupational issues within the community, such as in patterns and meanings of paid employment or lack of paid employment,[109-112] to studies of how particular groupings of people use their time,[113-116] to broader theses linking occupational concepts to ecological sustainability[117] and occupational behavior of other primates.[118]

Health Promotion

This section of the chapter will consider occupational therapists' interest in health promotion. These interests are not unconnected, because the evolving fascination of the study of humans as occupational beings grew with changing societal views about health and well-being and with the emerging objective of the WHO for "the attainment by all peoples of the highest possible level of health."[119] Although WHO was established in 1946 as a "specialist agency for health," the World Federation of Occupational Therapists did not join it until 1959. In a 1963 report in the *British Journal of Occupational Therapy,* Henderson points out that WHO "pursues an unlimited ideal and an immense task," but does not discuss the role of occupational therapists in helping to achieve this task.[120] Indeed, despite the broad health aims of the WHO, most occupational therapists, in line with most other health disciplines, continued to espouse a role more attuned to reductionist, illness models aimed at individuals, rather than holistic, wellness models aimed at the health of communities.

However, the WHO's interest in approaches to improve health and quality of life was in line with community interest, which escalated from the early 1960s, along with exploration of alternative lifestyles.[121,122] In common with many modern historians, some occupational therapists have speculated on reasons for this community interest and have suggested that it erupted from the illness-oriented medical model for several reasons, such as the advances in technology and the concurrent escalation of health care costs, the increase of health care knowledge generally leading to the dominant role of physicians being challenged, and technological development producing a societal reaction toward simpler, more natural remedies for disease control.[123] Johnson suggests that the interest was part of the human potential and countercultural movements, in which many groups, particularly women and minorities, reacted to social forces that seemed to ignore their individual, perceived needs.[124] She also cites growing dissatisfaction with medicine and perceived dehumanization in the medical care system as important factors, along with increasing recognition of ways in which the world was being polluted.

So, at about the same time that Reilly was arguing, from an occupational perspective, for occupational therapists to recognize the links between occupation and health, a group of leaders in the field with a preventive and health promotion perspective were encouraging them to aim, through occupation, at "maintaining optimum health rather than...intermittent treatment of acute disease and disability."[125] Wilma West (Figure 8-15) envisaged that health and medical care in the future would "emphasize human development by programs designed to promote better adaptation, rather than technologically oriented programs offering specific solutions to specific disabilities." She also held that each occupational therapist should function as a "health agent [rather than therapist] with responsibility to help ensure normal growth and development," considering more fully the "socio-economic and cultural as well as biological causes of disease and dysfunction," but all in a "new mold" rather than a recast of an earlier prototype.[125,126] Shortly afterwards, at the 5th International Congress of the World Federation of Occupational Therapists, in 1979, she proposed a health model for occupational therapy practice based on the assumption that health care in the decade ahead would be as concerned with prevention as with rehabilitation. Therefore, she advocated increasing involvement of both client and community in more effective methods to enhance and enrich development of physical, mental,

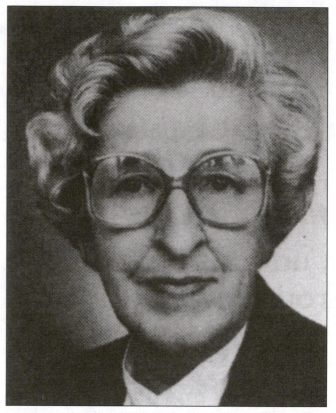

Figure 8-15. Wilma West. American Occupational Therapy Association. *A Professional Legacy: The Eleanor Clarke Slagle Lectures.* **Rockville, Md: Author; 1985. Reproduced courtesy of the American Occupational Therapy Association Inc, Bethesda, Md.**

emotional, social, and vocational abilities, and suggested a "timely translation" of occupational therapists' "long time focus on activities of daily living for the disabled to advocacy of the balanced regimen of age appropriate, work play activities for man in the pre-disease/disability phase."[127] Her view that such a role required only a "broader application of existing knowledge about the effects of activity—or its absence—on health" was an invitation to occupational therapists to revisit and use their underlying philosophy in a way advocated in this text.

At the same congress, and along similar lines, Florence Cromwell stated a need for occupational therapists to think about the global trend toward preventive rather than curative programs, about world health care, and about searching for more universal systems of care by considering, for example, how different nations combat the problems facing them.[128] She said that occupational therapists should move into the arena of well care, as specialists in human behavior in ordinary environments where patients live, work, and play.

Some therapists such as Wiemer discussed prevention as an aspect of the occupational therapist's role in community health.[129] Indeed, Geraldine Finn addressed *The Occupational Therapist in Prevention Programs* as the topic of her Slagle lecture in 1971.[130] In an update of that paper, she observed that, for the majority of therapists who practiced in the community at that time, there was a trend to select programs and services at the levels of secondary and tertiary prevention, an observation that still holds some truth. To encourage occupational therapy involvement in primary prevention, in line with Reilly, she proposed the development of a model of practice addressing the issue of the significance of occupation to human life. She argued that, as primary prevention is directed toward an understanding of both the relationship between the basic structural elements of society and health and of what keeps people in a state of health, occupational therapists should make their contribution with a greater understanding of the effects of occupation on health.[131] These views were compatible with emerging conceptualizations about the nature of health held by other leaders in the field at that time, such as Mosey and Fidler. Mosey defined health needs as "inherent human requirements that must be met for an individual to experience a sense of physical, psychological and social well-being,"[132] and Fidler held that health is the ability to carry out activities that are essential for developmentally appropriate self-maintenance and meeting of intrinsic needs according to the social context.[100]

West's prophecies and encouragement were optimistic: few real changes to practice eventuated, perhaps because of economic constraints, which affected health care budgets and curbed the development of new trends toward prevention that were not yet a priority in health planning. Also, as Grosman suggests, the work itself may appear less defined, less sophisticated, less measurable, and more isolated in the face of the massive social, economic, and political conditions that interfere with health.[133] The latter issues seem similarly daunting to present-day post-graduate students considering these issues, despite a recognition that these particular conditions are those that require most emphasis if change is to occur.[134] Laukaran suggests as other reasons limited opportunities or lack of professional incentives for service in positions not designated for occupational therapists; competition with other professionals; and inability to cross boundaries to work in community institutions.[81] These are compounded by long-held values, growing from occupational therapists' association with clinically based medicine, that occupational therapy is concerned with ill rather than well (or even all) people and that existing occupational therapy models (developing from those values) limit practice and result in gaps in knowledge and theory.[81] Such values limit occupational therapists' ability to recognize occupational dysfunctions, such as alienation, deprivation, and imbalance, as risk factors that can lead to disease, disability, and death and has meant that such dysfunction has not been identified as a primary prevention focus. Neither has it been appreciated that people in need of "preventive occupational therapy services," for example, are unlikely to be "referred through medical channels, since they are not diseased but are disengaged from daily life."[135]

It is also conceivable that a major change of focus toward community health was inhibited in part because occupational therapists were caught in the 1970s in a conflict between history, tradition, and value systems, changes in the health care system, and consumer expectations within society.[136] The 1970s were a time of crisis because, although the deterioration of its philosophical base was starting to be recognized, the rejection of occupation as central to occupational therapy practice was at its greatest,[137] leaving it with no common unifying concepts.[12] Margaret Smith, a British occupational therapist, in a keynote address to the 15th Federal Conference of the AAOT in 1988 described the 1960s and 1970s as "the age of confidence," but a major disappointment of the era as "the very reason for our being, the therapy of occupation...went right out the window."[137] The situation was made more complex because at the same time alternative ideas about life and health permeating the Western world generated fears that reductionism, which occupational therapy had accepted, could not provide all the answers in health care.[52,87]

The strength of the interest in health promotion among its members led the

American Association of Occupational Therapists, at the end of the turbulent 1970s and again a decade later, to put out position papers addressing the issues. However, in defining how occupational therapists may be instrumental in health promotion, the position papers still articulate a model aimed more at the individual than at communities. For example, a 1979 paper states that:

Occupational therapists value the nature and importance of goal-directed, productive interchange in the maintenance of health and prevention of disability, as well as in rehabilitation of the handicapped.

The occupational therapist's training instills a respect for the realities of life, for the tasks of living, and for the time it takes the individual to develop modes of coping with those tasks. Occupational therapy makes its unique contribution to health care through accent on fulfillment in human activity, and a special contribution to understanding the significance and worth of human enterprise.[138]

Although many occupational therapists remain concerned about the low level of occupational therapist involvement in health promotion and community health, it is apparent that interest has been ongoing with leading theorists within the profession continuously addressing the topic. For example, Elnora Gilfoyle in *Transformation of a Profession* advocates that occupational therapists increase their "awareness to include social, economic, and political factors" toward new understandings of "the value of occupation and the patients' occupational process in promoting their own health."[139] Johnson and Kielhofner point out that "occupation is a necessary prerequisite to health," arguing that "when social systems or other conditions deprive the individual of satisfying engagement in occupation, there is a clear threat to the mental and physical integrity of the person" and that the responsibility of occupational therapists of the future will be to "remediate the conditions of work and play, and the social, economic, and other factors that disrupt normal patterns of occupation."[62] Interest is also apparent from the number of articles in occupational therapy journals that relate to the topic. For example, 12 of 64 articles (19%) in six *Occupational Therapy in Health Care* journals dated between 1984 and 1989 dealt with topics that can be classified as "health promotion" or "disease prevention," and a further 12 can be classified as "health issues from a sociocultural perspective."

The last quarter of this century has provided time for the development of theories of a unique view of health promotion from an occupational therapy perspective, but practice still lags behind ideas. A shortage of experienced occupational therapists working as role models and developing frames of reference for younger therapists who are keen to work in the community but are not yet ready for a leadership role has been identified as a constraint to community health practice. That weakness has been compounded by a lack of knowledge about occupational therapy by community service administrators, lack of professional visibility and identity, role confusion, and lack of occupational therapy input into the planning of community services.[140-147]

In America today, occupational therapy practice in the community is limited to the provision of services that are reimbursable according to the 1991 Medicare guidelines.[148] In Britain, although many therapists' work is based in the community, their role is also determined by legislation relating to disability and community care.[149] Canadian occupational therapists seem to be currently leading occupational therapy initiatives within community health, which is reflective of the health promotion initiatives of their country as a whole[150,151] and their recognition that occupational therapy has "the potential to become a major contributor in assisting [the] national vision to become a reality."[152] Even there, Madill, Townsend, and Schultz, who found that occupational therapy's client-centered approach meshes well with health promotion as outlined in the Ottawa Charter, propose that substantial occupational therapy educational programs are required to reflect the developments in the field. They note, in particular, the need to generalize "client-centered issues to the broader social and economic environment," suggesting that occupational therapists have a role in community action, prevention, the workplace, and in public education.[153]

In Australia, Burnett, in a recent review of Australian community health centers, found a paucity of both occupational therapists and literature.[154] Indeed, all of the factors that inhibit the move to community-based practice, identified earlier, would seem to have had some bearing on occupational therapy programs, from the time when community initiatives started nationwide during the 1970s up to the present day. Because effective amounts of resources have not been directed away from curative services, jobs within community health are scarce for health professionals such as occupational therapists, while jobs in already established, better resourced services are still available. This effectively continues to limit the potential of occupational therapy in Australia to working with ill or disabled people, although employment opportunities for occupational therapists in conventional health services are becoming fewer as economic rationalism dehumanizes health services and reduces lengths of stay.

Occupational therapists do work in the community, but largely in jobs that are related to the management of disability rather than in programs aimed at occupation and health. Because of lack of understanding of the scope of occupational therapy, community agencies may only consider therapists for jobs if particular ill health problems are seen as needing to be addressed within any particular community, or may not consider employing them at all. For example, in a survey conducted in South Australia in 1993, the one occupational therapist employed in a metropolitan community health center was highly valued, and her skills and philosophies were seen as appropriate. In centers that had never employed an occupational therapist, those surveyed were unsure of occupational therapists' skills, convinced their philosophical base was inappropriate, and 60% would not consider employing one if funds were available.[143,144,155]

It is somewhat ironic that the notion of "an interaction between occupation and health" is more in line with the new public health in which occupational therapists do not (on the whole) work than it is with conventional medicine where they do work. Although compatible with earlier models of health care and entirely compatible with those proclaimed by public health in documents such as the Ottawa Charter, the idea of "health and occupation" is largely incompatible with the orientation of the services currently provided by conventional medicine and receives little, if any, consideration in community centers.

Additionally, although occupational therapists are exposed to population health issues during their education, they are not trained to consider research or intervention from this perspective and so are unable to translate their core concept in the most meaningful way. Not recognizing this, many try to adapt frames of reference developed for and suited to conventional medicine. Alternatively, they may address health promotion problems from a perspective identified by other disciplines, thereby providing less effective programs than they could, and thus losing their distinctive focus. They become unsure that what they can contribute to health promotion is of value.

This reinforces most therapists continuing with clinical models, in conventional settings, and may be why occupational therapists have, in the past, demonstrated a bias toward programs for individual client problems. From my own experience, particularly from being involved with student education about the topic, there is still an element of excitement and status associated with conventional hospital-based services that is appealing to young students entering the profession. This is built upon, during their training, by most fieldwork experience taking place in conventional settings because of fewer opportunities to experience community, health promoting practice, along with exposure to the many traditional practice frames of reference. The idea of a relationship between occupation and health is addressed in many of these frames of reference, but current economic conditions mean that there is little opportunity to implement them in clinically based services, and the community health frames of reference they consider do not focus on training in population-based measures of intervention, in part, because of lack of time. In the past few years the final fieldwork experience in South Australia for graduating students has been undertaken in community agencies or places where occupational therapy may not have a well-established presence. There they develop programs based on agency (client) need in a research and evaluation mode. This has been extremely effective in changing attitudes and recognizing potential.

It is hardly surprising, in most cases, that rather than trailblaze in isolated community agencies, therapists still opt for the security of institutional positions. There are hints of change, however. Papers presented at the 1995 AAOT Conference suggest a broadening of interest toward programs aimed at health, such as a "model of occupational harmony," applicable to diverse cultures, in which a balance of life roles is taken as the essence of health and well-being,[156] and to programs aimed at political lobbying. Dwyer, for example, who focused on the needs of non-English speaking and indigenous people, proposed that to enable them "to exercise their civil and political rights, it could be claimed that they need to be in a state of 'holistic health.' So to be politicized and politically active could be indicative of a state of wellness, physically and mentally."[157] Similarly, it can be argued that occupational therapists, because of a restriction of their potential within the medical model, have not enjoyed holistic health and wellness as a profession and that this has inhibited their political activism. They are unlikely to be aware of this effect, for as Fay argues "human history is the story of people who, in trying to satisfy their desires and their ideals, create social institutions and cultures but are not able or willing to see that that is what they have done."[74] Those occupational therapists who have taken up the challenge of living and working in the "new land" of community development have found it exciting, challenging, and fulfilling. Such therapists are thriving, "have rediscovered their purpose for being, and are making valuable contributions to their 'new society'" so that none would "return to the hostile, inequitable, under-resourced old world from which they came."[158]

Two surveys, both undertaken in 1989, have explored the perceptions and attitudes of Australian occupational therapists toward health promotion and public health. The first was a survey of 378 Australian occupational therapists which found that attitudes that reflect the "new public health model," such as client-therapist interaction, client responsibility, and holistic attitudes to health care prevail, especially with experienced therapists, older than 30.[159] The second, a national survey of a random sample of Australian occupational therapists, also found that occupational therapists hold positive attitudes toward health promotion, the benefits they perceive as ema-

| | | Response | |
		Number	Percentage
Satisfied with Amount	No	180	72.0%
of Health Promotion	Yes	47	18.8%
Done in Job	Don't Know	23	9.2%
	Total	250	100.0%
Constrained by time to develop/ implement program		118	46.8%
Constrained by heavy workload		118	46.8%
Constrained by limited staff and resources		99	39.3%
Constrained by employing agency policy		37	14.7%
Constrained by fear of invading individuals' rights		15	6.0%
Other constraints		18	7.1%

Table 8-1. Constraints to Providing Health Promotion in Current Work.

nating from it, and their belief that occupational therapists should be involved in it and have a special contribution to make.[160] Close to 72% of respondents said they were not satisfied with the amount of health promotion they were able to do in the course of their work because they were constrained by lack of time to develop or implement programs, heavy workloads, limited staff and resources, employing agency policies, and fear of invading individual rights (Table 8-1).

The respondents suggested that the benefits of increasing health promotion programs would include healthier community and individual lifestyles, home and community problems being better addressed, targeted programs for risk groups, programs for relatives, increased client responsibility for their own health, and a reduction in ill health and hospital/institution admissions (Table 8-2).

While the recognition of their potential for health promotion and of the need to translate the core concept of "occupation and health" into community action is strong, respondents believed some change of emphasis in occupational therapy undergraduate education is required (Table 8-3).

Summary

In summary, occupational therapy's assumptions about the relationships between occupation and health have changed throughout the profession's development. This has been, in large part, because of its smallness, its gender imbalance, its dependence on medicine, its difference, and the difficulty of explaining or understanding its promise without an appreciation of its origins and rich philosophical history. In recent years, as feminist and other social action has challenged and changed some traditional values and as an appreciation has grown of the value of its difference, occupational therapists have begun to articulate theory that has the potential to offer a unique contribution in many arenas, including public health. This can only occur, however, if the

| | Response | |
	Number	Percentage
Healthier community and individual lifestyles	173	68.7%
Home and community problems better addressed	133	52.8%
Allow targeted programs for risk groups	136	54.0%
Provide health promotion programs for relatives	128	50.8%
Promote client responsibility for own health	174	69.0%
Reduce ill health and hospital/institution admissions	153	61.0%

Table 8-2. Benefits if Health Promotion Programs Were Increased.

| | Response | |
	Number	Percentage
Need education on risk factors	78	31.0%
Need education on principles of lifestyle modification	104	41.3%
Need training in counseling skills	136	54.0%
Need education on public policy regarding health	97	38.5%
Need multidisciplinary health professional education	113	44.8%
Need multidisciplinary intersectorial education	79	31.3%
Need other education and training	50	20.0%

Table 8-3. Further Education Requirements.

profession changes its overwhelming focus toward individuals with disability to one that recognizes, researches, and develops practice centered on the occupational needs of all people, communities, and cultures. In a way, similar to the increased understanding of the whole population regarding the relationship of nutrition to health, it is only when there is a general appreciation that engagement in occupation is a principle mechanism for health that real changes can occur. Occupational therapists are still limited, however, by their small numbers, lack of understanding by others of their potential contribution, and by political, social, and economic factors that restrict their practice to within a diminishing institutional scene. Also necessary is an acceptance of the importance of this idea by public health, along with opportunities for occupational therapists to undertake population studies to test and measure the idea and implement appropriate strategies.

The next and final chapter will discuss how occupational therapists could contribute to community and public health if these restrictions were overcome and if they themselves accepted the value of a public health focus. They could do this by taking a strong educational and political stance aimed at social action for change relating to maximizing the effects of occupation on health and well-being for the wider community, as well as individuals with disability.

References

1. Bockhoven JS. Occupational therapy: a neglected source of community rehumanisation. In: *Moral Treatment in Community Mental Health*. New York, NY: Springer Publishing Co, Inc; 1972:218,220.
2. Willis E. *Medical Dominance, The Division of Labour in Australian Health Care*. Sydney, Australia: George Allen and Unwin; 1983.
3. Turner BS. Knowledge, skill and occupational strategy: the professionalisation of paramedical groups. *Community Health Studies*. 1985;5(1):38-47.
4. Dunton WR Jr. Occupation as a therapeutic measure. *Medical Record*. 1913;83:388-389.
5. Dunton WR Jr. History of occupational therapy. *Modern Hospital*. 1917;8:380-381.
6. Woodside HH. The development of occupational therapy 1910-1929. *American Journal of Occupational Therapy*. 1971;XXV(5):226-230.
7. Dunton WR Jr. *Prescribing Occupational Therapy*. 2nd ed. Springfield, Ill: Charles C Thomas; 1928.
8. Serrett KD. *Philosophical and Historical Roots of Occupational Therapy*. New York, NY: The Haworth Press Inc; 1985:19-20,22.
9. Yerxa EJ, Gilfoyle E. Research seminar. *American Journal of Occupational Therapy*. 1976;30:509-514.
10. Rogers JC. Order and disorder in medicine and occupational therapy. *American Journal of Occupational Therapy*. 1982;36(1):29-35.
11. Yerxa EJ. 1966 Eleanor Clarke Slagle Lecture. Authentic occupational therapy. *American Journal of Occupational Therapy*. 1967;XXI(1):1-9.
12. Gillette N, Kielhofner G. The impact of specialisation on the professionalisation and survival of occupational therapy. *American Journal of Occupational Therapy*. 1979;33(1):20-28.
13. Pattison HA. The trend of occupational therapy for the tuberculous. *Archives of Occupational Therapy*. 1922;1:19-24.
14. Griffin S. Conflicts in professional practice. *Australian Occupational Therapy Journal*. 1988;35(1):5-12.
15. Hopkins HL, Smith HD, eds. *Willard and Spackman's Occupational Therapy*. 5th ed. Philadelphia, Pa: JB Lippincott; 1978:4.
16. Anderson B, Bell J. *Occupational Therapy: Its Place in Australia's History*. Sydney, Australia: NSW Association of Occupational Therapists; 1988:2,5,39,147,154,156,158,200-202,221,223.
17. Frank G. Opening feminist histories of occupational therapy. *American Journal of Occupational Therapy*. 1992;46(11):989-999.
18. Dunton WR Jr. *A Manual for Nurses*. Philadelphia, Pa: WB Saunders; 1915.
19. Fuller D. Introduction. In: Tracey SE. *Studies in Invalid Occupations: A Manual for Nurses and Attendants*. Boston, Mass: Whitcomb and Barrows; 1913:5.
20. Litterest TAE. Occupational therapy: the role of ideology in the development of a profession for women. *American Journal of Occupational Therapy*. 1992;46:20-25.
21. Cott NF. The bonds of womanhood: "women's sphere" In: *New England 1780-1835*. New Haven, Conn: Yale University Press; 1977.
22. Slagle EC. Training aides for mental patients. *Archives of Occupational Therapy*. 1922;1:11-17.
23. Jacobs K. *Occupational Therapy: Work Related Programs and Assessments*. Boston, Mass: Little, Brown and Co; 1985.
23a. Hollis I. *Hand Therapy at Chapel Hill*. Lecture given at South Australian Institute of Technology, 1980.
24. Shannon PD. The derailment of occupational therapy. *American Journal of Occupational Therapy*. 1977;31(4):229-234.
25. Jantzen A. Some characteristics of female occupational therapists. Part 1—descriptive study. *American Journal of Occupational Therapy*. 1972;26:19-26.
26. Brunyate RW. From the president—after fifty years what stature do we hold? *American Journal of Occupational Therapy*. 1967;21:262-267.
27. Matthewson M. Female and married: damaging to the occupational therapy profession. *American Journal of Occupational Therapy*. 1975;29(10):601-605.
28. Acquiviva FA. AOTA's ad hoc commission on occupational therapy manpower: Part 1: summary of findings. *American Journal of Occupational Therapy*. 1986;40(7):455-457.
29. MacKinnon JR. Current supply and future requirements for occupational therapy manpower in British Columbia. *Canadian Journal of Occupational Therapy*. 1985;52(5):251-257.
30. Taylor S. Summary of national survey of occupational therapy labour force 1981. *Australian Occupational Therapy Journal*. 1983;30(4):161-164.
31. Freidson E. *Profession of Medicine: A Study of the Sociology of Applied Knowledge*. New York, NY: Harper and Row; 1970.
32. Freidson E. Foreword. In: Gritzer G, Arluke A, eds. *The Making of Rehabilitation: A Political Economy of Medical Specialisation 1890-1980*. Berkeley, Calif: University of California Press; 1985:XIV-XV.
33. Gritzer G, Arluke A, eds. *The Making of Rehabilitation: A Political Economy of Medical Specialisation*

1890-1980. Berkeley, Calif: University of California Press; 1985:107-108,158.

34. Rothberg JS. Territorial imperatives and the boundaries of professional practice in rehabilitation. *Archives of Physical Medicine and Rehabilitation.* 1971;52:397-412.

35. Larson MS. *The Rise of Professionalism: A Sociological Analysis.* Berkeley, Calif: University of California; 1977.

36. Millerson G. *The Qualifying Associations: A Study in Professionalisation.* London, England: Routledge; 1964.

37. Johnson TJ. *Professions and Power.* London, England: Macmillan; 1972.

38. Berlant JL. *Profession and Monopoly: A Study of Medicine in the United States and Great Britain.* Berkeley, Calif: University of California Press; 1975.

39. Goode W. Theoretical limits of professionalisation. In: Etzioni A, ed. *The Semiprofessional and Their Organisation.* New York, NY: The Free Press; 1969:266-313.

40. Griffin SD, Rapaich Z. A survey of occupational therapy as a professional group. Unpublished manuscript, School of Occupational Therapy, Cumberland College of Health Sciences, Sydney, Australia, 1979. Cited in Griffin S. Conflicts in professional practice. *Australian Occupational Therapy Journal.* 1988;35(1):5-12.

41. Reilly M. 1961 Eleanor Clarke Slagle Lecture. Occupational therapy can be one of the great ideas of 20th century medicine. *American Journal of Occupational Therapy.* 1962;16:1-9.

42. Roberts CA. Healing the sick-responsibility or privilege—for the patient or the professional therapist. *Canadian Journal of Occupational Therapy.* 1962;29:5-14.

43. Barton G. Occupational therapy. *Trained Nurse Hospital Review.* 1915;54:138-140.

44. Swain LT, Taylor M. Occupational therapy for the orthopaedic patient crippled by chronic disease. *Occupational Therapy and Rehabilitation.* 1925;IV(3):171-175.

45. Canton EL. Psychology of occupational therapy. *Occupational Therapy and Rehabilitation.* 1923;2:347.

46. Wolfe RJ. *History of Occupational Therapy 1800-1920.* Lecture notes. University of Southern California; 1979.

47. Fidler GS. From crafts to competence. *American Journal of Occupational Therapy.* 1981;35:567-573.

48. Fidler GS. Psychological evaluation of occupational therapy activities. *American Journal of Occupational Therapy.* 1948;1:284-287.

49. Fidler GS. The activity laboratory: a structure for observing and assessing perceptual, integrative and behavioral strategies. In: Hemphill B, ed. *The Evaluation Process in Psychiatric Occupational Therapy.* Thorofare, NJ: Charles B Slack; 1982.

50. Fidler GS, Fidler JW. *Introduction to Psychiatric Occupational Therapy.* New York, NY: Macmillan; 1954.

51. Fidler GS, Fidler JW. *Occupational Therapy: A Communication Process in Psychiatry.* New York, NY: Macmillan; 1963.

52. Kielhofner G, Burke JP. Occupational therapy after 60 years. *American Journal of Occupational Therapy.* 1977;31(1):675-689.

53. Russell JI. *The Occupational Treatment of Mental Illness.* London, England: Bailliere, Tindall and Cox; 1938.

54. Jones MS. *An Approach to Occupational Therapy.* London, England: Butterworths; 1960:312.

55. Guillebaud CW. Foreword. In: Jones MS. *An Approach to Occupational Therapy.* London, England: Butterworths; 1960.

56. Krusen FK. History and development of physical medicine. In: Watkins AL, ed. *Physical Medicine in General Practice.* Philadelphia, Pa: JB Lippincott; 1946:5,8.

57. Cooke GR. The Arts and Craft Society of Queensland, part 2: whatever happened to it? *Craft Australia.* 1986;Summer:73-76.

58. Brintnell ES, Cardwell MT, Robinson IM, Madill HM. The fifties and sixties: the rehabilitation era: friend or foe. *Canadian Journal of Occupational Therapy.* 1986;53:27-28.

59. Piersol GM. Editorial, the doctor shortage in physical medicine. *American Journal of Physical Medicine.* 1956;35(8).

60. Rusk HA. Tomorrow is not yesterday. *Archives of Physical Medicine and Rehabilitation.* 1966;47(5).

61. Kubie L. *The Riggs Story.* New York, NY: Hoebart Press; 1960.

62. Kielhofner G. *Health Through Occupation: Theory and Practice in Occupational Therapy.* Philadelphia, Pa: FA Davis Co; 1983:36,191.

63. Fidler G. Some unique contributions of occupational therapy in treatment of the schizophrenic. *American Journal of Occupational Therapy.* 1958;12(9):36.

64. Dargan F. Taking stock. *Bulletin.* 1955;July.

65. Thornton G, Rennie H. Activities of daily living: an area of occupational therapy expertise. *Australian*

Occupational Therapy Journal. 1988;35(2):49-58.

66. Frankfurt H. Freedom of will and the concept of a person. *Journal of Philosophy*. 1971;67(1):5-20.

67. Bennett J. *Linguistic Behavior*. New York, NY: Cambridge University Press; 1976:Chapter 3.

68. Taylor C. *Human Agency and Language*. Philosophical papers, series I. New York, NY: Cambridge University Press; 1985:13-114.

69. Tucker RC, ed. *The Marx-Engels Reader*. 2nd ed. New York, NY: Norton; 1978.

70. Rousseau JJ. Discourse on the origin of inequity. Cole GDH, trans. London, England: Dent; 1968.

71. Horkheimer M. Kritische Theorie (1968). Translated in O'Connell MJ. *Critical Theory: Selected Essays*. New York, NY: Harder and Harder; 1972.

72. Marcuse H. *Eros and Cvilisation*. London, England: Sphere Books; 1969.

73. Habermas J. *Knowledge and Human Interests*. McCarthy T, trans. Boston, Mass: Beacon Press; 1973.

74. Fay B. *Critical Social Science: Liberation and Its Limits*. Ithaca, NY: Cornell University Press; 1987:53,57.

75. Lerner M. *America as a Civilisation*. New York, NY: Simon and Schuster 1957.

76. Fromm E. *The Fear of Freedom*. London, England: Routledge; 1960.

77. Solomon P, et al. *Sensory Deprivation*. Cambridge, Mass: Harvard University Press; 1961.

78. Reilly M. The challenge of the future to an occupational therapist. *American Journal of Occupational Therapy*. 1966;20:221-225.

79. Reilly M. The modernisation of occupational therapy. *American Journal of Occupational Therapy*. 1971;25:243-246.

80. Reilly M. A response to: defining occupational therapy: the meaning of therapy and the virtues of occupation. *American Journal of Occupational Therapy*. 1977;31(10):673.

81. Laukaran VH. Toward a model of occupational therapy for community health. *American Journal of Occupational Therapy*. 1977;31:71.

82. Reilly M. The education process. *American Journal of Occupational Therapy*. 1969;23:299-307.

83. Reilly M. *Play as Exploratory Learning*. Beverly Hills, Calif: Sage Publications; 1974.

84. Van Deusen J. Mary Reilly. In: Miller BRJ, Sieg KW, Ludwig FM, Shortridge SD, Van Deusen J. *Six Perspectives on Theory for the Practice of Occupational Therapy*. Rockville, Md: Aspen Publications; 1988.

85. Kielhofner G, Burke JP. A model of human occupation. Part 1, conceptual framework and content. *American Journal of Occupational Therapy*. 1980;34:572-581.

86. Kielhofner G. General systems theory: implications for theory and action in occupational therapy. *American Journal of Occupational Therapy*. 1978;32(10):637-645.

87. Kielhofner G, ed. *A Model of Human Occupation, Theory and Application*. Baltimore, Md: Williams and Wilkins; 1985.

88. Yerxa EJ, Clark F, Frank G, et al. An introduction to occupational science: a foundation for occupational therapy in the 21st century. *Occupational Therapy in Health Care*. 1989;6(4):3.

89. Clark FA, Parham D, Carlson ME, et al. Occupational science: academic innovation in the service of occupational therapy's future. *American Journal of Occupational Therapy*. 1991;45(4):300-310.

90. Yerxa EJ. Occupational science: a new source of power for participants in occupational therapy. *Journal of Occupational Science: Australia*. 1993;1(1):3-10.

91. Polatajko H. Muriel Driver Memorial Lecture. Naming and framing occupational therapy: a lecture dedicated to the life of Nancy B. *Canadian Journal of Occupational Therapy*. 1992;59:189-200.

92. Fossey E. The study of human occupations: implications for research in occupational therapy. *British Journal of Occupational Therapy*. 1992;55(4):148-152.

93. Mocellin G. An overview of occupational therapy in the context of the American influence on the profession. *British Journal of Occupational Therapy*. 1992;55(1):7-12 and 55(2):5-60.

94. Mosey AC. Partition of occupational science and occupational therapy. *American Journal of Occupational Therapy*. 1992;46(9):851-853.

95. Mosey AC. Partition of occupational science and occupational therapy: sorting out some issues. *American Journal of Occupational Therapy*. 1993;47(8):717-723.

96. Clark F, Zemke R, Frank G, Carlson M, Dunlea A. Further thoughts on the pitfalls of partition: a response to Mosey. *American Journal of Occupational Therapy*. 1995;49(1):73-81.

97. Nelson DL. Occupation: form and performance. *American Journal of Occupational Therapy*. 1988;42(10):633-641.

98. Cynkin S, Robinson AM. *Occupational Therapy and Activities Health: Toward Health Through Activities*. Boston, Mass: Little, Brown and Co; 1990.

99. Christiansen C, Baum C, eds. *Occupational Therapy: Overcoming Human Performance Deficits*. Thorofare, NJ: SLACK Inc; 1991.

100. Fidler GS, Fidler JW. Doing and becoming: purposeful action and self actualisation. *American Journal*

of Occupational Therapy. 1978;32:305-310.

101. Fidler GS. *Overview of Occupational Therapy in Mental Health.* Prepared by the American occupational therapy task group of the American Psychiatric Association on psychiatric therapies, 1981.

102. Mosey AC. *Psychosocial Components of Occupational Therapy.* New York, NY: Raven Press; 1986:6.

103. Moore JC. Behavior, bias and the limbic system. The 1975 Eleanor Clarke Slagle Lecture. *American Journal of Occupational Therapy.* 1976;30(1):11-19.

104. Llorens LA. The 1969 Eleanor Clarke Slagle Lecture. Facilitating growth and development: the promise of occupational therapy. *American Journal of Occupational Therapy.* 1970;XXIV(2):93-101.

105. do Rozario L. Purpose, place, pride and productivity: the unique personal and societal contribution of occupation and occupational therapy. Keynote address, *Australian Association of Occupational Therapists 17th Conference proceedings.* Darwin, 1993:51.

106. Townsend E. 1993 Muriel Driver Memorial Lecture. Occupational therapy's social vision. *Canadian Journal of Occupational Therapy.* 1993;60(4):174-183.

107. Gilfoyle EM. 1984 Eleanor Clarke Slagle Lecture. Transformation of a profession. *American Journal of Occupational Therapy.* 1984;38(9):575-584.

108. Schemm RL, Corcoran M, Koldner E, Schaff R. A curriculum based on systems theory. *American Journal of Occupational Therapy.* 1993;47(7):623-634.

109. Jensen H. What it means to get off sit down money: community development employment projects. *Journal of Occupational Science: Australia.* 1993;1(2):12-19.

110. Farnworth L. Women doing a man's job: female prison officers working in a male prison. *Australian and New Zealand Journal of Criminology.* 1992;25(3):278-296.

111. Pettifer S. How engagement in occupation other than paid employment influences the health and well-being of people who are long term unemployed. Master's degree in health science (occupational therapy), University of South Australia. Thesis in progress.

112. Farnworth L. An exploration of skill as an issue in employment and unemployment. *Journal of Occupational Science: Australia.* 1995;2(1):22-29.

113. MacKinnon J, Avison W, McCain G. Rheumatoid arthritis, occupational profiles and psychological adjustment. *Journal of Occupational Science: Australia.* 1994;1(4):3-10.

114. Stanley M. An investigation into the relationship between engagement in valued occupations and life satisfaction for elderly South Australians. *Journal of Occupational Science: Australia.* 1995;2(3):100-114.

115. Yerxa EJ, Locker SB. Quality of time used by adults with spinal cord injuries. *American Journal of Occupational Therapy.* 1990;4:318-326.

116. Pentland W, McColl MA, Harvey A, do Rozario L, Neimi I, Barker J. *The Relationship Between Time Use and Health, Well-Being, and Quality of Life: Multidisciplinary Research Meeting.* Kingston, Canada: Queens University; 1993.

117. Thomas K. *How Do Social Development Facilitators Encourage Ecological Sustainability?* University of South Australia. PhD thesis in progress.

118. Wood WH. *Environmental Influences upon the Relationship of Engagement in Occupation to Adaptation Among Native Chimpanzees.* University of Southern California, 1995. Doctoral thesis.

119. Article 1 of the constitution of the World Health Organisation (First) International Health Conference. New York, NY, June 19 to July 22, 1946. In: Commonwealth Department of Community Services and Health. *World Health Organisation: A Brief Summary of Its Work.* Canberra: Australian Government Publishing Service; 1988:3-10.

120. Henderson CLE. World Health. *British Journal of Occupational Therapy.* 1963;26(4):3-4.

121. Neville R. *Play Power.* London, England: Cape; 1970.

122. Roszak T. *The Making of a Counter Culture.* New York, NY: Doubleday; 1969.

123. Brown KM. Wellness: past visions, future roles. In: Cromwell FS, ed. *Sociocultural Implications in Treatment Planning in Occupational Therapy.* Haworth Press; 1987.

124. Johnson JA. *Wellness: A Context for Living.* Thorofare, NJ: SLACK Inc; 1986.

125. West W. The occupational therapists changing responsibilities to the community. *American Journal of Occupational Therapy.* 1967;21:312.

126. West W. The 1967 Eleanor Clarke Slagle Lecture. Professional responsibility in times of change. *American Journal of Occupational Therapy.* 1968;XXII(1):9-15.

127. West W. The emerging health model of occupational therapy practice. *Proceedings of the 5th International Congress of the WFOT,* Zurich, 1970.

128. Cromwell FS. Our challenges in the seventies. Occupational therapy today—tomorrow. *Proceedings of the 5th International Congress.* Zurich, 1970:232-238.

129. Wiemer RB. Some concepts of prevention as an aspect of community health: a foundation for development of the occupational therapists role. *American Journal of Occupational Therapy.* 1972;26(1):1-

9.

130. Finn GL. The 1971 Eleanor Clarke Slagle Lecture. The occupational therapist in prevention programs. *American Journal of Occupational Therapy.* 1972;26(2):59-66.

131. Finn GL. Update of Eleanor Clarke Slagle Lecture: the occupational therapist in prevention programs. *American Journal of Occupational Therapy.* 1977;31(10):658-659.

132. Mosey AC. Meeting health needs. *American Journal of Occupational Therapy.* 1973;27:14-17.

133. Grosman J. Preventive health care and community programming. *American Journal of Occupational Therapy.* 1977;31(6):351-354.

134. Class discussion in subjects "occupational science" and "health promotion for occupational therapists." Master's Degree in Health Science (Occupational Therapy), University of South Australia, 1992-1995.

135. Johnson J, Kielhofner G. Occupational therapy in the health care system of the future. In: Kielhofner G, ed. *Health Through Occupation: Theory and Practice in Occupational Therapy.* Philadelphia, Pa: FA Davis Co; 1983:191.

136. Johnson JA. Humanitarianism and accountability: a challenge for occupational therapy on its 60th anniversary. *American Journal of Occupational Therapy.* 1977;31(10):631-637.

137. Smith ME. Why research? Tales of the unexpected. *Australian Occupational Therapy Journal.* 1989;36(1):4-13.

138. American Association of Occupational Therapists. Position paper on the role of occupational therapy in promotion of health and prevention of disabilities. *American Journal of Occupational Therapy.* 1979;33:50-51.

139. Gilfoyle EM. The 1984 Eleanor Clarke Slagle Lecture. Transformation of a profession. *American Journal of Occupational Therapy.* 1984;38(9):575-584.

140. Dasler PJ. Deinstitutionalising the occupational therapist. In: Cromwell FS, ed. *Occupational Therapy in Health Care.* Vol 1. New York, NY: Haworth Press; 1984:31-40.

141. Sabari JS. Professional socialisation: implications for occupational therapy education. *American Journal of Occupational Therapy.* 1985;39(2):96-102.

142. MacKinnon JR. Current supply and future requirements for occupational therapy manpower in British Columbia. *Canadian Journal of Occupational Therapy.* 1985;52(5):251-257.

143. Stephenson L, Vanclay F. Deinstitutionalisation of occupational therapy and health care administrators knowledge. *Australian Occupational Therapy Journal.* 1989;36(4):193-199.

144. Brintnell ES, Madill HM, Wood PA. What do they think we do? OT functions as percieved by administrators and allied health professionals. *Canadian Journal of Occupational Therapy.* 1981;48(2):76-82.

145. Baum CM. Growth, renewal and challenge: an important era for occupational therapy. *American Journal of Occupational Therapy.* 1985;39(12):778-784.

146. Tiara ED. After treatment what? New roles for occupational therapists in the community. In: Cromwell FS, ed. *Occupational Therapy in Health Care.* Vol 2. New York, NY: Haworth Press; 1985:13-23.

147. Tompson M. Muriel Driver Memorial Lecture: ripples to tidal waves. *Canadian Journal of Occupational Therapy.* 1989;56(4):165-170.

148. Jackson B. Home based occupational therapy: then and now. *American Journal of Occupational Therapy.* 1992;36(1):84-85.

149. Richards S. Community occupational therapy: past dreams and new visions. *British Journal of Occupational Therapy.* 1992;55(7):257-259.

150. Townsend E. Developing comunity occupational therapy services in Canada. *Canadian Journal of Occupational Therapy.* 1988;55(2):69-74.

151. McColl M, Malcolm C. Community occupational therapists and volunteers: a survey of utilisation and satisfaction. *Canadian Journal of Occupational Therapy.* 1985;52:52-66.

152. Edwards J. National perspective: health promotion. An opportuniy for occupational therapy. *Canadian Journal of Occupational Therapy.* 1990;57(1):5-7.

153. Madill H, Townsend E, Schultz P. Implementing a health promotion strategy in occupational therapy education and practice. *Canadian Journal of Occupational Therapy.* 1989;56(2):67-72.

154. Burnett T. Occupational therapy in community health centres. *Proceedings of the 16th Federal Conference of the Australian Association of Occupational Therapists.* Adelaide, 1991.

155. Dean P. Occupational therapy in community health in South Australia. *S.A. A.O.T. State Conference Proceedings,* 1995.

156. Wicks A. Occupational harmony—the essence of well-being: a model for occupational therapy. *The Australian Association of Occupational Therapists 18th Federal and Inaugural Pacific Rim Conference Proceedings.* Hobart, Tasmania, 1995.

157. Dwyer P. Holistic health and politicisation in multicultural Australia in the 21st century. *The Australian Association of Occupational Therapists 18th Federal and Inaugural Pacific Rim Conference*

Proceedings. Hobart, Tasmania, 1995.

158. Twible R. Journeying to a new land of hope—a promise for our survival. Keynote address. *The Australian Association of Occupational Therapists 18th Federal and Inaugural Pacific Rim Conference Proceedings*. Hobart, Tasmania, 1995.

159. Adamson BJ, Sinclair-Legge G, Cusick A, Nordholm L. Attitudes, values and orientation to professional practice: a study of Australian occupational therapists. *British Journal of Occupational Therapy*. 1994;57(12):476-480.

160. Wilcock AA. Australian occupational therapists' views on health promotion: a national survey. Submitted to *Australian Occupational Therapy Journal*. 1997.

Suggested Reading

Bockhoven JS. Occupational therapy: a neglected source of community rehumanisation. In: *Moral Treatment in Community Mental Health*. New York, NY: Springer Publishing Co, Inc; 1972.

Christiansen C, Baum C, eds. *Occupational Therapy: Overcoming Human Performance Deficits*. Thorofare, NJ: SLACK Inc; 1991.

Fidler GS, Fidler JW. Doing and becoming: purposeful action and self actualisation. *American Journal of Occupational Therapy*. 1978;32:305-310.

Finn GL. The 1971 Eleanor Clarke Slagle Lecture. The occupational therapist in prevention programs. *American Journal of Occupational Therapy*. 1972;26(2):59-66.

Frank G. Opening feminist histories of occupational therapy. *American Journal of Occupational Therapy*. 1992;46(11):989-999.

Gilfoyle EM. 1984 Eleanor Clarke Slagle Lecture. Transformation of a profession. *American Journal of Occupational Therapy*. 1984;38(9):575-584.

Gritzer G, Arluke A, eds. *The Making of Rehabilitation: A Political Economy of Medical Specialisation 1890-1980*. Berkeley, Calif: University of California Press; 1985.

Jones MS. *An Approach to Occupational Therapy*. London, England: Butterworths; 1960.

Kielhofner G. *Health Through Occupation: Theory and Practice in Occupational Therapy*. Philadelphia, Pa: FA Davis Co; 1983:36,191.

Laukaran VH. Toward a model of occupational therapy for community health. *American Journal of Occupational Therapy*. 1977;31:71.

Llorens LA. The 1969 Eleanor Clarke Slagle Lecture. Facilitating growth and development: the promise of occupational therapy. *American Journal of Occupational Therapy*. 1970;XXIV(2):93-101.

Miller BRJ, Sieg KW, Ludwig FM, Shortridge SD, Van Deusen J. *Six Perspectives on Theory for the Practice of Occupational Therapy*. Rockville, Md: Aspen Publications; 1988.

Polatajko H. Muriel Driver Memorial Lecture. Naming and framing occupational therapy: a lecture dedicated to the life of Nancy B. *Canadian Journal of Occupational Therapy*. 1992;59:189-200.

Reilly M. 1961 Eleanor Clarke Slagle Lecture. Occupational therapy can be one of the great ideas of 20th century medicine. *American Journal of Occupational Therapy*. 1962;16:1-9.

Rousseau JJ. Discourse on the origin of inequity. Cole GDH, trans. London, England: Dent; 1968.

Shannon PD. The derailment of occupational therapy. *American Journal of Occupational Therapy*. 1977;31(4):229-234.

Townsend E. 1993 Muriel Driver Memorial Lecture. Occupational therapy's social vision. *Canadian Journal of Occupational Therapy*. 1993;60(4):174-183.

West W. The emerging health model of occupational therapy practice. *Proceedings of the 5th International Congress of the WFOT*, Zurich, 1970.

Yerxa EJ. 1966 Eleanor Clarke Slagle Lecture. Authentic occupational therapy. *American Journal of Occupational Therapy*. 1967;XXI(1):1-9.

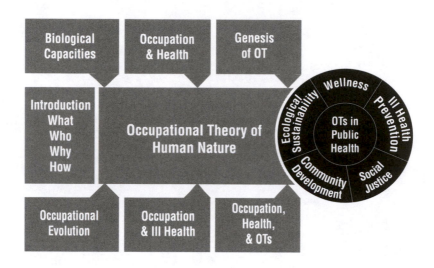

Chapter 9
Occupational Therapy and Public Health

This chapter presents the reader with ideas about:
- A potential role for occupational therapy in public health
- Examples that illustrate some of the potential
- An action-research approach to future practice in public health based on an occupational perspective of health
- Different approaches to health from an occupational perspective encompassing wellness, preventive medicine, social equity, community development, and ecological sustainability models
- A new synthesis of occupational therapy approaches compatible with the profession's philosophical and theoretical base
- Systematic and logical integration of the World Health Organization objectives and the "new public health" direction toward "health for all" into occupational therapy practice

This final chapter brings together the major ideas that have emerged from the explorations of humans as occupational beings; of occupational evolution; of the part occupation plays in ill health, health, and well-being; and of the theories, values, and skills that occupational therapists have to offer to promote health. It suggests that occupational therapists with a well-developed concept of the relationship between people's engagement in occupation and health are a primary source of expertise for research and for developing public health practice based on the relationship. Examples are given of existing programs provided by occupational therapists and suggest an action-research framework that, by extending their contribution to take in the broad notions about the relationship between occupation and health discussed in earlier chapters, can be used in many different models of health promotion. Five different models are considered in detail.

A Potential Role for Occupational Therapy

In Chapter 8, it was made clear that many occupational therapists consider their role to extend beyond the amelioration of illness to the promotion of optimal states of health in line with World Health Organization (WHO) philosophies and that they could play an important role in public health as it is currently conceived. However, if occupational therapists are to deliver the promise of the understanding of humans as occupational beings as part of the total picture of an evolving ecology, they should not conform to the present biases of public health as they have to conventional medicine. They must bring to public health their concept of the "occupational human" and be prepared to challenge and analyze public health research directions and strategies from this perspective. At present, because the distinct contribution occupational therapists could bring to health promotion is barely recognized by other public health workers, the understanding of the complex interaction between occupation and health is lost. Bockoven, a psychiatrist taking a multidisciplinary look at community mental health in the 1970s, considered that "acknowledgment of the critical moral importance of occupation in human life demands an in-depth review by the health professions of their own value judgments and practices with respect to identifying which are the means and which are the ends of our endeavors." He argued that occupational therapy is "a neglected source of community rehumanization" which was "blocked from perceiving either the depth or the breadth of its role as a moral and scientific force. This role has even more central importance to future human development than could possibly be claimed by any existing scientific specialty which neither has nor claims a moral basis." He considered that occupational therapists are the health professionals most skilled to advance this concept because they have "acquired a body of moral perspectives and occupational lore of unique value to society" which "can be more effectively utilized if it is not limited to being a service solely for sick people."[1]

The following examples from Australia and North America provide an indication of some recent programs offered by occupational therapists that address concerns of public health, but because they are little known about, are unacknowledged contributions:

- Until its closure, the Mount Lyell Copper Mine in Tasmania employed an occupational therapist full-time in occupational health and safety practice. Rudge provided education on health and safety for all levels of the workforce, ergonomic assessment and adaptation of heavy vehicles and mining equipment being used in geographically hostile environments, monitored work methods and practices of employees, and set up an on-site rehabilitation center. She reported challenges such as "a working environment knee deep in muddy, dark, noisy tunnels," "mastering mining terminology and technology," and "gaining an understanding of the implications of living in an isolated mining town."[2]

- In the New South Wales coal mining industry, Arvier and Bell provide a back injury management and prevention program and report an encouraging trend "in the types of clients attending back programs since the service first began...from miners with long-term or chronic injuries, through to uninjured workers who are anxious to learn something of back care."[3]

- Schwartz provided an industrial accident/injury primary prevention program for a group of 110 workers at a major Texas grocery distribution center, similar to traditional "back school" training, but based upon educational psychology principles. Workers and supervisors were trained in environmental modification, work simplification, and proper body mechanics in small groups at their actual work stations. Results of the program were positive, and the program has continued to expand into a comprehensive accident/injury prevention project within the company.[4]

- In contrast to these work-related programs, Deily describes the development and operation of a home safety program for older adults in Virginia. A disproportionately high number of older adults are involved in home accidents at considerable cost to individuals and the nation. The program provided education about ways to modify the environment or activities of daily living to lessen the risk of accidental injury, safety improvements for individual homes, and community education.[5] In South Australia, occupational therapists at the Noarlunga Community Health Service also played a major role in a recent state "prevention of falls in the elderly" program.

- In a more traditional health setting, Stout outlines an Automotive Safety for Children Program based at a children's hospital in Indianapolis, which meets the demands of federal and state legislation, as well as societal trends, for enabling the safe transportation of children with physical handicaps.[6]
- A parent-child activity group was introduced and developed by an occupational therapist as part of a community outreach program that focused on preschool children at risk for developing psychiatric disorders. The program was instituted collaboratively by a major teaching hospital and a local day care center in New York and used play and group process.[7]

These examples clearly illustrate scope for occupational therapists in preventive medicine to reduce work hazards from an occupational health and safety perspective, to retard the effects of disability, to work with clients and relatives to help reduce at-risk behaviors, and to enable practice of safe and satisfying activities, which may retard progression of disorders and early death.

Some occupational therapists also use community development approaches, particularly in socially disadvantaged countries. Kerry Thomas, a South Australian occupational therapist, for example, during a few years as regional training adviser for Southeast Asia, described an integrated rural development project in Pakistan in which she was responsible for training the local trainers and that included health care training, health education with school-aged children, agro-forestry, poultry rearing, vocational training, and marketing of local crafts, such as carpets. The process of community development was slow because the villagers were mostly illiterate and they needed to see the results of activities of people who were participating before many of them became enthusiastic. Training and education were practical, assisted by role plays, storytelling, and locally made pictures because of the low literacy skills.[8]

While this type of overseas program demonstrates the principles of community development in empowering local people toward self-reliance,[9] occupational therapists closer to home have been using the same principles and theories on a smaller scale. The following Australian examples demonstrate a range of such programs:

- Work with remote and rural Aboriginal communities, such as in the Top End of the Northern Territory, using community-based rehabilitation models, and with the Tjalku Warra community to improve conditions and promote independence, healthier lifestyles, and improved quality of life.[10-12]
- Planning and implementing a Community Integration Policy Project aimed at increasing access for disabled people to Melton Shire Council's programs, employment opportunities, decision-making processes, and physical facilities. The project progressed through analysis of all the Shire's functions, at all levels, and across all departments, staff development sessions, policy development, and implementation.[13]
- Participation in a Community Liaison Team at Manly Hospital "to assist raising the communities ideas about nursing homes, to support community groups, and to assist patients discharged from formal treatment to involve themselves in the community."[14]

- Design, development, and implementation of a quality-of-life project with the elderly for the Department of Veterans Affairs, Sydney, based on Nominal Group Technique.[15] Consumer participants (422 people from 11 locations over 6 weeks) identified issues that affected the quality of their everyday lives,[16] and the process empowered them to establish a "Getting Out and About Club."[17]

Communal "doing" for the common and individual good has always been part of human activity. In modern societies of the 20th century, this has become superseded by governmental initiatives that lack a genuine community base. Occupational therapists, as community development workers, use their philosophical beliefs by enabling people to recognize the needs of others as well as their own, and to take action, to do something, about meeting those needs more effectively. For example, Support, a group learning project, was conceived and designed by patients who completed a 24-hour occupational therapy stress management program offered at a community mental health day treatment center in New York. The patients had become a very close-knit group because of the nature and intensity of therapeutic activities. As they moved to ex-patient status and to a self-directed group they perceived a need to strengthen their community networks. They anticipated familial and community stressors and sought resources to provide knowledge and practice for themselves and their families in the management of those stressors.[18] Programs of this type extend occupational therapy into the sociopolitical arena.[17]

Action-Research Approach in Public Health

In the last quarter of the 20th century, public health has been defined by Last, who might be called a biographer of public health, as "the combination of sciences, skills, and beliefs that is directed to the maintenance and improvement of the health of all the people." He suggests that it is a "dynamic discipline," which has to be responsive to a "rapidly changing social and biological environment" where many factors set public health goals, such as the "historical and cultural context, available facts about perceived human need, social values, and scientific and technical capability to intervene effectively."[19]

For public health to accept the conceptualization of occupation as a powerful influence on health, it is necessary to suggest a direction that occupationally based public health can espouse. Articulation of this direction forms the main thrust of this chapter. I propose an action-research approach that grew from the exploration of ideas presented in this text, many of which already have a place in occupational therapy as demonstrated in the examples given above. However, this new synthesis extends these ideas and provides a more integrated view of occupational therapy as an important tool in public health practice. It requires therapists, among others, to re-assert occupation's fundamental role, to change their attitudes, to extend the domain of their concern to include all people (sick or well), and a commitment to action-research that is applied to groups, communities, and the global population, as well as individuals.

The starting point is a clear description of the key features and factors to be incorporated into this alternative approach to health promotion. These are:

- A balance of physical, mental, and social well-being attained through valued occupation
- Enhancement of species' common and individually unique capacities and potential

- Occupational and social support and justice for all people and communities
- Community cohesion through politically supported and socially valued, well-balanced, occupational opportunity
- Research and action aimed at enabling, mediating, and advocating for healthy public policy that is responsive to human needs rather than materialistic wants all within, and as part of, a sustainable ecology
- Health care aimed at the maintenance and enhancement of physical, psychological, spiritual, and social functioning of individuals and communities toward maximum potential and quality in everyday living, in interaction with the natural world that sustains all creatures, and in a way that ensures its healthy survival

These six points cover most of the five major directions of the Ottawa Charter, mentioned earlier, namely to develop personal skills, create supportive environments, strengthen community action, build healthy public policy, and reorient health services toward the pursuit of health.

I advocate an action-research approach in line with critical social science, which recognizes people as "participants in the sociohistorical development of human action and understanding."[20] Action-research aims at facilitating social change through self-reflective inquiry and consciousness raising which enlightens participants about equity and hegemony issues, collective sharing of critical self-reflections, dialogue, and questions, leading to collective planning and action.[21] Comstock suggests that such research includes "repeated movement" through several phases—the interpretive, the empirical-analytical, the critical-dialectical, and the practical-educational and political-action phases—in its progress toward increased understanding and social action.[20] This approach is suggested because critical social science has beliefs in common with my occupational perspective, specifically the assumption that "humans are active creatures" and that people shape both natural and social environments through their activity. Because people are largely unaware of themselves or their cultures as "the 'objects' they have created," their activity "is carried out in a disorganized and often self-defeating way," which can result in less than optimum conditions or opportunities.[22] To overcome the problems associated with this lack of awareness, it is essential to use approaches that raise consciousness, as well as provide support for reflection and informed action. Environments and health services can be shaped through participatory action-research. If occupational therapists adopted such an approach, it would enable the communities they worked with to create a way of life, in balance with the ecology, in which individuals as well as their communities would be able to meet their needs for occupational satisfaction, increased well-being, and health.

This action-research model espoused includes four interlinking phases:

1. Research
2. Awareness and education
3. Activism
4. Occupational change by individuals and communities as well as at socio-techno-political levels

These phases are never complete, each one leading to the next, but available to be revisited to check or alter as new evidence suggests new possibilities. The phases may be fleshed out as follows. The research phase centers on exploring issues about occupational deprivation, alienation, imbalance, meaning, capacities, potentials, balance, and satisfaction, at individual, community, national, global, and ecological levels, using quantitative or qualitative methodologies. The awareness and education phase involves a multilevel educational strategy to raise consciousness of this way of viewing health, technology, societies, and global activities. The phase of activism aims at gradual social change toward human occupation (on a global scale), which is in line with biological needs, social justice, intra-species flourishing, and a sustainable ecology. The final phase is occupational change through socio-techno-political response to the global and local needs of people as part of the natural world rather than materialistic and power-based wants.

The interlinking involves ongoing research and exploration to monitor the effects, to feed back into education, activism, socio-techno-political change, and so on in a continuous spiral. The components of the approach are not compartmentalized, and interaction between them is ongoing, reflective, and dynamic, in order to investigate and act according to multiple truths in a way that is flexible and able to anticipate needs or meet them as they occur and that can take corrective action when required. The research and awareness-raising phases will now be considered separately. The action and occupational change phases will be considered within the five models discussed later.

Research Phase

The research phase would use whatever methodologies are most suited to explore the question. Public health has always favored an epidemiological approach, and this remains an approach of choice for clinically based aspects of occupation studies. Such empirical studies can be used to inform the action-research participants, and the public at large, and can be used in combination with other types of exploration. Occupational scientists, in contrast to public health epidemiologists, have favored qualitative approaches in order to explore the complexities of humans as occupational beings, their experiences, and the individual meaning given to engagement in occupation.[23] This preference is strong because of the fear that reductionist study will remain predominant to the detriment of in-depth work on the complexities of people interacting with their environment (Yerxa, personal communication, 1990). Indeed, the preference for qualitative research has arisen because of concern that occupational therapists have been overly influenced by the positivistic assumption that "all true knowledge is scientific, in the sense of describing the coexistence and succession of observable phenomena"[24] and that philosophical and theoretical observations are only significant if they are constructed from empirical, preferably numerical, data. This has limited occupational therapists' research, in the past, to explorations, such as surveys or clinical trials in the medical science tradition; as a result, many questions of a holistic nature, important from the profession's philosophical foundations, remain unanswered. Qualitative approaches have the potential to answer some of these questions because they "extend traditional views of 'truth' to include multiple realities, values, and meanings" from participants' points of view. Data can be collected, for example, by interviews, storytelling, time-diaries, experience sampling, observation, documenting conversations, interactions and activities, focus groups, searching out, and reviewing records and written documentation,[25] all of which can "produce meaningful descriptions and interpretations of social processes," "offer explanations of how certain conditions came into existence and persist," and provide "the basis for realistic proposals" for improving social environments.[26,27]

In the proposed action-research approach, no one methodology is favored, rather, appropriate combinations of research methods would allow for the research to be exploratory, descriptive, or explanatory, and for analysis to be empirical, interpretative, or critical.[25] Qualitative researchers, particularly, recognize the complementary value of quantitative and qualitative approaches rather than their incompatibility. In combination, they can add rigor and breadth and provide a more complete picture than either approach used alone.[28-30] Different blends will lead to new ways of knowing about humans as occupational beings and will help to provide different perspectives of people's experience of engagement in occupation, of the organization, and balance of occupations in lifestyle throughout lifespan, and the relationship of each to adaptation, social expectations, life satisfaction, and health.[23] Extended methods of inquiry will enable the study of underlying factors that prompt people to do the things they do, day by day, often or occasionally, why different social groups and cultures use time differently, and whether current sociocultural structures and institutions are based on values that will enable humans to continue evolving in directions that are appropriate and necessary to the ecology and our species' survival and well-being.

While occupational science should provide the major research base of an occupational health promotion approach, it will need to draw upon the expanding knowledge of the medical, social, and behavioral sciences, as well as the natural and biological sciences. Human occupation crosses all boundaries from genetic codes, cellular system formation, biological capacity, and personal ideas, through family, community, social, and political domains to have effects upon the world ecology. Within all these domains, there is a need for research to begin to understand and influence occupation choices toward healthier bodies, minds, lifestyles, environments, and national and international policies.

Education-Awareness Phase

Findings from this diverse research need to be accessible to the public at large. In action-research terms, they must lead to an education-awareness phase, including approaches that promote healthy behavior and lifestyle by increasing understanding of how engagement in occupation can prevent illness and promote health and well-being, and demonstrate how political, social, and technological structures facilitate or inhibit achievement of occupational satisfaction and potential. Strategies that could be used to increase political, public, community, or individual awareness include social planning, which, in turn, includes problem-solving based on data gathering and goal setting; social action, such as rallies and boycotts, conferences, workshops, seminars, in-service training, health fairs, brochures, and circulars in libraries; and group discussion and individual counseling in community agencies, health centers, schools, and the workplace, as well as in routine health provider-consumer interactions.

Behavior modification or mass propaganda principles that provide information about healthy living, such as health warnings on cigarette packs, assume that at least some people accessing the information will adjust behaviors as a result of the message. The effects of such programs can usually only be expected in the long-term and are difficult to measure, and, indeed, there are some who would deny this as a health education approach. Green et al suggest that health education requires voluntary participation of the consumer[31]; and for individuals to change habitual patterns of behavior, this is probably the most effective approach. Unless information is specifically sought by people motivated to use it, learning, which is cumulative, can only occur after repeated exposure to an idea. However, in the case of increasing awareness about the relationship between occupation and health, it may be necessary to use mass propaganda approaches, because the basic relationship is so little understood. For example, awareness can be raised following mass media exposure of the ideas in topical programs, in documentaries, and as themes in soap operas, in much the same way as other health messages, such as about nutrition or abortion, have been conveyed to the public.

Occupational therapists are not skilled at accessing the media, in part because their health message is not understood in a society that values a medical science "illness" approach to health. Even for the film "Gorillas in the Mist," Dianne Fossey, originally an occupational therapist, was portrayed as a physiotherapist. If occupational therapists do take up the challenge of public health practice, they will need to develop advocacy and public relations skills to ensure that their health education messages are accessible. Alternatively, their public health partners, experienced in disseminating information, could become their advocates. In their traditional role, most occupational therapists are skilled in health education because of their daily work with many at-risk and disadvantaged individuals and groups. For example, one occupational therapy educational strategy to assist people with psychosocial dysfunction to change habit patterns includes invalidation of current patterns of behavior, exploration of alternatives "through thought and action," followed by habituation and integration over time of the chosen alternative behavior.[32]

Undergraduate occupational therapists are trained in individual and group education and teaching skills, but, like many other health professions, would not see their primary role as health counselors or even health educators. A greater emphasis on this aspect of practice is required. Jungfer, a general practitioner who pioneered an integrated health service in South Australia, believed that every member of the health care team "must seize every teachable moment to explain fully to the patient the part he must play in maintaining his health," because reinforcement from many sources facilitates increased awareness.[33] Increased awareness enables people to decide for themselves the most appropriate action to promote healthy living, to understand and define their own health problems and needs, and to understand what action they can take using their own resources.

Some occupational therapists already provide specific programs aimed at increasing awareness and educating about health matters. Jaffe, for example, describes the Medical Marketplace health promotion and health education program in the American corporate world in which an occupational therapist was the principal investigator. The project was federally funded research designed to assess the effectiveness of a health consumer education and training program on the reduction of health care costs. The training was intended to increase the knowledge and skills of employees, making them wise and informed consumers of health services, to improve the quality of health care by helping consumers find appropriate care more quickly and directly, and to reduce employee health costs by eliminating the use of unnecessary or inappropriate services.[34] In a more traditional context, Breen describes an approach developed for use with elderly people in a nursing home where the concept of self-help arising from traditional programs, which encouraged patients to assist themselves in their daily needs to prevent deterioration and to promote recovery, was expanded into a formal program of patient education in health-enhancing strategies.[35] Both of these examples demonstrate valid approaches that are in line with conventional health promotion ideologies. In contrast, Rosenfeld suggests an approach based on

Kielhofner's Model of Human Occupation, which uses "didactic presentation of important lifestyle concepts, self-reflection, goal identification, and concrete planning" and includes examination of "the doing process and the development of personal competence, ...life roles, the use of time, and four planes of existence (physical, emotional, intellectual, and spiritual)."[36] He suggests that illness or dysfunction, which disrupt life processes, facilitate an occupational shift because "disruption leads to a novel and clear recognition of intricate occupational patterns, places, and circumstances that weave the fabric of life."[37]

The education-awareness phase of this public health action-research model requires more than occupational therapists providing information and more than participants in any one group engaging in a change-growth experience, important though these may be. The exploratory phase of the approach should be contextual as well as individual, and this phase should be context-dependent. The education-awareness phase should link structuralism and individualism, broader social processes with the problems people face in their daily lives, occupational behaviors, meanings and health outcomes, and should be viewed as an agent of sociopolitical structural change that can empower and enhance individual awareness of optimum physiological functioning, role performance, and personal potential.[38-40] It should, for example, encompass the occupational determinants that can contribute to health and well-being discussed in Chapter 5 or contribute to the preclinical health disorders, and ultimately to disease, disability, or death, as discussed in Chapter 6.

The third action phase of the approach will vary according to the problem but will be based on "doing" and on developing techniques and strategies that may facilitate improved personal, community, national, and international occupational health.

Five models, which are not mutually exclusive, are discussed here. See Table 9-1 for an overview. The models are wellness, preventive medicine, social justice, community development, and ecological sustainability, which are defined in accordance with ideas expressed by a majority of works about each approach. The five approaches represent significant ideas that have emerged during 8 years of study. An overview of the differing ideologies of each reveals how they might be integrated and what direction an action-research approach could take from an occupational perspective. This method of dividing out differing aspects of services aiming at health promotion provides us with ways of seeing (understanding), organizing (setting objectives and deploying resources), and doing (research, strategies, and programs). All are important and need not be separated in practice.

Wellness Model

The wellness model (Figure 9-1) is the first to be considered because, theoretically, it fits most closely with occupational therapists' traditional orientation and could be used in practice in arenas, such as conventional medical environments, where many occupational therapists still work. In 1954, Halbert Dunn, a physician, conceptualized and defined wellness as "an integrated method of functioning which is oriented toward maximizing the potential of which the individual is capable within the environment where he is functioning."[41] This, plus other definitions, which include words such as "meaning, purpose, philosophy of living, a state of being, and holism" are clearly compatible with occupational therapy philosophy,[42-45] but the following definition by Hettler, from the University of Wisconsin, is highlighted because it is appropriate to an action-research approach and my occupational theory. Wellness is

	Base	Definition	Occupation: Research Direction	Occupation: Action Approach
Wellness	• Individual • Illness/wellness • Reductionist/holistic • Medical/social/ behavioral sciences • Person-centered	An active process through which individuals become aware of and make choices toward a more successful existence.	Health and occupational satisfaction, creativity, meaning, purpose, choice, opportunity, balance, challenges, growth, equity, freedom, potential	Disseminate research findings Individual counseling Personal skill development toward occupational potential
Preventive Medicine	• Populations/ individuals • Illness • Reductionist • Epidemiology/ behavioral/medical/ social science • Informative	The application of Western medicine and social science to prevent disease, prolong life, and promote health in the community through intercepting disease processes.	Underlying occupational determinants: alienation, deprivation, imbalance	Disseminate research findings Individual and group occupational counseling and programs Social and individual change of occupational structures
Community Development	• Communities • Well-being • Holistic • Social/political science • Self-sustaining • Local resources • Person-centered • Participatory	Community consultation, deliberation, and action to promote individual, family, and community-wide responsibility for self-sustaining development, health, and well-being.	Participatory analysis of community occupational structure, local resources, community views on positive and negative occupational determinants	Disseminate research findings Facilitate occupational change and growth of community Development of community according to their perceived needs and using local resources
Social Justice	• Groups/communities • Inequities=ill health • Holistic • Social/political science • Person-centered • Participatory	Promotion of social and economic change to increase individual, community, and political awareness, resources, and equitable opportunities for health.	Participatory analysis of occupational disadvantage, underlying occupational determinants, and uncovering occupational injustice	Disseminate research findings Facilitate social action for change of occupational policies toward occupational equity and justice Social and political lobbying
Ecological Sustainability	• Global • Species' well-being • Holistic • Biological/natural sciences • Self-sustaining	Promotion of healthy relationships between humans, other living organisms, their environments, habits, and modes of life.	Effect of occupational factors including technology and economic structures on the ecology (locally and globally), alternative occupational constructs which allow for occupational nature of people and needs of all species	Disseminate research findings Facilitate social action for change toward sustainable occupational constructs of benefit to all species and occupational health of people

Table 9-1. Overview of Health Promotion Models.

"an active process through which individuals become aware of and make choices toward a more successful existence."[46]

According to Dossey, this health model assumes that every individual has innate capacities for healing, nurture, self-reflection, taking risks, and for making change toward wellness; that all people are searching for answers about the life process, meaning, and purpose; and that health is also about individuals being able to live according to their beliefs.[43] Wellness embraces a multidimensional concept of balance, referring to work, play, and rest; to nutritional balance; to balance between use of

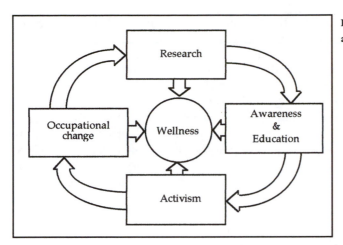

Figure 9-1. An action-research approach to wellness.

physical, psychological, intellectual, and spiritual capacities; as well as within self, environment, and culture.[47] The health model is seen by some as synonymous with health promotion and ill health prevention, especially in America where it has become a preferred approach at many industrial, business, and corporate work sites,[48-51] where programs aimed at preventing illness and at-risk behaviors are the most often described. Indeed, in this context, Opatz has defined health promotion as: "Systematic efforts by an organization to enhance the wellness of its members through education, behavior change, and cultural support."[52] Its acceptance in the corporate sector reflects the strong self-responsibility, individualist approach in American society. A different view suggests that this approach requires careful monitoring as too much emphasis on self-responsibility can lead to victim blaming, which may be unfounded in the light of epidemiological data that points to environmental and social conditions as major contributors to ill health. As Antonovsky argues:

> *...It is disingenuous to, however, to talk about getting enough sleep while disregarding the economic pressures on tens of millions of people, which compel them to moonlight or work extra shifts; to talk about eating well but say nothing of the powerful advertising industry; to talk of not smoking and drinking moderately yet be blind to to the manifold social stressors that lead people to use smoking and drinking as maladaptive coping responses.*[53]

European approaches, in contrast to American, emphasize union-initiated structural and legislative changes to work site health issues. According to a survey of 11,000 new members of 12 trade unions in the United Kingdom, along with better pay, improved health, and safety, equity and social justice were most often reported by members as what they wanted from union membership.[54]

In Australia, wellness is not recognized in public health circles as a serious model. Rather, it is viewed as a trendy concept, peripheral to medicine, that displays an encouraging indication of a change in public attitude toward health concerns. This reflects the conservatism of the health care system, in some ways as a result of the dominance of the Australian Medical Association in health matters. Individualized health promotion strategies are, on the whole, left to the private sector and alternative health providers. This peripheralizing of wellness maintains the dominance of an illness approach to individual health within conventional medicine and, once more, a health value that is in accord with occupational therapy is trivialized.

In the light of the complex, interactive nature of the relationship between occupation and health, it can be questioned whether an individual wellness approach has any value. I believe it can offer a useful starting point to increase awareness of individual needs and potential and how underlying influences affect health, particularly if research and action consider the context as well as the individual. Additionally, because the wellness model follows the tradition of the growth ideologies discussed earlier, it is an approach suited to all people, including those who are handicapped, disabled, and disadvantaged; person-centered rehabilitation programs and wellness approaches all aim at self-esteem, performance, roles, and quality-of-life skills to promote personal growth and well-being. It is, however, "essential to look below the surface signs to address real needs," Ryan and Travis argue, because "a person can be living a process of wellness and yet be physically handicapped, aged, scared in the face of challenge, in pain, imperfect...Diseases and symptoms are not really the problem. They are actually the body-mind's attempt to solve a problem."[55] Dossey explains that "when people are under varying degrees of stress or illness, they can lose their appreciation for life's purpose and meaning. It is at these times that the practitioner facilitates the journey toward understanding the wellness process."[43] This suggests that the wellness model may be a useful adjunct to conventional medicine,[56] to counteract the trend toward increasingly restricted acute care with a focus on high technology, which is expensive and expects a passive, rather than participatory, attitude from consumers.

Rehabilitation concerned with clients' personal skill development and aimed at maximizing potential and quality of life, which was an extension of conventional medicine, has declined in importance over the past 20 years to a token service. Now, occupational therapy in conventional medicine is being reduced as bed turnover increases and resources are stretched to cover other more acute and technologically sophisticated specialties. Even in 1966, Reilly recognized that it was becoming harder for occupational therapists to "advocate for patients to practice a healthy balance of work, rest, and play within the OT clinic, the institution as a whole, and eventually within the larger community environment,"[57] and Spencer suggested that the challenge of the 1980s was the transition of occupational therapy from hospitals to community.[58] In the clinic, occupational therapy interventions are becoming limited to formalized and predetermined assessment rather than life skill development and, increasingly, use compensatory and counseling approaches rather than facilitatory remedial approaches, which take longer. The types of program that are gradually being axed include evaluation of people's capacities, values, and occupational performance skills; health education relating to occupational balance; symptom reduction through engagement in occupation; retraining in the context of occupations of daily living; environmental modification; self-management; relaxation; stress management; and work simplification.

Limitation of practice occurs even in community agencies that conform to a conventional medical model, such as the regional Domiciliary Care Services in South Australia, which aim to assist people with long-term disabilities, regardless of age, at risk of premature or inappropriate admission to institutions. Limited resources for large numbers of referrals mean that occupational therapists have experienced difficulty in being able to practically implement their beliefs in health rather than ill health approaches. Domiciliary care service guidelines establish a clear focus on primary care and rehabilitation, but study undertaken in South Australia as early as 1987 revealed that, although 80% of the occupational therapists surveyed expressed a belief

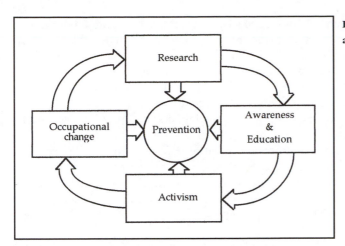

Figure 9-2. An action-research approach to prevention.

that domiciliary care provides an appropriate base for health promotion programs, which they were keen to offer, only 9% of occupational therapists were able to provide this type of intervention.[59]

Given these concerns, it is important to consider what direction the proposed action-research approach could take, if public health supported occupational therapy wellness programs. Research, education, and action for this approach could aim at the positive influences on well-being and occupational indicators of health status as shown in Figure 5-1. Other possibilities include:

- Exploration of attitudes and practice of health workers in hospitals, of health planners, of state and federal health bodies, of the public, and of consumers, with subsequent awareness-raising, action, and change
- Evaluation of the effects of focusing on illness, in the short-term, at the expense of long-term wellness using, for example, longitudinal clinical outcome studies of people with disability who experience wellness, growth, and increased potential programs against controls who do not
- Exploration of the degree of occupational wellness (balance, satisfaction, opportunity, self-actualization, etc.) experienced by accident victims, "fat file" patients, or outpatient attenders, followed by public education and action, such as the introduction of wellness groups in hospital wards or in general medical practice or community centers
- Possibly most important, programs aimed at discovering and enhancing the occupational potential of children according to their genetic strengths, while enabling them to recognize the links between what they do, how they feel, and the effects on social and ecological environments[60,61]

Preventive Medicine

The second model to be discussed, preventive medicine (Figure 9-2), is the most closely linked to public health, both historically and at present. Based on a wide variety of preventive medicine literature, I define it as "the application of Western medical and social science to prevent disease, prolong life, and promote health in the community through intercepting disease processes."

Like conventional medicine, it is a reductionist, illness model aimed at individuals, although it often uses population-based studies as a foundation for its approaches, which aim at protection against disease agents by methods such as immunization, vaccination, screening, and social and environmental engineering. It emphasizes early diagnosis with consequent retardation of disability and focuses on preventing illness rather than promoting wellness, although, as stated earlier, it is viewed by many (I believe, erroneously) as equivalent to health promotion. Last, for example, writes of the need for "...more effective health promotion programs aimed at smoking cessation, reduced alcohol use, nutrition, exercise, stress reduction, and control of violent behaviour..."[19]

Prevention of ill health through epidemiological research aimed at "early preclinical factors" (a medical science approach to public health) remains the strongest influence and attracts the most resources, despite a stated commitment to social health. An example of this commitment is provided in the Australian Commonwealth Department of Community Services and Health's brief summary of WHO's work, which states, at Clause 24, that:

> *In addition to the availability of suitable health services at a cost the country can afford, it (health for all by the year 2000) also means a personal state of well-being and a state of health that enables each person to lead a socially and economically productive life. Therefore, member states will continue to consider obstacles to health such as ignorance, malnutrition, poor housing, unemployment, and contaminated drinking water just as important as other considerations such as the lack of nurses and doctors, drugs, vaccines, or hospital beds.*[62]

Preventive medicine's strong commitment to epidemiology is demonstrated by Last's assertion that although the needs of public health workers, such as health educators, industrial hygienists, and sanitary engineers are different, all "share a common reliance on one scientific discipline, epidemiology." The most fundamental purpose of epidemiology, he says, is to "supply information, and ways to interpret it, for the diagnosis and measurement of the health problems of the population."[19] While occupational therapists do not focus on developing epidemiological research skills at the undergraduate level, they could focus intervention on epidemiological evidence provided by other researchers. However, the interventions should be interpreted and extended according to an occupational perspective. For example, substance abuse habits could be considered alongside occupational behavior, the negative effects of occupational deprivation, and the underlying determinants that lead to the deprivation. To do this, occupational therapists may use other research tools of a qualitative nature as adjuncts to epidemiology, just as public health workers interested in social health have done.

In order to realize the implications of the ideas raised in this text, it will be necessary to challenge many ideas that are central to political, social, and health ideologies. This is particularly so because in post-industrial societies with an economic-technological-power focus, rather than one aimed primarily at meeting the needs of humans in a way that recognizes ecological strengths and constraints, highly technical, illness-based health services are fostered and applauded. This type of service encourages people to continue stressful, regulated, time-dictated, and unnatural lifestyles because it offers to undo many of the obvious effects of consumer societies with spare parts and chemical remedies; it is essentially antidotal. The whole societal configuration inhibits, by default, the establishment of alternative systems that may help prevent illness. This implies that the theoretical foundations of this action-research approach

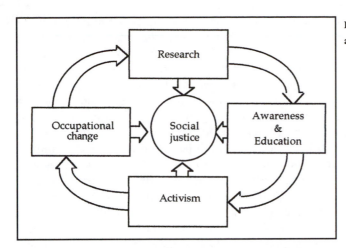

Figure 9-3. An action-research approach to social justice.

must address structural as well as individual prevention issues.

Occupational therapists have a surprisingly long history of interest in prevention, although many will be unaware that as early as 1934, in Canada, it was being recognized that occupational therapists had a potential role in the community in preventing ill health. At that time, Le Vesconte suggested that, in combination with social workers, occupational therapists should be involved in social and economic reorganization to that end.[63,64] Unfortunately, this direction got lost in medicalization of professional offerings and did not re-emerge until about the time of West's 1969 paper "The Growing Importance of Prevention." This introduced occupational therapists to the concept of involvement in primary and secondary prevention, to prevent the occurrence and progression of disease or injury, and to not being limited to working at a tertiary prevention level to minimize and reduce disability.[65]

Examples of the types of programs occupational therapists already offer were provided at the start of the chapter. The proposed occupational therapy action-research approach to prevention would extend contributions such as those, aiming at occupational institutions and activities such as division of labor, technology in daily living, and legislation that lead to "risk factors impinging on the individual" such as "lack of opportunity to develop potential," occupational imbalance, deprivation, and alienation as well as "early, preclinical health disorders" such as boredom, burnout, or sleep disturbance as shown in Figure 6-1. This may well include helping individuals to identify occupational factors that lead to:

- Stress, drug abuse, child abuse, women in transition, or other crises
- Practical and effective parenting
- Developmental screening
- Youth activities
- Elder citizens' activity groups and social clubs

Social Justice

The social justice model of health (Figure 9-3) is a participatory, community model that, in light of the literature, I define as the "promotion of social and economic change to increase individual, community, and political awareness, resources, and equitable opportunities for health."

Social justice is based on the belief that ill health is often an outcome of inequitable distribution of resources and power, resulting from factors such as the type of economy, national priorities and policies, and cultural values. It aims to change those underlying determinants of ill health.[66-69] In the Alma Ata and Ottawa Charter documents, social justice surfaces as one of the fundamental prerequisites of health. Both claim that for "health for all by the year 2000" it is essential to "close the gap between the 'haves' and 'have nots'" and to achieve "more equitable distribution of health resources within and among countries, including preferential allocation to those in greatest social need so that the health system adequately covers all the population."[70]

The relationship between social justice and health has been the subject of numerous investigations. In one of the most notable, Hart found that in the United Kingdom, the availability of good medical care tends to vary inversely with the need of the population served, and in areas where there is the greatest proportion of illness and death, both general practitioners and hospitals have the largest caseloads and the fewest resources.[71] A little later, *The Black Report* on "Inequalities in Health" in Britain gave an account of the inverse relation between health status and social location and called for a radical overhaul of health service activities and resources.[72] Similarly, in Australia, Broadhead found, in an investigation in which occupation, education, and affluence were used as variables of social status, that the four indicators of morbidity—recent illnesses, chronic conditions, days of reduced activity, and mental health—showed significant relationships to affluence for both sexes, after standardization for age.[73] According to Opit, in 1983, approximately 15% of the Australian population suffered from poverty and from lack of autonomy or power, with subsequent anxiety, depression, risk-taking, injudicious alcohol consumption, and premature death, all exacerbated by the inability to take advantage of the limited resources committed to their welfare. Those suffering most were Aboriginals, many single parents, the unemployed, large families with a single wage earner, the elderly, and many recent migrants, and the degree of deprivation and the numbers were increasing.[74] The rhetorical commitment to social justice and egalitarianism in most liberal economies cannot be achieved without structural change and "there is no sign that any Western democracy has the political will to make the massive redistribution involved in recommendations such as those of *The Black Report.*"[69]

In the interests of understanding the relationship between health and social justice, Gallagher and Ferrante call for a critical analysis of the cultural processes that shape both the medical care system and the broad social concern with medical care, because standard rehearsals of equity, in the liberal tradition, ignore the underlying determinants and processes of health experiences and the extent to which they arise from factors beyond individual control.[75-77] In terms of societal preconditions for need satisfaction, Doyal and Gough have identified civil and political rights, the right of access to "need satisfiers," and political participation. In occupational terms, underlying factors, such as the type of economy, national priorities and policies, and societal values as determinants of health status, have been identified. The action-research approach would focus debate on the underlying occupational factors, institutions, and activities that reduce occupational choice, satisfaction, balance, and meaning that prevent people from reaching their potential and that lead to the experience of occupational alienation and deprivation, early preclinical health disorders, disease, and disability.

Occupational therapists have an implicit concern with social justice as part of their philosophical base, but it has not been central in their documented approach to health promotion even though, from my own experience, more clients from socially disadvantaged groups than from affluent groups receive occupational therapy services. Townsend has suggested that occupational therapists need to become conscious of how "the social vision which forms the foundation of occupational therapy" is "narrowed to comply with dominant community, managerial, and medical approaches to disability and aging." She advances the idea that "enabling people to participate as valued members of society despite diverse or limited potential" is central within the vision.[78] According to Hodges, action toward social justice for, and with, the disabled does not occur.[79] Health promoting and risk notification programs "need to be capable of affirmatively motivating and empowering [them] to make appropriate, constructive responses" in order to protect the health of the disabled and pursue "their justified legal remedies."[80] These are obvious starting points for occupational therapists to become involved in social justice issues, to promote change to environments as well as people, and to influence the development of person-centered policies and laws.[78] Another direction involves being more responsive to "the concept of illness as a condition of the total human being, including the spiritual dimension." This would enable therapists to work "with conditions within the patients' primary systems...to bring about changes in conditions that are detrimental to health (such as poor living conditions, inadequate infant nutrition, or nuclear proliferation)." Johnson proposes the setting up of laboratories in which "patients acquire skills they need to influence change in their environments."[44] Such a laboratory could be envisaged as part of critical action and is in line with the action-research approach.

From an occupational point of view, interventions designed to approach social justice might involve developing community awareness about inequities in occupational opportunities through the use of social action involving community groups and the media, along with providing individual and community laboratories to practice relevant skills that lead to political lobbying for structural change. An example of how increasing community awareness can lead to social action comes from Kinnell's account of how rising levels of literacy, which resulted from the increased emphasis on education in England during the late 18th and early 19th centuries, fostered the growth of trade in children's books. Because the books dealt increasingly with themes such as the right to exercise individual moral judgment and social justice, this development was instrumental in disseminating radical ideas and raising the level of people's political consciousness and dissent.[81] This example suggests that information about occupational justice and health, packaged in an attractive and consumer-oriented manner, perhaps using the Internet or popular magazines, might be one way to approach consciousness raising on a population scale.

An occupationally just society would be one that provided opportunity for people to develop their own potential, rather than be expected to fit into socioeconomically established roles. Many people are straitjacketed into roles set by their communities—for example, there is enormous pressure on adolescents and even young children to do well at school in a restricted range of subjects to be fitted for particular jobs or to go to college. In many instances, a child's particular talents are set aside in the interests of potential material reward and educational and societal expectations. This scenario is not surprising within basic national frameworks characterized by "economic division of labor organized for private profit rather than human need"; a gender-based division of occupation "that separates privatized child rearing from recognized and remunerated work"; "paid labor markets that generate a marginalized underclass"; and a globalized international political economy that increasingly subjugates its poor-

Figure 9-4. An action-research approach to community development.

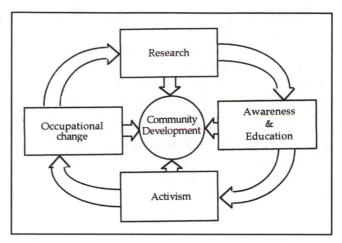

est workers and must then "engage in crisis management in the form of segmented social welfare concessions."[82,83] In addition, legislative changes that reduce risks, individuality, and experimentation also reduce occupational opportunity and satisfaction and can lead to occupational alienation, deprivation, and imbalance. Even social justice and equity models are, on the whole, biased toward current social, economic, educational, and health opportunities, which can lead to reduced occupational choice. Social justice approaches require expansion to encompass egalitarian ideas about individual and community uniqueness, and occupational therapists could take up this particular aspect of social justice.

Community Development

Community development is the fourth model (Figure 9-4) to be considered. From definitions, descriptions, and views found in community development literature, I define it as "community consultation, deliberation, and action to promote individual, family, and community-wide responsibility for self-sustaining development, health, and well-being."

It is a holistic, participatory model, aimed at facilitating a community's social and economic development, based on community analysis, use of local resources, and self-sustaining programs. It was widely used in African and Asian colonial administrations after World War II to stimulate local leadership and, later, in rural programs aimed at mass literacy and education.[84] In the 1960s, in the United States and the United Kingdom, community development strategies were adopted for use in socially disadvantaged urban areas to stimulate self-help and innovative solutions that were cost-efficient.[85,86] (In the United States, community development became national policy under Title II of the Economic Opportunity Act of 1964.)

Similarly, the move toward more community-based health care in Australia can be seen as a response aimed at the social and environmental origins of much ill health and, also, at meeting the growing interest in health issues by large sections of the community. In the 1970s, Australia introduced a Community Health Program that offered a framework for funding public and private group projects for community-based preventive, diagnostic, therapeutic, and rehabilitation services based in local centers and complemented by home care, day care, health education, mental health, and alcohol and drug abuse programs.[87] This resulted in a great variety of community-based services, some, like domiciliary care, with traditional health values, and others that tended to challenge vigorously conventional health ideologies, as some women's health groups did. Perhaps because of these wide-ranging community initiatives, it is common to confuse "health services based in the community" with "community development."

Health services in the community can adopt a community development approach by encouraging community consultation as the basis of the service and by being responsive to underlying social factors that affect health in the long-term. Such an approach is a means of enabling all people to become involved in planning, implementing, questioning, and changing circumstances within their own communities so that they are economically and socially advantaged. This, it is believed, leads to improved health and to improved community health care provisions. For this reason, the strengthening of community action is one of the five strategies for health promotion prescribed in the Ottawa Charter, which "accepts the community as the essential voice in matters of its health, living conditions, and well-being" and asserts that "empowerment of communities, their ownership, and control of their own endeavors and destinies" are "at the heart" of the community development process.[88] It is often the restrictions imposed by government funding bodies that inhibit the use of community development approaches and maintain a "top down" delivery of services.

Initiatives aimed at helping communities develop systems of primary health care that cater to their specific needs, use available resources, and are sustainable are used more commonly in economically disadvantaged countries with poorly developed health services than in post-industrial societies. Such programs may use various approaches, such as the prevention and control of diseases through immunization, the improvement of environmental conditions, the training of local health workers, and the development of skills to make most use of available resources for community growth. An example is provided by a reportedly very successful action-research project in two Egyptian villages, which took place between 1986 and 1990. Community members, and especially the women, learned to work within, and as part of, the organizational structure of their local government as they participated in the construction and improvement of local sanitation facilities. At the same time, they took part in health education concerned with the need for proper sanitation.[89]

Occupational therapists leading the profession in community development often work in programs similar to the one described above; an example is Thomas' work, outlined early in the chapter. Thomas, who has also worked in Ethiopia, Sudan, and Cambodia, as well as in community development programs with Aboriginal groups in Australia, promotes occupational therapy as "one of the best health-related bases" for entry into community development work, because its philosophy is compatible with "independence and self-reliance" and because of its "practical and functional approach," "broad-based training," and skills in "responsible problem-solving." However, she believes specialized post-graduate experience or training is required to enhance knowledge of community development processes and particularly to assist in analysis and mediation of political, economic, and social factors and consequences of interventions.[90]

One good starting point for more occupational therapists to use an action-research approach to community development is Community Based Rehabilitation, which is

Figure 9-5. An action-research approach to sustainable ecology.

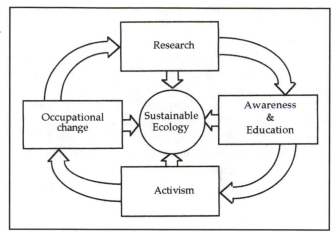

defined as "strategy within community development for the rehabilitation, equalization of opportunity and social integration of all people with disabilities." It is "implemented through the combined efforts of disabled people themselves, their families and communities, and the appropriate health, education, vocational, and social services."[91] The occupational perspective should be taken further, however, to include all people, not just those who are disabled. Opportunities for people differ from community to community. Exploration of the underlying reasons for these differences and how they impact on health and well-being needs to be undertaken using a community development, participatory approach. This is one of the most suitable approaches to increase awareness and promote action about the causes and effects of occupational alienation, deprivation, and imbalance, with the advantage of potential to also provide support and encouragement for the self-reliant, self-chosen occupation, which gives meaning, purpose, and social approval that, as earlier chapters demonstrated, are integral to health and well-being.

Ecological Sustainability

The last of the models to be considered is an ecological sustainability model of health (Figure 9-5). It is, perhaps, the least understood and the most vital in terms of the long-term health of all people. Aggregating several definitions, I define it as the "promotion of healthy relationships between humans, other living organisms, their environments, habits, and modes of life."

Based on biological and natural sciences, it, too, is an holistic model with much in common with social justice and community development.[92] Community development workers are recognizing the urgency of including ecological sustainability as part of just, people-centered initiatives.[93-97] For example, Atkinson and Vorratnchaiphan suggest that to redress the socioeconomic and ecological imbalance caused in Thailand by development evolving from European priorities, it is necessary to decentralize power and resources to local authorities and communities and for them to undertake action planning that focuses on improved management of the environment for the benefit of local people.[98]

The 1992 United Nations Conference in Rio de Janiero on Environment and Development focused world attention on the issue of ecological sustainability but, according to the sustainable development lobby, failed to consider adequately the necessary transformational changes.[99] The lobby argues that the policy prescriptions of a market industrial system based on economic rationalism are unable to deal with emerging world complexity and that that system will lead to a continuation of environmental degradation and an ever-widening gap between the "haves and the have nots."[100,101] Only 20% of humanity account for an estimated 75% to 80% of the human burden on earth's ecology, but enjoy its material rewards. The 20% of humanity who live in a state of absolute deprivation and the other 60% whose traditional lifestyles are disrupted by the promise of "economic growth" experience ongoing social and occupational injustice.

Indeed, "those who control accumulated financial credits seek out ecological stocks wherever environmental frontiers remain"[99] and effect the resubordination of countries that appear to be breaking through to developed status.[102] Such actions support the myth that human survival is an "economic and political science problem" that "assumes that man is free or could be free from the forces of nature."[92]

The alternative is a reduction of population growth, a restructuring of economic goals and societal values, reformation of resource policies to reflect community interests, a merging of the economic and biological in ecological decision-making, and changes to make human activity more sustainable.[92,101,103,104] Figures 9-6 and 9-7 illustrate the increasing problem of maintaining a sustainable ecology against global population growth, technological progress, and resource depletion. Curbing those three processes will require fundamental change to assumptions and values about wealth that are at the heart of business relationships.[105] The accumulation of monetary wealth is a major factor in alienating individuals from a sense of community and place, in the "homogenization of cultures and of unsustainability." Sustainability requires decentralization, which "distributes and roots economic power in place and community."[99]

Public health has long recognized that the health and well-being of people cannot be divorced from the environment. Its greatest triumphs were the identification and virtual eradication of some diseases that emanated from "sick environments." The sick environments were, on the whole, the result of human activity, the most obvious of which were the living and working conditions imposed by widespread industrialization, mentioned in earlier chapters. Improvement in these environments led to improved physical, mental, and social health. The ecological sustainability model, which is proactive as well as reactive, extends the public health approach from specific social environments to global, natural environments. New models for public health are emerging to address these concerns. Labonte, an international leader of the health promotion movement, for example, uses "econology" to describe a union between economy and ecology in theories which integrate health and sustainable development.[106,107]

Human occupation has been a primary force in ecological degradation and, therefore, requires urgent consideration and change aimed at ecological rehabilitation. Although occupational development served to protect people from the discomfort and unhealthy effects of natural phenomena,[108] people who live in cities and spend their days "doing" in the "technosphere of human creation"[109] have a loss of connection with ecological reality. For example, other animals and plants have become regarded and treated as if their only purpose were to serve humans. The widespread practices of replacing natural plants with exotics, hunting and fishing for sport rather than need, and the killing of any animal that dares to attack a human demonstrate

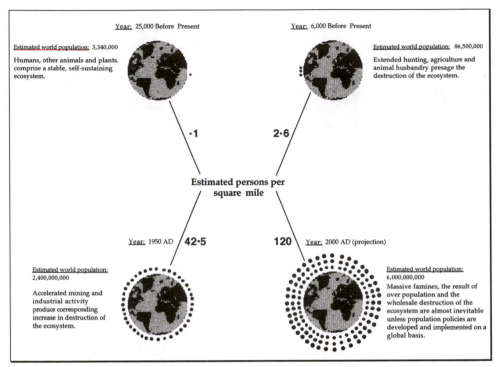

Figure 9-6. Human population growth throughout evolution. Adapted from Campbell BG. *Humankind Emerging.* **5th ed. New York, NY: Harper Collins Publishers; 1988:518-519.**

this propensity. In addition, the very successful public health initiatives that condemned animals as the carriers of disease, linked with the hygienic, "domesticity cult," separated humans still further from other species. It maintained the human superiority argument and gave permission for material wants to be considered more important than an ecological way of life in which all are dependent on each other. Darwinian theories failed to halt the segregation of people from other species, and even today, when researchers are demonstrating substantial health benefits of pets to humans, there remain many rules that restrict human-animal partnerships.[110-115] The philosophy of humanism is in question here. The drive to "rearrange both the world of Nature and the affairs of men and women so that human life will prosper," despite nature, is humanism gone awry.[108] Spiritual and occupational alienation, and consequent loss of well-being, are largely unrecognized sequelae. Many believe that, in the short-term, an ecological sustainability model is essential to decrease widespread spiritual alienation resulting from people's loss of contact with the natural world, which, it is supposed, may account for increasing levels of stress and violence, the use of drugs, and addictive responsiveness to marketing strategies.[116] In the long-term, an ecological sustainability model is also necessary to maintain the requirements for basic sustenance of life.

Loretta do Rozario, as a group leader in a Health Promotion Workshop (1990 World Federation of Occupational Therapists Congress), developed with her group the following ecological vision of occupational therapy:

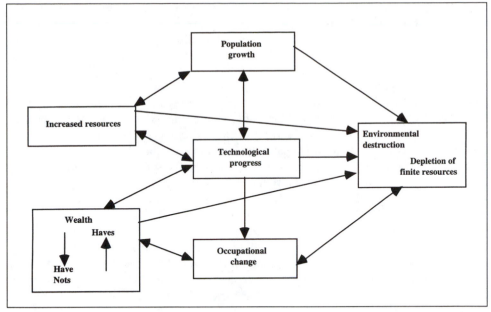

Figure 9-7. Interaction: population/technology/resources/wealth/occupation/the environment.

Occupational therapists will work towards the harmonious relationship of people with their environment, by empowering individuals and communities toward health, well-being, and sustainability through the use of interaction, occupation, and socio-political action.[117]

The occupational action-research approach should, as soon as possible, focus on how people can meet their creative potentials without damaging the environment, so that future health and well-being is ensured. Critical theorists could be potential allies in this process if they heed Bronner's call "to reconsider the notion of progress and human well-being."[118] Other research, education, and action would focus on discovering the natural balance of occupation in daily life, of the richness and wisdom of indigenous people with regard to occupation and the ecology, of natural ontogenetic timing of occupational drives and needs, and attributes of humanism, which include what promotes the health and potential of all species and environments.

Summary of Health Models

The five models discussed were chosen, in part, because different aspects of occupational health are demonstrated and, in part, because together they represent a holistic paradigm for health promotion practice. They also, in large measure, summarize the outcomes of the exploration undertaken in this history of ideas. Wellness is aimed at individual maintenance and improvement in health, including biological needs and physiological factors such as homeostasis, mental and spiritual growth toward potential, and self-actualization within socioculturally approved and supported mores. Individual patterns of occupation, occupational balance, satisfaction, creativity, choice, and opportunity to meet unique capacities and potential are important here. Preventive medicine is concerned with preventing people from experiencing negative health outcomes and with limiting risk factors that impinge upon the health of individuals and communities. Individual and community occupations and occupational institutions that erode health and lead to disability, disease, and death are central to this approach. Social justice approaches aspire to a more equitable experience of health, equitable access to conditions that are health giving, and to health services for all people. Occupational inequities and injustices prevail universally, affecting health outcomes negatively; action-research toward identifying and eradicating both inequities and injustice is required urgently. Community development approaches seek community health and well-being in a broad perspective that concentrates on sociocultural institutions and activities in conjunction with particular health strategies. Much of this approach is based on development of self-sustaining occupational infrastructures that will support community life so that its members experience increased and ongoing health and well-being. Ecological sustainability approaches strive toward the transformation of economic, political, sociocultural, and human values and actions to halt the destruction of the ecosystem so that the world and its interdependent life systems and organisms will survive healthily in the long-term. As the occupational nature of people is, in large part, to blame for the underlying factors that have led to the present unacceptable state of the ecology, the transformation of occupational behaviors, which meet both human and ecological needs, is essential.

A New Synthesis for Occupational Therapy

The action-research approach chosen corresponds with the philosophical tradition and directions of the founders of occupational therapy outlined in the 1917 objectives of the American National Society for the Promotion of Occupational Therapy. The exploratory-research phase is in tune with "the study of the effect of occupation upon the human being"; the education-awareness-raising phase is in accord with "the scientific dispensation of this knowledge"; and the action and community change phases have much in common with the notion of "the advancement of occupation as a therapeutic measure,"[119] if therapy is considered as "activity...intended to remedy or alleviate a disorder or undesirable condition."[120]

The major change necessary from current research in occupational therapy is to an emphasis on underlying sociocultural and ecological occupational issues and the use of critical research approaches, and from current practice is an emphasis on communities, occupational justice, and socioecological-political action. It is debatable whether occupational therapists will make such changes, although they have the philosophical persuasion and the potential to contribute a wide-ranging and holistic occupational perspective in the arena of public health. As Bockoven foresaw, if this occurs "the occupational service worker" will be "divorced from medicine" with a:

> *Base of growth outside the hospital. He will belong to the educational and economic life of the community, to which he will contribute a much-needed kind of knowledge, and in which he will be a force in fostering respect for occupations.*[1]

This expansion of role would recompense for the failure to act on the challenge posed to human's occupational natures by industry and capital at the time of the profession's genesis, as discussed in Chapter 7. I believe that failure to recognize the underlying factors that continue to influence the relationship between occupation and health and failure to accept responsibility for research and action in this domain would be negligent. However, there is a major problem. Occupational therapy continues to be largely unrecognized as a scientific discipline with a distinctive and important contribution to make to public health, and for it to articulate and follow a direction different from dominant paradigms implies that the profession has "to stick its neck out." A leading Australian social commentator suggests that although in current society there is a "need to encourage new ideas, dissident views, debates, and critics," those who argue have had "to speak the same language and work from similar sets of assumptions to those in power."[121] Does this mean that occupational therapists' different views will not be heard unless they modify them? What of making use of the Ottawa Charter's occupational directions? People listening to new ideas often only interpret from their own perspective. In the case of the Ottawa Charter, although it recognizes that health is inextricably bound up with what people do, it has been interpreted within public health from its own dominant paradigms, and the occupational elements have been largely disregarded. This leaves a major question as to whether public health will welcome or even recognize the potential contributions of occupational therapy's distinct and different viewpoint.

I started my research with a strong belief in a relationship between occupation and health and a conviction that occupational therapists could make a unique and valuable contribution to public health. However, it was not until after several years of study that I came to understand the relationship in terms of a theory of human nature and occupational therapists' potential contribution in the broad approach outlined here. Within the confines of my study, it was possible to explore only some of the more obvious connections and philosophical associations such a theory implies. These have, however, tested the theory in many directions and, in the main, supported its contentions.

A theory of human nature must consider the biological characteristics that all humans share. As well, because I was relating the theory to health and survival, it appeared wise to subject it to other notions about health and survival of a biological nature that have been subjected to rigorous study by scientists of many disciplines. For this reason, I explored ideas held by evolutionary scientists and geneticists and considered the theory in terms of neuroscientific understanding of human behavior. This furthered my belief that physiological systems support and promote occupational behavior to such an extent that the need "to do" is so natural, so much a part of being, that humans have failed to recognize it as an entity. Instead, they have reduced the holistic concept of occupation by dividing it and then made it more complex by endowing specific aspects with particular value.

The value and the division of occupation has altered with its evolution and because of cultural diversity, in part, because humans' occupational nature has immense variability, so that no two people have the same occupational potential or needs, and these are susceptible to and developed according to environmental demands. Despite the variability, it was possible to tease out four major functions of occupation, which form a three-way link with survival and health:

1. Provide for sustenance, self-care, and shelter
2. Safety from and superiority over predators and the environment
3. Balanced exercise of personal capacities
4. The enabling of individual development so that each person and the species will flourish

The variability between people and cultures made it important to subject cultural evolution to an occupational perspective: this reinforced a view held by many that human action (occupation) shapes culture and is, in turn, shaped by culture. People's potential for new and different pursuits, for exploring ways of making their lives easier and giving themselves time for chosen occupations, has led to a situation in which the products and results of human occupation appear to have assumed a greater importance than "natural" human need or the health and survival of the ecosystem on which humans depend.

An exploration of the history of ideas that surround health, well-being, and ill health was a natural extension of the issues and concerns arising from Chapters 2, 3, and 4. It uncovered underlying determinants that have resulted from humans' occupational natures, from the economic base of societies, the ways of structuring them, and the values that emanate from them. The institutions and activities resulting from these foundations and their effect upon the occupational experience of individuals and communities can lead to positive or negative health outcomes. Although some of these have been recognized by world and public health authorities, there is little action to promote the positive or inhibit the negative from an occupational perspective.

In an analysis of the foundation philosophies of occupational therapy and a review of its unique but repressed history, a picture emerges of a profession with particular strengths in conceptualizing humans from an occupational perspective. Not only that, they have other assets that have been represented in health promotion rhetoric as essential, such as a person-centered, enabling approach that considers environmental as well as physiological factors. In reviewing attitudes to a change of emphasis toward a health promotive approach, most therapists appear to be already committed in that direction. Yet, despite all this in their favor, community agencies are hesitant to employ them, and I know of no departments of public health with occupational therapists on their team.

Occupational therapists, while interested in health promotion, may not be willing to change direction to the extent of the approach suggested. It is possible that a modified or less extensive approach may be more appealing. However, I am convinced that the study of health, from this perspective, requires serious and immediate consideration, research, and action at individual, community, and environmental levels. Action-research developed from the same conceptual base as occupational therapy and is an obvious choice of methodology, alongside epidemiology, to explore the underlying determinants of health and ill health from an occupational perspective.

Dubos observed that humans are faced with a future in which "the biosphere of his inheritance, [and] the technosphere of his creation are out of balance, indeed potentially in deep conflict."[109] The debate about the conflict between nature and nurture remains critical. Occupation is central in both. This is a matter that will affect health scientists a long way into the future, but will not be solved if the occupational nature of humans is not considered.

References

1. Bockhoven JS. Occupational therapy: a neglected source of community rehumanization. In: *Moral Treatment in Community Mental Health.* New York, NY: Springer Publishing Co, Inc: 1972:219.
2. Rudge MA. Occupational therapy in the underground mining industry. *The Australian Association of Occupational Therapist's 15th Federal Conference.* Sydney, Australia; 1988.
3. Arvier R, Bell A. Back injury management and prevention in the New South Wales coal mining industry. *The Australian Association of Occupational Therapists 15th Federal Conference.* Sydney, Australia, 1988.
4. Schwartz RK. Cognition and learning in industrial accident injury prevention: an occupational therapy perspective. In: Johnson JA, Jaffe E, eds. Health promotive and preventive programs: models of occu-

pational therapy practice. *Occupational Therapy in Health Care*. 1989;6(1):67-85.

5. Deily J. Home safety program for older adults. In: Johnson JA, Jaffe E, eds. Health promotive and preventive programs: models of occupational therapy practice. *Occupational Therapy in Health Care*. 1989;6(1):113-124.

6. Stout JD. Occupational therapists' involvement in safe transportation for the handicapped. In: Johnson JA, Jaffe E, eds. Health promotive and preventive programs: models of occupational therapy practice. *Occupational Therapy in Health Care*. 1989;6(1):45-56.

7. Olson L, Heanery C, Soppas-Hoffman B. Parent-child activity group treatment in preventive psychiatry. In: Johnson JA, Jaffe E, eds. Health promotive and preventive programs: models of occupational therapy practice. *Occupational Therapy in Health Care*. 1989;6(1):29-43.

8. Thomas K. A letter from Nepal. In: Wilcock AA, ed. *Health Promotion and Occupational Therapy*. Workbook: World Federation of Occupational Therapists Congress, Melbourne, Australia, 1990.

9. Burkley S. *People First: A Guide to Self Reliant Participatory Rural Development*. London, England: Zed Books; 1993.

10. Glynn R. Some perspectives on cross-cultural rehabilitation with remote area Aboriginal people. *Australian Occupational Therapy Journal*. 1993;40(4):159-162.

11. Pondaag B. Working with the Tjalku Warra community: a project report. *The Australian Association of Occupational Therapists 15th Federal Conference*. Sydney, Australia, 1988.

12. Walker V. An occupational therapist's contribution to Aboriginal health worker training. *The Australian Association of Occupational Therapists 15th Federal Conference*. Sydney, Australia, 1988.

13. Johnson V. The occupational therapist as a tertiary consultant in a local government agency. *The Australian Association of Occupational Therapists 15th Federal Conference*. Sydney, Australia, 1988.

14. Munro J. Community liaison team, Manly District Hospital. *The Australian Association of Occupational Therapists 15th Federal Conference*. Sydney, Australia, 1988.

15. Delbecq AL, Van de Ven AH, Gustaffson DH. *Group Techniques for Program Planning*. Glenview: Scott, Foresman and Company; 1975.

16. Twible RL. Consumer participation in planning health promotion programmes: a case study using the Nominal Group technique. *Australian Occupational Therapy Journal*. 1992;39(2):13-18.

17. Twible RL. Journeying to a new land of hope: a promise for occupational therapy. *The Australian Association of Occupational Therapists 18th Federal and Inaugural Pacific Rim Conference Proceedings*. Hobart, Tasmania, 1995.

18. Hill L, Brittell TD, Kotwal J. A community mental health group designed by clients. In: Johnson JA, Jaffe E, eds. Health promotive and preventive programs: models of occupational therapy practice. *Occupational Therapy in Health Care*. 1989;6(1):57-66.

19. Last JM. *Public Health and Preventive Medicine*. Conn: Appleton and Lange; 1987:3,4,6.

20. Comstock D. A method for critical research. In: Bredo E, Feinberg W, eds. *Knowledge and Values in Social and Educational Research*. Philadelphia, Pa: Temple University Press; 1982:377.

21. McCutcheon G, Jung B. Alternative perspectives on action research. *Theory Into Practice*. 1990;29(3):147.

22. Fay B. *Critical Social Science: Liberation and Its Limits*. Ithaca, NY: Cornell University Press; 1987:47-53.

23. Yerxa EJ, Clark F, Frank G, et al. An introduction to occupational science: a foundation for occupational therapy in the 21st century. *Occupational Therapy in Health Care*. 1989;6(4):1–17.

24. Quinton A. Positivism. In: Bullock A, Stalleybrass O, Trombley S, eds. *The Fontana Dictionary of Modern Thought*. 2nd ed. London, England: Fontana Press; 1988:669.

25. Wilcock AA. Biological and socio-cultural perspectives on time-use studies. In: Pentland WE, Harvey A, Lawton MP, McColl MA, eds. *The Application of Time Use Methodology in the Social Sciences*. Plenum. In press.

26. Denzin NK. *Interpretive Interactionism: Applied Social Research Methods Series*. Vol 16. Newberry Park, Calif: Sage Publications; 1989:23.

27. Becker HS, Horowitz IL. Radical politics and sociological observation: observations on methodology and ideology. In: Becker HS, ed. *Doing Things Together: Selected Papers*. Evanston, Ill: Northwestern University Press; 1986:83-102.

28. Tripp-Reimer T. Combining qualitative and quantitative methodologies. In: Leininger M, ed. *Qualitative Research Methods in Nursing*. Orlando, Fla: Grune and Stratton; 1985:179.

29. Silverman D. *Qualitative Methodology and Sociology*. Vt: Gower Publishing Co Ltd; 1985:17.

30. De Landsheere G. History of educational research. In: Keeves JP, ed. *Educational Research, Methodology and Measurement*. Oxford, UK: Permagon Press; 1988:10.

31. Green L, Kreuter M, Deeds S, Partridge K. *Health Education Planning: A Diagnostic Approach*. Calif: Mayfield Publishing Co; 1980:8.

32. Kielhofner G, Barris R, Watts J. Habits and habit dysfunction: a clinical perspective for psychosocial occupational therapy. *Occupational Therapy in Mental Health*. 1982;2:1-21.

33. Jungfer C. Prevention—an attitude of mind. *Australian Family Physician*. 1979;8:219-221.

34. Jaffe ER. Medical consumer education: health promotion in the workplace. In: Johnson JA, Jaffe E, eds. *Occupational Therapy: Program Development for Health Promotion and Preventive Services*. New York, NY: The Haworth Press; 1989.

35. Breen VW. Education with activity: a health promotion program in a nursing home. *Occupational Therapy in Health Care*. 1989;6(1):101-111.

36. Rosenfeld MS. Occupational disruption and adaptation: a study of house fire victims. *American Journal of Occupational Therapy*. 1989;43:89-96.

37. Rosenfeld MS. Lifestyle education and revision for the worried well. *Work*. 1992;2(3):21-27.

38. Crawford R. You are dangerous to your health: the ideology of victim blaming. *International Journal of Health Services*. 1979;7:663-680.

39. French J, Adams L. From analysis to synthesis: theories of health education. *Health Education Journal*. 1986;45(2):71-74.

40. Colquhoun D. *Health Education Politics and Practice*. Geelong, Victoria: Deakin University; 1992.

41. Dunn H. *High Level Wellness*. Arlington, Va: RW Beatty; 1954.

42. Brown KM. Wellness: past visions, future roles. *Sociocultural Implications in Treatment Planning in Occupational Therapy*. New York, NY: The Haworth Press; 1987:155-164.

43. Dossey BM, Guzzetta CE. Wellness, values clarification and motivation. In: Dossey BM, Keegan L, Kolkmier LG, Guzzetta CE. *Holistic Health Promotion. A Guide for Practice*. Rockville, Md: Aspen Publishers; 1989:69-70.

44. Johnson J. Wellness and occupational therapy. *American Journal of Occupational Therapy*. 1986;40(11):753-758.

45. West W. The emerging health model of occupational therapy practice. *Proceedings of the 5th International Congress of the WFOT*. Zurich, 1970.

46. Hettler W. Wellness—the lifetime goal of a university experience. In: Matarazzo JD, et al, eds. *Behavioural Health. A Handbook of Health Enhancement and Disease Prevention*. New York, NY: John Wiley and Sons; 1990:1117.

47. Howard RB. Wellness: obtainable goal or impossible dream. *Post Graduate Medicine*. 1983;73(1):15-19.

48. Zechetmayr M. Wellness programs and employee assistance programs in industry. *Arena Review*. 1986;10(1):28-42.

49. Conrad P. Wellness in the workplace: potentials and pitfalls of worksite health promotion. *Milbank Quarterly*. 1987;65(2):255-275.

50. Conrad P, Walsh DC. The new corporate health ethic: lifestyle and the social control of work. *International Journal of Health Services*. 1992;22(1):89-111.

51. Walsh DC, Jennings SE, Mangione T, Merrigan DM. Health promotion versus health protection? Employees' perceptions and concerns. *Journal of Public Health Policy*. 1991;12(2):148-164.

52. Opatz JP. *A Primer of Health Promotion: Creating Healthy Organizational Cultures*. Washington, DC: Oryn Publications; 1985:7.

53. Antonovsky A. The sense of coherence as a determinant of health. In: Matarazzo JD, et al, eds. *Behavioural Health. A Handbook of Health Enhancement and Disease Prevention*. New York, NY: John Wiley and Sons; 1990:124.

54. Whitston C, Waddington J. Why join a union? *New Statesman and Society*. 1994;7(329):36-38.

55. Ryan RS, Travis JW. *The Wellness Workbook*. Calif: Ten Speed Press; 1981:xv.

56. Levenstein S. Wellness, health, Antonovsky. *Advances*. 1994;10(3):26-29.

57. Reilly M. The challenge of the future to an occupational therapist. *American Journal of Occupational Therapy*. 1966;20:221-225.

58. Spencer EA. From hospital to community—the health care challenge of the 1980s. In: Johnson JA, Jaffe E, eds. *Occupational Therapy: Program Development for Health Promotion and Preventive Services. Occupational Therapy in Health Care*. New York, NY: The Haworth Press; 1989.

59. Wilcock AA. Domiciliary care, occupational therapists and health promotion. *The Proceedings of the Australian Association of Occupational Therapists 15th Federal Conference*. Sydney, Australia, 1988.

60. Losada CA. Some values in occupational therapy. *Occupational Therapy in Rehabilitation*. 1936;15:285-289.

61. Bowden S. Development of a research tool to enable children to describe their engagement in occupation. *Journal of Occupational Science: Australia*. 1995;2(3):115-123.

62. Commonwealth Department of Community Services and Health. *World Health Organization: A Brief*

Summary of Its Work. Canberra: Australian Government Publishing Service; 1988:10.

63. Le Vesconte HP. The place of occupational therapy in social work planning. *Canadian Journal of Occupational Therapy.* 1934;2:13-16.

64. Le Vesconte HP. Expanding fields of occupational therapy. *Canadian Journal of Occupational Therapy.* 1935;3:4-12.

65. West W. The growing importance of prevention. *American Journal of Occupational Therapy.* 1969;23:223-231.

66. Moscovitch A, Drover G. *Inequality: Essays on the Political Economy of Social Welfare.* Toronto, Canada: University of Toronto Press; 1981.

67. Veatch RM. Justice in health care: the contribution of Edmund Pellegrino. *The Journal of Medicine and Philosophy.* 1990;15:269-287.

68. Young IM. *Justice and the Politics of Difference.* Princeton, NJ: Princeton University Press; 1990.

69. Bunton R, Macdonald G, eds. *Health Promotion: Disciplines and Diversity.* London, England: Routledge; 1992:171.

70. World Health Organization. *Formulating Strategies for Health for All by the Year 2000.* 1979.

71. Hart JT. The inverse care law. *The Lancet.* 1971;Feb 27:405-412.

72. Report of a 1977 working party, chaired by Sir Douglas Black, Hart JT. The Black report: a challenge to politicians. *The Lancet.* 1982;Jan 2:35-36.

73. Broadhead P. Social status and morbidity in Australia. *Community Health Studies.* 1985;IX(2):87-98.

74. Opit LJ. Economic policy and health care: the inverse care law in Australia. *New Doctor.* 1983.

75. Gallagher EB, Ferrante J. Medicalisation and social justice. *Social Justice Research.* 1987;1(3):377-392.

76. Le Grand J. Equity, health and health care. *Social Justice Research.* 1987;1(3):257-274.

77. Sen A. *Commodities and Capabilities.* Amsterdam: Elsevier; 1985.

78. Townsend E. 1993 Muriel Driver Memorial Lecture: occupational therapy's social vision. *Canadian Journal of Occupational Therapy.* 1993;60(4):174-184.

79. Hodges A. Health promotion and disease prevention for the disabled. *Journal of Allied Health.* 1986;Nov.

80. Needleman C. Ritualism in communicating risk information. *Science, Technology and Human Values.* 1987;12(3-4):20-25.

81. Kinnell M. Sceptreless, free, uncircumscribed? Radicalism, dissent and early children's books. *British Journal of Educational Studies.* 1988;36(1):49-71.

82. Denzin NK. *Symbolic Interactionism and Cultural Studies.* Oxford, UK: Blackwell; 1992:145.

83. Fraser N. *Unruly Practices.* Minneapolis, Minn: University of Minnesota Press; 1989:107.

84. Marris P. Community development. In: Kuper A, Kuper J, eds. *The Social Science Encyclopedia.* London, England: Routledge; 1985:137-138.

85. Marris P. *Community Planning and Conception of Change.* London: Routledge; 1982.

86. Marris P, Rein M. *Dilemmas of Social Reform.* 2nd ed. Harmondsworth, England: Penguin; 1974.

87. Milio N. *Making Policy: A Mosaic of Australian Community Health Policy.* Australia: Department of Community Services and Health; 1988.

88. World Health Organization, Health and Welfare Canada, Canadian Public Health Association. *Ottawa Charter for Health Promotion.* Ottawa, Canada; 1986.

89. el Katsha S, Watts S. Environmental health interventions in Egyptian villages. *Community Development Journal.* 1994;29(3):232-238.

90. Thomas K. Comments on working in Sudan and Ethiopia. In: Wilcock AA, ed. *Health Promotion and Occupational Therapy.* Workbook: World Federation of Occupational Therapists Congress, Melbourne, Australia, 1990.

91. World Health Organization, ILO, UNESCO. *Definition of Commuity Based Rehabilitation.* Geneva, Switzerland: WHO; 1994.

92. Potter VR. Bioethics, the science of survival. *Perspectives in Biology and Medicine.* 1970;14:127-153.

93. International Institute for Environment and Development. Whose Eden? Empowering local communities to manage their wildlife resources. *IIED Perspectives.* 1994;13:3-5.

94. Korten DC. *Sustainable Livelihoods: Redefining the Global Social Crisis.* New York, NY: People Centred Development Forum; 1994.

95. Korten DC. *Sustainable Development Strategies: The People Centred Consensus.* New York, NY: People Centred Development Forum; 1994.

96. Robertson J. *People Centred Development: Principles for a New Civilisation.* New York, NY: People Centred Development Forum; 1994.

97. Vavrousek J. Human values for sustainable living. Edial. *The Network.* The Centre for our Common Future; 1993.

98. Atkinson A, Vorratnchaiphan CP. Urban environmental management in a changing development context: the case of Thailand. *Third World Planning Review*. 1994;16(2):147-169.

99. The Asian NGO Coalition, IRED Asia, People Centred Development Forum. *Economy, Ecology and Spirituality: Toward a Theory and Practice of Sustainability*. 1993.

100. Schroyer T. Research programs from the Other Economic Summit (TOES). *Dialectic Anthroplogy*. 1992;17(4):355-390.

101. MacNeill J. Strategies for sustainable development. *Scientific American*. 1989;261(3):155-165.

102. Bello W. *Dark Victory: The United States, Structural Adjustment, and Global Poverty*. London, England: Pluto (in association with the Institute for Food and Development Policy and Transnational Institute); 1994.

103. Egger G, Spark R, Lawson J. *Health Promotion Strategies and Methods*. Sydney, Australia: McGraw-Hill; 1990:107.

104. Corson WH. Changing course: an outline of strategies for a sustainable future. *Futures*. 1994;26(2):206-223.

105. Stead WE, Stead J. Can humankind change the ecological myth? Paradigm shifts necessary for ecologically sustainable business. *Journal of Organizational Change Management*. 1994;7(4):15-31.

106. Labonte R. Econology: integrating health and sustainable development. Part one: theory and background. *Health Promotion International*. 1991;6(1):49-64.

107. Labonte R. Econology: integrating health and sustainable development. Part two: guiding principles for decision making. *Health Promotion International*. 1991;6(2):147-156.

108. Ehrenfeld D. *The Arrogance of Humanism*. New York, NY: Oxford University Press; 1981:10.

109. Dubos R. *Only One Earth*. London, England: Doubleday; 1988.

110. Moore JC. 1975 Eleanor Clarke Slagle Lecture: behaviour, bias, and the limbic system. *American Journal of Occupational Therapy*. 1976;30(1):11-19.

111. Vombrock J. Cardiovascular effect of human-pet interventions. *Journal of Behavioural Medicine*. 1988;ii(5):509-517.

112. Hundley J. The use of pet facilitated therapy among the chronically mentally ill. *Journal of Psychosocial Nursing*. 1991;29(6):23-26.

113. Harris M. Pet therapy for the homebound elderly. *Caring*. 1990;9(9):48-51.

114. Chinner T. An exploratory study on the viability and efficacy of a pet facilitated therapy project within a hospice. *Journal of Palliative Care*. 1991;7(4):13-20.

115. Fick KM. The influence of an animal in social interactions of nursing home residents in a group setting. *American Journal of Occupational Therapy*. 1993;47(6):529-533.

116. Southeast Asian contribution to the Earth Charter. *In Our Hands*. Southeast Asia Regional Consultation on a People's Agenda for Environmental Sustainable Development: Towards UNCED and Beyond. SEARCA. Philippines, 1991.

117. do Rozario L. Keynote address. Purpose, place, pride and productivity: the unique personal and societal contribution of occupation and occupational therapy. *Australian Association of Occupational Therapists 17th Conference Proceedings*. Darwin; 1993.

118. Bronner SE. *Of Critical Theory and Its Theorists*. Oxford, UK: Blackwell; 1994:349.

119. Certificate of Incorporation of the National Society for the Promotion of Occupational Therapy, Inc. (1917). *Then and Now: 1917-1976*. Rockville, Md: American Occupational Therapy Association; 1967:4-5.

120. *Funk and Wagnall's Standard Desk Dictionary*. New York, NY: Harper and Row Publishers;1984:701.

121. Cox E. A truly civil society: lecture 1: broadening the views. *The 1995 Boyer Lectures*. Australia: Radio National Transcripts; 1995:Nov 7.

Suggested Reading

Brown KM. Wellness: past visions, future roles. *Sociocultural Implications in Treatment Planning in Occupational Therapy*. New York, NY: The Haworth Press; 1987.

Dubos R. *Only One Earth*. London, England: Doubleday; 1988.

Fay B. *Critical Social Science: Liberation and Its Limits*. Ithaca, NY: Cornell University Press; 1987:47-53.

Hart JT. The inverse care law. *The Lancet*. 1971;Feb 27:405-412.

Johnson J. Wellness and occupational therapy. *American Journal of Occupational Therapy*. 1986;40(11):753-758.

Korten DC. *Sustainable Development Strategies: The People Centred Consensus*. New York, NY: People Centred Development Forum; 1994.

Korten DC. *Sustainable Livelihoods: Redefining the Global Social Crisis*. New York, NY: People Centred Development Forum; 1994.

Labonte R. Econology: integrating health and sustainable development. Part one: theory and background. *Health Promotion International.* 1991;6(1):49-64.

Labonte R. Econology: integrating health and sustainable development. Part two: guiding principles for decision making. *Health Promotion International.* 1991;6(2):147-156.

Reilly M. The challenge of the future to an occupational therapist. *American Journal of Occupational Therapy.* 1966;20:221-225.

Townsend E. 1993 Muriel Driver Memorial Lecture: occupational therapy's social vision. *Canadian Journal of Occupational Therapy.* 1993;60(4):174-184.

West W. The growing importance of prevention. *American Journal of Occupational Therapy.* 1969;23:223-231.

World Health Organization, ILO, UNESCO. *Definition of Commuity Based Rehabilitation.* Geneva, Switzerland: WHO; 1994.

Glossary

action research: Research aimed at social change through self-reflective inquiry undertaken by participants within any shared situation to increase understanding of the ideologies and practices of their particular situation and to empower and improve them through action. It is usually described as a dynamic, spiraling process with ongoing observation, reflection, planning, and action, and is aligned with critical research.

agrarian: A way of life centered on an agricultural economy.

alienation: A state in which through historically created human possibilities a person, community, or society is estranged to an activity or its results or products, the nature in which it lives, other human beings, and to self.

artifact: A purposefully formed object; any object used, modified, or made by humans.

Arts and Crafts movement: A 19th century English social and aesthetic movement, largely antimachines. Founded by William Morris and his Pre-Raphaelite associates.

atomistic societies: Societies such as many in the "West" which are based on individualism, external connections, causal and reductionistic explanations, rule orientation, and artificial frameworks.

Australopithecus*:** A genus of fossil primates that lived 1 to 5 million years ago in Southern and Eastern Africa, co-existing for some of this time with early forms of humans (see ***Homo). They walked erect and had teeth resembling those of modern humans, but the brain capacity was less than half that of modern *Homo sapiens*.

biotope: The smallest subdivision of a habitat, characterized by a high degree of uniformity in its environmental conditions, plants, and animal life.

Broca's area: Part of the human cerebral cortex involved in speech production. It is situated in the left frontal lobe and named after Paul Broca, a French surgeon.

Calvinism: Christian doctrine as interpreted by John Calvin (1509-1564), a French-born Swiss Protestant church reformer and theologian. It central doctrine is predestination.

capacities: Innate and sometimes undeveloped potential, aptitude, ability, talent, trait, or power of individuals for anything in particular.

Cartesian dualism: Separation of mind and soul from body and brain. The former can exist without the latter and withstand its corruption and death (term based on the work of René Descartes, see **Descartian**).

coercion: Constrain into obedience.

community development: Community consultation, deliberation, and action to promote individual, family, and community responsibility for self-sustaining development and well-being.

Copernicus, Nicolaus (1473-1543): Polish cleric and astronomer who formulated the heliocentric theory of the solar system. This theory, which replaced the earth as the center of the universe against all established authorities of his time, caused a complete change of outlook in many spheres, known as the Copernican revolution.

copying-fidelity: Reproduction of exact copies.

critical research: A research approach oriented toward advocacy and criticism in order to unmask the ideological roots in self-understanding which constrains equity and supports hegemony, and to empower individuals/groups toward greater autonomy, social justice, and emancipation. It is openly ideological, political, and socially analytical.

critical social science: An interpretive critique of society, especially of the theoretical bases of its organization.

cybernetics: The study of communication and control between humans, machines, and organizations. The human ability to adapt and make decisions is imitated in the design of computer-controlled systems. Cybernetics has also been used as a link between the physical and life sciences, for instance in using information theory to explain how messages are transmitted in nervous systems and in genetic processes.

cytoarchitectonic maps: Maps of the brain in terms of the structure and function of cells.

delayed return economies: Time investment in the future is part of daily life.

Descartian (link with Cartesian dualism): René Descartes (1596–1650), French philosopher and mathematician. After a Jesuit education and military service, he settled in Holland. Descartes' *Discourse on Method* (1637) introduced themes which he developed in his greatest work, the *Meditations* (1641). Asking "How and what do I know?" he arrived at his famous statement "Cogito ergo sum" ("I think, therefore I am"). From this he proved to his own satisfaction God's existence (he was a Roman Catholic) and hence the existence of everything else. He believed that the world consisted of two different substances—mind and matter (the doctrine of Cartesian dualism).

division of labor: The separation of tasks. It may take several forms such as social division of labor according to the economics of different societies and communities; division of labor by gender, which is a basic structural element in human social organizations which originates from differences in human physiology; and division of labor between workers who perform only a partial operation in production and what is produced is a social product of the collective workers.

DNA (deoxyribonucleic acid): The chief ingredient of chromosomes, DNA is necessary for the organization and functioning of living cells.

ecological sustainability: To uphold and support the ecology and ecosystems by practices which maintain, and continue to maintain, the natural environment and the relationships of different species.

ecology: The scientific study of organisms in their natural environment, including the relationships of different species with each other and the environment.

ecosystem: A biological community and the physical environment associated with it.

electrophoresis: A technique for the analysis and separation of colloids; used extensively in studying mixtures of proteins, nucleic acids, carbohydrates, enzymes, etc. In clinical medicine it is used for determining the protein content of body fluids.

epidemiology: The basic science of public health and preventive medicine. Originally the study of epidemic diseases and their control.

epigenesis: The development of an organism from an undifferentiated cell, consisting in the successive formation and development of organs and parts that do not pre-exist in the fertilized egg.

ethology: The study of animal and human behavior. Central to the ethologist's approach is the principle that animal behavior (like physical characteristics) is subject to evolution through natural selection, through the development of the individual, and, in humans, in cultural history.

existentialism: A philosophical movement which rejects the metaphysical and centers on an individual person as a being in the world. It has as a major tenet that every person is unique, and cannot be explained in reductionist physiological terms. It aims toward a comprehensive concept of human existence and uses phenomenological methods to grasp the "essence" of peoples' consciousness, feelings, moods, experiences, and relationships.

favism: Familial Mediterranean fever. Hereditary biochemical lesion of the erythrocytes and consequent enzyme deficiency.

fecundity: The fertility of an organism. Normally all organisms, assuming they reach reproductive age, are sufficiently fecund to replace themselves several times over. Darwin noted this, together with the fact that population numbers nevertheless tended to remain fairly constant. These observations led him to formulate his theory of evolution by natural selection.

feminism: A doctrine and movement advocating the granting of the same social, political, and economic rights to women as the ones granted to men.

flow: A state of consciousness when people are so involved in an activity that nothing else seems to matter; of optimal experience, transcendence, and enjoyment when individuals are challenged but engaged within the scope of their abilities.

founder effect: The genetic consequences of founding a new population with few individuals. The founder population will most likely differ genetically from its parent population because it will contain only a fraction of the total genetic variation. Any recessive gene will increase in frequency.

Galileo, Galilei (1564–1642): Italian mathematician, physicist, and astronomer whose work anticipated and revolutionized the experimental methods of scientific inquiry. His support of Copernicus' work on the solar system led to 8 years of house arrest by the Inquisition.

gene: A unit of heredity composed of DNA. In classical genetics, a gene is visualized as a discrete particle, forming part of a chromosome, that determines a particular characteristic.

gene flow: The exchange of genes among populations either directly by migration or by diffusion of genes over many generations.

general systems theory: A theory put forward by von Bertalanffy which, in the broadest sense, refers to a collection of general concepts, principles, tools, problems, and methods associated with all kinds of systems.

genetic drift: The random change of gene frequencies over time which happens in all populations but can take place rapidly in small populations.

genome: The complete set of genetic information in every living organism. Human genome consists of 3,000 million matching pairs of nucleotides.

hegemony: Domination or leadership, especially the predominant influence of one state over another.

high longevity: Long life.

history of ideas: Discipline that studies the history and development of ideas and theories in terms of their origins and influences.

holism: Philosophical theory that wholes are greater than the sum of their parts. In health care, treating of the whole person rather than the symptoms of a disease.

First used in modern times by JC Smuts in 1928.

hominid: Of the primate family including humans and their fossil ancestors (Latin *Homo homin*=man).

Homo: The genus of primates that includes modern humans (modern *Homo sapiens* sometimes known as *Homo sapien sapiens,* the only living representative) and various extinct species, of which four or five are usually recognized although the number is uncertain.

- *H. habilis:* the earliest species (small and large forms, probably two species)
- *H. erectus:* descended from *H. habilis*
- *H. sapiens:* descended from *H. erectus*
- Neanderthal man (*H. sapiens Neanderthalensis* or *H. Neanderthalensis)*

Homo erectus: A direct ancestor of modern man who appeared about 1.5 million years ago and lived to 300,000 years ago. Fossils of *H. erectus,* which are sometimes called *Pithecanthropus* (ape man), are similar to present-day man except that there was a prominent ridge above the eyes and no forehead or chin. They had crude stone tools and used fire.

Homo habilis: The oldest *Homo.* Fossils of *H. habilis* were found in the Olduvai Gorge in Tanzania. Estimated to have lived 2.3 to 1.5 million years ago. Gracile or delicate-boned toolmaker.

Hormic School of Psychology: An early psychological school of thought centered on vital or purposeful energy, and related to Jung's view of the importance of an individual's search for meaning in life.

humanism: A non-religious philosophy based on belief in potential of human nature rather than in religious or transcendental values.

immediate return economies: Hand-to-mouth subsistence existence.

individualism: A social theory that emphasizes the importance of the individual.

kin selection: Natural selection of genes that tends to cause the individuals bearing them to be altruistic to close relatives. These relatives have a higher probability of bearing identical copies of those same genes than do other members of the population. Thus, kin selection for a gene that tends to cause an animal to share food with a close relative will result in the gene being spread through the population because it (unconsciously) benefits itself. The more closely two animals are related, the higher the probability that they share some identical genes and therefore the more closely their interests coincide. Parental care is a special case of kin selection.

!Kung San: Hunter-gatherer peoples who live on the northern fringe of the Kalahari Desert. Their language has a characteristic clicking sound which is represented by ! prefixing Kung.

long distance exchange: The exchange of objects as currency a long distance from where the objects are found or made. Seashells found hundreds of miles inland are a particularly good example.

Marxist structuralism: A philosophy of science or method of inquiry, which has affinities with Realism. It investigates "systems" in terms of totality, self-regulation, and transformation.

Mendelian genetics: The theory of heredity that forms the basis of classical genetics, proposed by Gregor Mendel (1822–1884) in 1866. Mendel suggested that individual characteristics were determined by inherited "factors."

moral treatment: The first systematic treatment which commenced in the last decade of the 18th century providing responsible care for an appreciable number of people with mental illness. "Moral" was used in this early context as the equivalent of "emotional" or "psychological" (from the same root as morale) and also has to do with custom, conduct, way of life, and inner meaning.

mutation: Genetic change which, when transmitted to offspring, gives rise to heritable variations (Latin *muto*=change).

neo-Darwinism: see **synthetic Darwinism**.

neophilia: Love for, great interest in what is new; novelty.

nepotism: Favoritism shown to relatives, especially in conferring offices.

neural Darwinism: Gerald Edelman's theory of the biological development of the brain within an individual's lifespan, rooted in Darwinian notions of natural selection. See also **neuronal group selection**.

neuronal group selection: The central theory of Edelman's neural Darwinism. It has three major tenets: a dynamic selection process which sets up the neuroanatomical characteristics of individuals during development; patterns of responses selected from this anatomy during experience; and physiology and psychology which give rise to behavior through re-entry, a process of signaling between brain maps. See also **re-entrant signaling**.

new public health: Global Public Health initiatives of recent years based on the Declaration of Alma Ata and the Ottawa Charter for Health Promotion. Emphasis is on primary health care, illness prevention, and health promotion.

Occident: Europe and America as distinct from the Orient (Latin *occidens -entis*=setting, sunset, west).

occupation: All "doing" that has intrinsic or extrinsic meaning.

occupational alienation: Sense of isolation, powerlessness, frustration, loss of control, estrangement from society or self as a result of engagement in occupation which does not satisfy inner needs.

occupational balance: A balance of engagement in occupation which leads to well-being. For example, the balance may be among physical, mental, and social occupations; between chosen and obligatory occupations; between strenuous and restful occupations; or between doing and being.

occupational deprivation: Deprivation of occupational choice and diversity because of circumstances beyond the control of individuals or communities.

occupational imbalance: A lack of balance or disproportion of occupation resulting in decreased well-being.

occupational justice: The promotion of social and economic change to increase individual, community, and political awareness, resources, and equitable opportunities for diverse occupational opportunities which enable people to meet their potential and experience well-being.

occupational potential: Future capability, to engage in occupation toward needs, goals, and dreams for health, material requirement, happiness, and well-being.

occupational science: The rigorous study of humans as occupational beings.

occupational technology: Means and tools by which material things are produced in a particular civilization which change ways of "doing."

ontogeny: The development of an individual from egg to adult throughout the life span.

organic communities: Societies in which natural functions, role perspectives, mutual interdependence, and intrinsic relationships are paramount.

Paleolithic: The earliest part of the Stone Age that began some 2.6 million years ago in Africa with the first recognizable stone tools, known as Oldowan, from Olduvai Gorge in Tanzania.

phenylketonuria: A hereditary disorder characterized by brain damage and mental retardation due to an inability to develop an essential enzyme, phenylalanine hydroxylase.

phrenology: An approach to the study of neurology first proposed by Gall (1758-1828) in which it was proposed that the shape of the skull indicated the development and various mental functions of the underlying brain.

phylogeny: The evolutionary history of species.

physiological neophilia: Everything new is attractive in puberty.

polymorphism: Diversity occurring within biological populations.

pragmatism: A philosophy of the late 19th and 20th centuries which interprets truth in terms of practical effects. "Meaning" can best be understood by examining its consequences on human activity.

praxis: Doing, acting, action, practice; free, universal, creative, and self-creative activity. Can be any kind of activity, but often used for business or political activity, accepted practice or custom, and as a descriptor in action research.

preventive medicine: The application of Western medical and social science to prevent disease, prolong life, and promote health in the community through intercepting disease processes.

proto humans: Early members of the *hominidae* family such as *Australopithecus* (Greek *protos*, proto=first).

public health: Protection of the community or public at large from illness, disease, and epidemics.

radiator theory: A theory proposed by Dean Falk, an anthropologist, that the evolution of increased brain size was dependent on adequate cooling through heat dispersal. This theory is based on the differences in cranial vessels and drainage patterns (foramen in the skull) between australopithecines and early *Homo* brains. These patterns become increasingly elaborate over evolutionary time.

reciprocity: Mutual action, exchange, practice of give and take.

reductionism: A philosophical stance associated with empiricism and scientific "disciplines" in which understanding is achieved through the study of parts and their effects on each other.

re-entrant signaling: A term used by Edelman in his theory of neural Darwinism. Brains contain multiple maps that automatically adapt their boundaries to changing signals to categorize and make sense of perceptions. The maps are connected by parallel and reciprocal connections. Re-entrant signaling occurs along these connections. This means that, as groups of neurons are selected in a map, other groups in different maps may also be selected at the same time. Re-entrant signaling is the process by which correlation and coordination of such selection events are achieved (from Edelman).

Reformation: A religious movement in 16th century Europe. Attempts to reform the Roman Catholic church resulted in the establishment of independent Protestant churches.

Renaissance Utopians: Utopians who emerged at the time of the Renaissance in the 14th through 16th centuries. Most were multitalented and interested in humanities. Utopians aimed toward an imagined perfect place, perfect society, or state of things.

self-actualization: Full humanness; the development of the inner nature and biological potential (destiny) of people. Self-actualizing people are not selfish but altruistic, dedicated, self-transcending, and social.

sexual dimorphism: The male and female of a species are distinctly different (e.g., in size or shape).

social Darwinism: A largely discredited doctrine of the late 19th and early 20th centuries which applied (mostly erroneously) Darwin's theory of biological evolution to societies.

social justice: The promotion of social and economic change to increase individual, community, and political awareness, resources and opportunity for health and well-being.

sociobiology: The study of animal behavior, especially social behavior, from the perspective of evolution by natural selection.

stochastic: Any process in which there is a random variable.

synthetic Darwinism: A modern synthesis of Charles Darwin's arguments of natural selection with Gregor Mendel's mechanisms of heredity. This was accomplished in the 1940s by a group of evolutionists and geneticists and accounts for the origin of genetic variation as mutations in DNA as well as rearrangement of genetic structures in a process known as recombination. Also known as **neo-Darwinism**.

temporality: Of time (Latin *tempus -por*=time).

topobiology: A term used by Edelman in his theories about brain evolution because many transactions leading to shape are place dependent (*topo*=place).

Wernicke's area: A region of the human brain in the left parieto-temporal region involved in the comprehension of speech. Named after neurologist Carl Wernicke (1848-1905).

Index

action-research approach
  community development, 238f
  definition, 224–225
  prevention, 233f
  public health, 224–226
  social justice, 235f
  sustainable ecology, 240f
  wellness, 231f
action-research model
  phases, 225–229
activity
  definition, 24–26
activity analysis, 193
adaptive nature
  occupational therapy, 198–199
Addams, Jane
  biographical sketch, 174–175
agrarian lifestyle
  vs. hunting and gathering, 79
agrarian revolution, 77–80
agriculture
  human occupation, 77–80
arts and crafts movement, 175–177
association areas, 33
atomistic societies, 151

balanced lifestyles, 139
behaviors, observed
  ontogenetic development, 34
Better Health Commission of Australia, 3
biological capacities and characteristics,
  13, 41–64
biological mechanism
  survival and health, 115
biological needs
  health mechanism, 115
biological processes
  gender, 47
  ontogenesis, 47–48
  race, 46–47
biological-sociocultural issues
  combination, 11–12
bipedalism, 33
  capacities, 48–50
brain, 31, 72

evolution, 43, 143
function, 42–45, 105–106
sizes, 32
structures, 42–45, 53–54
survival and health, 30

case histories
  occupation influence
    health, 4–5
charm, 98
circumstances
  vs. choices, 120
cities, 80–81
cognitive capacity, 120
coherence, 103
commerce, 84–85
community development
  action-research approach, 238f
  health promotion model, 230f,
    238–240
community well-being, 107
confidence, 103
consciousness
  capacities, 56–58
craftsman, 84
creativity
  capacities, 58–61
cultural capacities, 33–34
cultural evolution
  occupational technology, 35
culture, 25
  language, 55

Declaration of Alma Ata, 109
diagnosis
  occupational theory
    human nature, 35–36
disfigurement, 135
drives concept, 115–117

ecological sustainability
  health promotion model, 230f,
    240–243
ecological vision
  occupational therapy, 242–243

ecological well-being, 107–108
education awareness phase
    action-research model, 227–229
electronic era, 87
ethology, 12
evolution
    agriculture, 77–80
    brain, 43, 143
    human population growth, 242f
    industry, 82–86
    occupational deprivation and imbalance, 149
    occupations, 71–90
    post-industry, 86–90
    societies in education, 75
    theories, 27
extrinsic needs, 204

feminism, 174–175
flow, 98–99

gathering and hunting lifestyle, 141
    health and occupation, 110–114
    morbidity results, 113
    mortality patterns, 113
    occupations, 72–77
    vs. agrarian lifestyle, 79
gender
    capacities, 47
gender bias
    occupational therapy, 190–191
general systems theory, 108
genetic variations
    human capacities, 45
growth models of health, 5
    occupational therapy, 204

habit, 178–179
hand function
    capacities, 50
happiness, 98
healing views, 114–115
health, 4
    definition
        Australian Aboriginal Health
            Organization, 107
        occupational perspective, 110

Ottawa Charter for Health
    Promotion, 109
    WHO, 97–98
gathering and hunting, 110–114
growth models, 5
occupation influence, 121–124
    case histories, 4–5
occupation relationship, 106t
occupational perspective, 14, 97–124
survival
    occupation, 245–246
well-being
    self-initiated occupation, 6
health and occupation
    concepts, 8–9
    medical science influence, 10–11
health and well-being
    occupational species nature,
        123–124
health mechanism
    biological needs, 115
health, positive
    well-being, 99–100
health promotion
    occupational therapy, 205–212
health promotion models, 229–244
health related fitness, 141
health-related functions
    occupation, 5–6
health views, 114–115
healthy balance, 137
healthy survival
    occupational theory
        human nature, 36–37
history
    occupational therapy, 165–181
history of ideas, 8–10
    exploration, 246
    pit falls, 9
holism, 108–109
holistic health, 108
homeostasis
    capacities, 63–64
homeostatic perspective
    needs, 117
Hull House, 174-176
human capacities

bipedalism, 48–50
    consciousness, 56–58
    creativity, 58–61
    definition, 41–42
    genetic variations, 45
    hand function, 50
    homeostasis, 63–64
    language, 52–56
    needs, 119
    occupational natures, 48
    prevention disorder, 118
    race and gender, 46–47
    range availability, 33
    sleep, 61–63
    visual system, 51–52
human characteristics
    complexities, 7
human mental capacities, 58–61
human nature
    occupational theories, 21–37, 245
human population growth evolution,
    242f
hunting and gathering lifestyles, 141
    health and occupation, 110–114
    morbidity results, 113
    mortality patterns, 113
    occupations, 72–77
    vs. agrarian lifestyle, 79

ill health
    occupational deprivation, 147
    occupational risk factors, 14–15,
        131–155
illness prevention
    public health researchers, 131
incapacity
    well-being, 105
individual potential development
    occupations, 111–112
industrialization, 87, 170–171
industrial society, 82–86
industry, 82–86
information
    organization, 143–144
intellectual capacity, 120
intrinsic needs, 204

labor, 76
    definition, 23–24
    vs. leisure, 80
language
    capacities, 52–56
learning experiences, 33
leisure
    definition, 24
    vs. labor, 80
Lewin's three stages
    theory development, 21
lifestyles
    agrarian, 77–80
    gathering and hunting, 72–77
limbic system function
    occupational behavior, 204
loss of near relation, 135

materialism, 87–88
maternal neglect, 148
maturation, 204
medical model
    occupational therapy, 4, 188
medical science
    influence, 10–11
    public health, 131–133
medical science influence
    health and occupation, 10–11
mentally healthy people
    National Mental Health Association
        of America
        definition, 101–102
mental well-being, 101–104
    occupation, 103–104
Meyer, Adolph
    biographical sketch, 172–174
mind, 106
moral treatment, 165, 167–170
morbidity results
    gathering and hunting, 113
    occupational history, 134–136
mortality patterns
    hunting and gathering, 113
motor skill related fitness, 141

needs
    capacities, 119

health role, 117–120
   occupational, 11
needs concept, 115–117
need to do
   occupational theory
      human nature, 31–33
neurological rehabilitation, 6
non-omnipotence, 120

occupation, 3
   definition, 22–23, 72
   functions, 89–90, 245–246
   gathering and hunting, 110–114
   health influences, 121–124
   health relationship, 106t
   health-related functions, 5–6
   history and elements, 8–9
   survival, 29–30
      health, 245–246
occupation and health
   concepts, 8–9
occupation influence
   health
      case histories, 4–5
occupation rediscovered, 199–204
occupation, self-initiated
   well-being
      health, 6
occupation, traditional
   scientific methods, 7
occupational alienation, 149–153
   definition, 149
   illustration, 150
occupational behavior, 86–87, 131
   biological basis, 31
   exercise regimen, 140–141
   foundation, 13, 41–64
   limbic system function, 204
occupational deprivation, 6, 145–149
   definition, 145
   ill health, 147
occupational environments
   variety, 7
occupational evolution, 13–14, 71–90
occupational factors
   health and well-being, 122f
occupational gender bias, 148–149
occupational health

public health, 133–134
occupational health and wellness
   examples, 194-196
occupational history
   morbidity patterns, 134–136
occupational human, 221–222
occupational imbalance, 137–145
   definition, 137–138
occupational indicators
   health and wellness, 121
occupational nature
   variability, 245
occupational needs, 89
occupational perspective
   health, 14, 97–124
   health and well-being, 123f
   health definition, 110
   mental well-being, 103–104
   physical well-being, 101
   social well-being, 104
occupational pursuits, 81
occupational risk factors, 137–155
   ill health, 14–15, 131–155
occupational science, 6–7
occupational species nature
   health and well-being, 123–124
occupational structure
   population size, 136–137
occupational theory
   history, 27–29
   human nature, 12–13, 26–37
      concepts, 29–35
      diagnosis, 35–36
      healthy survival, 36–37
      need to do, 31–33
      prescription, 36
occupational therapy, 4
   advantages, 202–203
   basic ideologies, 187
   definition
      Australian Association of
         Occupational Therapists, 166
      World Health of Occupational
         Therapists, 166
   early education and criteria, 180–181
   ecological vision, 242–243
   foundation philosophies, 246
   genesis, 15, 165–181

growth model of health, 204
health and well-being, 165
health promotion, 205–212
history, 189
hypothesis, 1
influences, 180f
medical model, 4, 188
new synthesis, 244–246
occupation and health, 15–16,
    187–212
philosophical base, 179–181
potential role, 221–224
preventive medicine, 223
principal dynamics, 188–189
public health, 16, 221–246
    community based examples,
        223–224
    industrial based examples,
        222–223
public health perspective, 165
social vision, 204
strengths, 246
view
    occupation and health, 187
occupations
    gathering and hunting, 72–77
    individual potential development,
        111–112
    physical well-being, 101
ontogenesis, 47–48
ontogenetic development
    observed behaviors, 34
organization
    information and stimulation, 143–144
Ottawa Charter for Health Promotion,
    109–110

pain, 135
patronage
    occupational therapy, 191–192
personal skills
    development, 225
physical activity, 139
    protective effect, 140
physical fitness
    vs. psychological fitness, 102t
physical health
    definition and measure, 115

physical well-being, 100–101
physiological reflexes, 34
pleasure principle, 119
population size
    occupational structure, 136–137
positive health
    well-being, 99–100
post-industry, 86–90
pragmatism, 178–179
praxis
    definition, 23
prescription
    occupational theory
        human nature, 36
    occupational therapy, 188–189
prevention
    action-research approach, 233f
prevention disorder
    capacities use, 118
preventive medicine
    health promotion model, 230f,
        233–235
    occupational therapy, 223
professionalism
    occupational therapy, 192
prosperity, 98
protect
    needs, 117–118
psychological fitness
    vs. physical fitness, 102t
public health
    action-research approach, 224–226
    definition, 224
    medical science, 131–133
    occupational health, 133–134
    occupational therapy, 16, 221–246
        community based examples,
            223–224
        industrial based examples,
            222–223
public health perspective
    occupational therapy, 165
public health researchers
    illness prevention, 131
race
    capacities, 46–47
reductionism
    occupational therapy, 192–197

rehabilitation
    occupational therapy, 197–198
Reilly, Mary, 1, 7
    biographical sketch, 199–201
research phase
    action-research model, 226–227

scientific methods
    occupation, traditional, 7
semantics, 53
Simple-Lifers, 175
Slagle, Eleanor Clarke
    biographical sketch, 178
sleep
    capacities, 61–63
social justice
    action-research approach, 235f
    health promotion model, 230f,
        235–238
social vision
    occupational therapy, 204
social well-being, 104
sociocultural adaptations, 34
sociocultural influences, 120
sociocultural values
    hunting and gathering, 77
stimulation
    organization, 143–144
stress, 153–155
    definition, 151
        moderating factors, 154
        related illnesses, 154–155
structure
    brain, 42–43
style, 98
super-capacity, 56
survival
    biological mechanism, 115
    occupation, 29–30
        health, 245–246
survival mechanisms, 33
sustainable ecology
    action-research approach, 240f
syntax, 53

theory
    definition, 26
theory development
    Lewin's three stages, 21
therapeutic occupations, 171–172
time, 25
tool making, 73
tool technology, 72
towns, 80–81
twin studies
    behavior, nature and nurture, 45–46

visual system
    capacities, 51–52

warn
    needs, 117–118
well-being, 4
    combination of all, 105–107
    definition, 98–100
    health
        self-initiated occupation, 6
    incapacity, 105
    individual, 100–107
    material associations, 98
    occupational species nature, 123–124
wellness
    action-research approach, 231f
    health promotion model, 229–233
West, Wilma
    biographical sketch, 205–207
work
    definition, 23
    health, 118
    physiological and mental functions,
        118
World Health Organization (WHO), 3

Yerxa, Elizabeth, 7
    biographical sketch, 201–202